THE THEORETICAL INTERPRETATION OF ELECTROENCEPHALOGRAPHY (EEG)

The Important Role of Spontaneous Resting EEG and Vigilance

Electroencephalography for Neuropsychiatrists, Psychiatrists, Neurologists, Clinical Psychologists, Neuropsychologists, Psychophysiologists, and Neuroscientists

by
Gerald Ulrich, M.D.
University Medicine / Charité
Berlin (Germany)

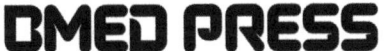

www.bmedpress.com

Dedicated to my grandchildren

Leonie
Armin
Anton
Linus
Johann
Jana
and Lilli v. Einem, the cat

13509 Berlin, Im Brachfeldwinkel 15
March 2013

For more information about this book:

BMED Press LLC
5402 South Staples St.
Suite 200
Corpus Christi, Texas 78411
Phone: (817) 400-1639
www.bmedpress.com

Copyright © 2013 by Gerald Ulrich, M.D.
All Rights Reserved

10-digit ISBN: 978-0-9827498-2-1
13-digit ISBN: 0982749821

All rights reserved.
No part of this book may be reproduced without
written permission of the publisher.

CONTENTS

Preface		1
Chapter 1	*A Critical Review of the Present Status of the EEG in Psychiatry*	5
Chapter 2	*The EEG in Psychiatry – Only Screening for Neurological Disorders – or more?*	9
Chapter 3	*Conditions for the Development of the Psychiatric EEG*	13
3.1	Framework	13
3.2	Methodology	14
3.3	Terminology	15
3.3.1	"Normal" versus "Abnormal"	16
3.3.2	*Allgemeinveränderung* (General Slowing Down of Frequencies)	18
3.3.3	*Krampfbereitschaft* (Proneness to Epileptic Seizures)	20
3.3.4	One Feature - Many Terms	26
3.4	Theoretical Foundations	30
3.4.1	Systems Physiology, Cybernetics and Biorhythms	30
3.4.2	The Spontaneous Resting EEG (SR-EEG) as a non-stationary process	33
3.4.3	EEG and Vigilance	36
3.4.4	The Importance of the SR-EEG as a Macroindicator of Cerebral Global Function (CGF)	67
3.4.5	EEG and Maturation: General points of view	69
3.4.6	EEG and Maturation : Individual Indicators	71
3.4.7	EEG and Psychophysiology	99
3.4.8	About the impossiblity of an external validation of psychopathologically defined psychiatric diagnoses	105

Chapter 4		Qualitative Features of the Psychophysiological EEG : General Principles of Pathological Dissolution of the Organization of Brain Electrical Activity *(**Pathologischer Funktionswandel**)*	**117**
	4. 1	From the Physiomorphic (PM) to the Diffuse Dysrhythmic EEG (DD)	118
	4. 3	From the Diffuse-Dysrhythmic EEG (DD) to Brain-Electrical Inactivity	146
	4. 4	Involutional Psychosyndromes and Healthy Aging	159
	4. 5	Dynamic Rigidity (DR) and Dynamic Lability (DL) with Exogenous Psychosyndromes	169
	4. 6	Dementia of the Alzheimer Type (DAT)	177
	4. 7	Depressed Syndromes and Disturbed Dynamics of EEG-vigilance	185
	4. 8	Manic Syndromes and Lowered EEG-Vigilance	196
	4. 9	Schizophrenic Psychoses	202
	4. 10	Epileptic Psychoses	210
	4. 11	The EEG in Meditation	221
	4. 12	Multiple Sclerosis	222
Chapter 5		*Changes in the EEG Induced by Psychotropic Substances: The Basics*	**225**
	5.1	Neuroleptics	232
	5. 2	Thymoleptics	244
	5.3	Lithium	250
	5.4	Carbamazepine	255
	5.5	Tranquilizers, Hypnotics, Narcotics	259
	5.6	Alcohol	263
	5.7	Opioids, Psychoanaleptics, Psychodysleptics	267
	5.8	Psychotomimetics	274
	5. 9	Nootropics	275
Chapter 6		*The Quantified EEG (QEEG): Its Present Scientific Status and Eddington's Parable*	**277**
	6. 1	Promises, Fictions, Disappointments: A Documentation from the Literature	278
	6. 2	The Reasons for the Present Deadlock of QEEG	286
	6. 2. 1	The "Normality"- Problem	286

6.2.2	The Deliberate Assumption of Stationarity of the SR-EEG and the Central Limit Theorem	287
6.2.3	The unrecognized *A*rterial *P*ulse *I*mpedance *A*rtifact (APIA)	288
6.2.4	The Non-consideration of the Dynamics of SR-EEG as Macroindicator of Cerebral Global Function (CGF)	292
6.2.5	The Misunderstanding of Head's Theoretical Construct of ***Vigilance***	292
6.2.6	The Primary Quantification of SR-EEG	295
6.2.7	The Abuse of EEG for Neuroanatomical Demarcation of Neophrenological "Moduls"	297

Chapter 7 *Limits and Possibilities of QEEG in Clinical Psychiatry* **299**

7.1	About the Quantification of Qualities: General Principles	300
7.2	Longitudinal, Serial, Dynamical, or *I*psative *T*rend *A*ssessment (ITA)	304
7.3	Validity and Reliability of ITA as well as examples of use	311
7.3.1	Senile Dementia (SD) or Dementia of Alzheimer Type (DAT or AD)	312
7.3.2	Acute Alcohol Withdrawal (detoxification)	319
7.3.3	Depressive Syndromes	322
7.3.4	Manic Syndromes	324
7.3.5	Schizophrenic Psychoses	327
7.3.6	Attention-Deficit-Hyperactivity-Disorder (ADHD)	330
7.3.7	Other Psychiatric Disorders: Obsessive Compulsive Diosorder (OCD) and Borderline Personaliy Disorder (BPD)	333
7.4	Non-linear Complexity Analysis: An important supplement and extension to traditional linear q-EEG analysis	334

Chapter 8 *Outlook* 337

References 345

Index 405

PREFACE

In the introduction of my monography, *Psychiatrische Elektroenzephalographie* (ULRICH, 1994), I cautioned the reader that the book might perhaps offend proponents of clinical EEG. Thus, I deemed it appropriate to refer to the fundamental conviction of the famous swiss philosopher of science and psychologist Jean PIAGET(1896-1980). PIAGET (1974) emphasized that two scientists can only be interested in a clear-cut ***discordance*** when attempting to find a solution to a certain problem from two opposing premises, provided they were not prevented by a weakness of character! This is because one may learn somewhat about the facts and their interpretations only through thematisation of discordance.

Hans BERGER – at the time chairholder of the psychiatric university clinic in Jena, originally introduced the human EEG as a new technique for psychiatric diagnosis and research. Some experts pointed out that the gradual fading of the associated great expectations towards a scientific breakthrough was not associated with the unproductiveness of the method itself but rather with its inadequate handling. Since many criticisms have remained valid across the last two decades, a renewed thematization seems to be inescapable. Additionally, recent developments that are detrimental to the psychiatric EEG provoke further critical comments.

The statement that one can acquire an international reputation as an EEG expert without having the least knowledge of the visuo-morphologically defined patterning of the EEG recorded under the so-called, well-defined resting conditions (Spontaneous Resting EEG, **SR-EEG**) is still valid. Likewise unchanged is an explicit atheoretical or empiristic method-centred actionism, which follows the generally accepted let's-try-it-and-see strategy.

Neurology adopted the human EEG for psychiatric diagnostics and research shortly after BERGER had advocated it. Thereby, specific potentials within the scope of epilepsies played a decisive role; thus, the EEG became a central tool of the just developing neurological electrodiagnostics. Its usage for subdividing the wake-sleep cycle into successive stages was essentially in the hands of experimentally working psychologists. For clinical purposes it played only a subordinate role. Within psychiatry, attempts have been made to isolate features that would indicate nosological specifity. The gain was for the most part disappointing. Thus, the EEG soon emerged as an undisputed diagnostic method in clinical neurophysiology directed by neurology. BERGER originally wanted the EEG to be perceived as the core method in psychophysiology – this term being coined by him to denote a new basic discipline of psychiatry – faded into obscurity. Clinical neurophysiology was not distinguished from clinical psychophysiology probably due to the notoriously lacking methodological consciousness in psychiatry. Thus, it should be clarified that neurophysiology aims at objective measures, which can only be obtained from the position of the external observer. Clinical psychophysiology, in contrast, aims at correlating those objective data with subjective ones, which can only be obtained by observing the outer and inner behavior of a human being. In other words, clinical neurophysiology rests upon objective context-independent information in the sense of "brain physics," whereas clinical psychophysiology tries to conciliate this kind of objective information with behavioral context-dependent information in the sense of genuine psychology. The acknowledgement of this basic difference between neurophysiology and psychophysiology has, of course, decisive methodological consequences.

Unlike neurophysiology, psychophysiology may not be analogous with physics. Psychophysiology brings together two logically or epistemologically incommensurable types of data, one results from the objective third-person perspective and the other from the subjective first-person-perspective. Therefore, both types of data can only be conciliated from a metaperspectival point of view.

The greatest scientific contribution of the English neurologist Henry HEAD (1861-1940) involved the awareness of the distinction between neuro- and psychophysiology. Consequently, he coined and introduced *vigilance* as a theoretical term (or construct) in order to bridge the divide between the rows of the objective and the subjective data. It has to be stressed that *vigilance* was an outcome of clinical observations. To HEAD the construct seemed to be indispensable for explaining certain clinical phenomena, for instance, the spontaneous recovery of the CNS following damage or the characteristically fluctuating performances in the recovery phase.

In contrast to neurophysiology, psychophysiology treats a living system considering its permanent interactional process with environment. Since process is by definition a permanent change, one has to consider an ever-changing level of the hierarchically organized CNS, a view going back to the great English neurologist JACKSON (1835-1911). This applies not only to the actual act of interaction but also to the so-called resting state, which is by no means inert or inactive. If a spontaneous repetition of a similar structure is observed, one may speak about a self-organizing process of cyclic order.

To clarify the issue, it has to be added that the informational content of the EEG is not only an indicator of circumscribed or distributed brain lesions. Merit has to be given to Dieter BENTE (1921-1983) for initiating the development of the psychophysiological or psychiatric EEG by conceiving the Spontaneous Resting EEG (**SR-EEG**) as a systemic macroindicator of the organizational level of the Cerebral Global Function (**CGF**) and its dynamics. Moreover, it has to be considered that the unique time resolution of the EEG equalizes that of psychological processes.

BENTE'S work is based on the theoretical construct of *vigilance* introduced by HEAD about 40 years earlier. It should be mentioned that BENTE borrowed from ideas of the French EEG school of Mdm. LAIRY (e.g., LAIRY & DELL, 1957) who under the influence of the neo-Jacksonian psychiatrist EY (1900-1977) speculated about a relationship between **CGF** and the dynamic patterning of the **SR-EEG**.

As history shows, the psychophysiological or psychiatric EEG can only be advanced under the guidance of neuropsychiatrists with clinical as well as methodological and epistemological competences. From BENTE'S works and that of his co-workers and successors, it becomes clear that the EEG should no longer be devalued as a dispensible second line auxiliary tool for the diagnosis of neurological lesions. It has a privileged status with respect to the investigation of psychological and psychopathological functioning.

As an important point endangering its future perspectives, the fashionable trend towards visualization techniques having achieved a monopoly within brain research should not be ignored. Whereas neuroimaging doubtlessly represents an enormous progress in neurological diagnoses, its broad dominance with respect to neuroscientific research has promoted a revitalization of a thinking, which seemed to have become obsolete since at least the 1930s and which is now known as **Neophrenology**. Neophrenology has its roots in the pseudoscience of so-called Phrenology invented by the Viennese neuroanatomist GALL (1758-1826) who claimed to recognize characterological properties from defined palpable protrusions of the skull.

Instead of a f-MRI based delimitation of a *mosaic of rigidly encapsulated moduls*, a phrase coined by FODOR (1984) in his influential book entiteled *The Modularity of*

Mind, future psychophysiology should be oriented towards the experimentally well-founded alternative view of the CNS as a hierarchically organized unity consisting of spatially as well as functionally disparate substrata the integration of which is warranted by a superordinate rhythm in the 40 cps range.

Following BERGER, clinical psychiatry must rediscover the EEG as a field of clinical practice as well as of fertile future research.

The Author
Berlin, March, 2013

CHAPTER 1

A Critical Review of the Present Status of the EEG in Psychiatry

The EEG has made a disappointing contribution to psychiatry since BERGER'S (1882 -1941) startling discovery 80 years ago. A major breakthrough seemed to come to the fore with the general availability of the digital recording and quantification techniques in the early 1990s. However, the new possibilities were scarcely used to answer open questions in clinical psychiatry. Instead, all electrophysiological capacities were suddenly occupied by the so-called pharmacoelectroencephalography (**Pharmaco-EEG**), which was massively subsidized by pharmaceutical companies. Pharmaco-EEG consisted essentially of the spectral analytical characterization of new synthesized compounds, which was required for official authorization as a marketable drug. Thereby, economic interests supplanted scientific questions. Clinical psychiatrists, who refused the lucrative services that purchasers offered, turned away from EEG research. The original idea, according to which the clinical effects could be extrapolated from the spectral-analyzed EEG of medicated healthy young men, soon turned out to be erroneous, particularly because with the introduction of the atypical neuroleptics and the serotonin agonists (SSRI), Pharmaco-EEG became obsolete. Due to this failure, interest in EEG as a psychiatric research tool decreased across-the-board. Nevertheless, there was a short lasting resurgence of the clinical EEG, so-called **EEG mapping,** in the 1980's. Because of its picture-like appearance, EEG mapping was misunderstood as a novel brain imaging method. In this context, several authors published articles on the possibility of an objective diagnosis of psychiatric diseases by certain quantifications of multichannel recordings. The software offerings were promoted by allegedly comprehensive and high quality "Normative Data Bases", which were patented and thus not verifiable to others, even to the customers. As one would expect from principle reasons (see Chapter 4), such promises showed up as generally untenable. EEG mapping was soon replaced by the new brain imaging techniques, which were quite rightly celebrated in neurology and neurosurgery as a major diagnostic improvement. However, neuroradiologists, being unaware of psychiatry as such, utilized these methods.

This historical review across 80 years of psychiatric EEG research elucidates the reasons why the EEG could reach a dead-end without having gotten a real chance to proof its scientific potential.

Before the digital revolution, research questions were deduced from meticulous clinical preoccupation with individual patients. However, the technical means that would investigate them adequately were missing. Afterwards, the lack of meaningful questions (e.g. KOSSLYN, 1992) hampered the progress. Those who continued to use the EEG as a research tool were unable or unwilling to recognize the dead-end because they adhered to the Let's-try-it-and-see strategy, which has become increasingly popular. This new research strategy suffers from the empiristic self-deception that meaningful research can and even should be done without previous assessment of sensual qualities and theory-guided experimentation. Instead, only pure objective facts should matter. Such a view has to be contradicted decisively! Each science first needs a sound theory, which is necessarily coarse without differentiating details. An EEG-based psychophysiology, for example, needs a theoretical justification for relating two logically incommensurable types of data, i.e., brain electrical EEG patterns on the one hand and the manifold of inwardly and outwardly directed individual behaviors on the other. The former belongs to the domain of **physiology** (or **function**) to be assessed quantitatively as objective data while the latter belongs to the domain of **psychology** (or **performance**) to be assessed qualitatively as individual subjective data. The objective and the subjective domains of description are mutually irreducible as well as complementary. Both are needed to provide an entire or valid description of a person. To ignore one of them or to reduce the one to the other is tantamount to the epistemological sin of "categorical fallacy". The restriction of objectively measurable phenomena is the hallmark of the classical mechanistic and materialistic physics or natural sciences.

The English neurologist Henry HEAD (1861-1940) proposed to bridge the gap between physiology and psychology by means of the **theoretical construct of "vigilance"**. HEAD'S thinking was inspired by discussions with his famous friends from Cambridge University, Alfred North WHITEHEAD (1861-1947), mathematician and logician, and the biologist William BATESON (1861-1926). When experimenting with nerve-muscle preparations of frogs, he was especially engaged by another friend, the physiologist

C.S. SHERRINGTON (1857-1952), to be described in more detail hereafter. When stimulating the muscle in a serial manner, the intensity of contractions showed a dependency on the number of repetitions. Finally yet importantly, he sought an explanation for a well-known clinical phenomenon, i.e., the qualitative changeability of neurological and psychopathological symptoms as a function of test repetition. This was in conflict with the paradigm of fix-wired centers (see the newer doctrine of "rigidly encapsulated modules;" FODOR, 1984). From a systemic point of view, this spontaneous changeability refers to more than only one global state of brain functioning.

An intriguing example from daily life is the obvious inability to infer reliably the intensity of tiredness from physiological parameters. All correlation studies agree with respect to low correlation coefficients between EEG parameters on the one side and the values obtained by self-rating scales on the other ($rs < 0.20$). HEAD (1923) postulated that a third overriding factor, namely the actual level of the continually changing system's **vigilance,** unified both domains.

The French psychiatrist and philosopher Henri EY (1900-1977) an ardent follower of JACKSON (1835-1911), integrated both organic and psychodynamic factors in his *Psychiatrie Organo-Dynamique*. Inspired by EY'S ideas, his pupils LAIRY, BLANC, and DELL as well as the German Neuropsychiatrist BENTE (1922-1983) postulated that the EEG was an indicator of the degree of HEAD'S vigilance. In spite of convincing empirical proof of the veracity, this exciting new idea essentially went unheeded. This becomes conspicuous, for example, in the common equation of "**Psychophysiology**" and "**Neurophysiology**". He who excludes subjectivity from science or reduces psychology (performance) to physiology (function) is dealing with only one logical category, namely that of objective data. He is therefore conducting neurophysiology. To him HEAD'S theoretical term must be not only superfluous, but also nonsensical. "Psychophysiology" should be reserved to a science, which incorporates the entire system, i.e., both psychological performance (i.e., inner or outer behavior) and physiological function. However, relating two logically incommensurable but also complementary types of data requires HEAD'S theoretical construct. Otherwise, the logically inadmissible mutual reduction from the one domain to the other is unavoidable.

The famous theoretical physicist Niels BOHR (1885-1962), based on his complementaristic way of thinking, which he had derived from quantum theory, postulated that a human could only be understood in its entirety by a duality of perspectives. On the one hand, human has to be described as a biochemical machine, which of course is functioning due to the classical natural sciences. On the other hand, a human being is creative as he/she aligns his/her behaviors with certain values.

CHAPTER 2

The EEG in Psychiatry –
Only Screening for Neurological Disorders – or more?

Those who more than 80 years after the first publication of "Über das Elektrenkephalogramm des Menschen" by BERGER in 1929 compare BERGER'S aspirations with the actually achieved must come to the conclusion that the contribution of the EEG to psychiatric theory and practice has been very meagre mainly for two reasons. The first is that one cannot draw any psychiatrically relevant conclusions from an EEG. Secondly, thus far we have not been able to extract the information actually contained in the EEG. The prevailing opinion supports the first proposition. In German-speaking countries, one can still sense the lingering authority of JUNG (1950, 1953, 1967).

"For the present, the psychiatric application of the EEG remains limited to epilepsy and its peripheral area, to the exclusion of basic organic brain disorders and to shock therapy. For psychiatry in the more specific sense the EEG has not yet yielded many positive results. " and further: *"Neither for schizophrenia nor for manic-depressive disorders do we know of any changes in the EEG that can be used for diagnostics"* (JUNG, 1950, p. 291, translated from German).

On the other hand, we can quote KENNARD (1952. p. 440) who stated at approximately the same time as JUNG:

"The bulk of records seen in psychiatric EEG laboratories are quite different from those of other clinical services. At these meetings, it used to be true that those of us who read such records were grouped to discuss in a minority among ourselves. We have been consistently unable to explain ourselves to then other groups."

It is not in the least because the differences mentioned by KENNARD were unspecified and unsecured biometrically that JUNG'S view eventually gained dominance worldwide.

KUENKEL (1980) identified methodological imperfections as the reason for the unsuccessful search for "disorder-specific" patterns in EEGs. He complained, among other things, about the insufficient explanation of the terms "normality" and "abnormality."

In the English literature, it is also generally agreed that the usefulness of the EEG in psychiatry consists in the exclusion of neurological malfunctions ("organic screening", e.g., LOW, 1979; HALL et al. 1980; STRUVE, 1984; TAYLOR et al. 1985; SMALL, 1987; GARBER et al. 1989; HUGHES, 1997)

In her manual article cited above, SMALL tried to redefine the value of the EEG for psychiatry based on the DSM III with a quintessential conclusion:

"In summary, the importance of the EEG ... is primarily to rule out organic mental disorders" (p. 533).

WARNER et al. (1990) opened the discussion on whether empirical proof exists for the usefulness of such neurological screening. They considered an EEG finding as useful if it changed the diagnosis and/or the therapy. A retrospective study including 698 psychiatric in-patients showed that this was true in only two cases. The authors therefore drew the following conclusion:

"Its clinical use as a screening tool remains questionable. There exists, without any doubt, the need for further empirical clarification, since the rationality of the common practice is questioned."

Those who see opportunities for the psychiatric EEG to compliment or complete neurological screening oppose the general opinion. A questionnaire distributed to the psychiatric departments of German university hospitals in 1991 confirmed our suspicion that the EEG is used almost exclusively for neurological screening. We also learned that only a minority of psychiatric departments disposes of their own EEG labs. The EEG examinations usually take place at the EEG lab of a neighboring neurological hospital or at a central neurophysiological facility.

At this point, it must be mentioned that the way to evaluate general and specific EEG features is determined by the characteristics of the population under observation. This means that what seems irrelevant from a neurological perspective can be essential from the psychiatric perspective. On the other hand, considering neurological populations, frequent and important characteristics will not easily be recognized in psychiatric populations, or they will remain without clinical meaning. The popular but erroneous opinion that an electroencephalography that is independent from the observed matter and stands on its own under the name "clinical neurophysiology" has clearly hampered progress, still needs to be proved.

Whether we will be able to promote the development of a genuine psychiatric EEG depends considerably, under these circumstances, both on how convincingly we can present our arguments and on the openmindedness of our readers. In the following, we first ask the reasons for the prevailing pessimistic opinion. We can distinguish between external reasons that are based on institutional realities and internal, i.e., methodological-scientific ones. By pointing out the existing obstacles for the development, we state the conditions that are necessary for a future psychiatric EEG. A methodological framework that allows the justification of relating EEG and psychiatry is of central importance. The ensuing discussion of the conditions for the development would seem, at times, too theoretical. This would be especially true for readers with previous knowledge of electroencephalography and certification by a professional organization, since they would be expected to question essential areas of supposedly secure knowledge in their entirety. However, the success of our undertaking depends on our ability to initiate a critical discussion of established viewing and thinking habits. The well-known demand to first present facts before proceeding to theory leads to a vicious cycle. In contrast with prevailing opinion, facts or diagnoses do not necessarily speak for themselves. They must always be interpreted, and that requires a theoretical basis. This holds true whether or not the researcher is aware of his basic theoretical assumptions.

CHAPTER 3
Conditions for the Development of the Psychiatric EEG

3.1 FRAMEWORK

To avoid any misunderstanding at the outset, we want to stress that it is not our primary intention to question the usefulness of the EEG for neurological screening. Rather, we are convinced that from the EEG it is possible to extract information that is relevant to psychiatry. The reason for the prevailing pessimistic attitude herein is due, in part, to unfavorable external circumstances that from the beginning prevent the creation of the necessary base of experience. The situation seems hopeless when recording and interpretation occur apart from psychiatry. When a colleague from the neurological department next door is also responsible for the EEG of psychiatric patients, the result of course will be a purely neurological screening. A psychiatric department without its own EEG lab gives up, from the beginning, the possibility to use the EEG as a research tool. Since the complete dependence on external diagnosticians prevents one from gaining and accumulating own insights, the demand for the development of a genuine psychiatric EEG can only be met with rejection, disbelief or, at best, scepticism. However, even when the psychiatric department has its own EEG lab, an increase in knowledge is not guaranteed. Seemingly without fail, communication barriers arise between clinician on the one hand and EEG interpreter on the other. All too often, both sides want to protect their own territory. Inevitably, such territorial protection limits the experience and knowledge horizon. Thus, the misinterpretation of the EEG as an objective routine lab test is common among clinicians, as it is analogous with the determination of electrolyte or transaminases. Unabated and particularly valid for the electroencephalography in psychiatry remains until today what Matthews (1973) summarized several decades ago:

"The greater part of the work of most EEG departments consists of doing single records in patients referred by physicians almost wholly ignorant of the value and limitations of the technique, or who even openly admit to using EEG as a form of supportive psychotherapy (p.207-212)".

Failure to correct the tendencies that instrumentalize the EEG interpreters themselves must have a negative effect on the interaction among colleagues and consequently on the willingness to communicate with each other. On the other hand, the autistic drawing up of EEG descriptions and interpretations that ignores the interests of the physician is the rule rather than the exception. Although the separation of the written record into description and evaluation is generally accepted, many EEG interpreters do not view this kind of evaluation as beneficial for the physician, but rather as a summary of the previous long-windedly explained individual facts. The unfortunate lack of missing clinical experience of the EEG interpreter often fosters this behavior. Voluminous explanations irrelevant to the doctor in charge create legitimate doubts about their usefulness. Thus, the EEG as a whole is discredited.

3. 2 METHODOLOGY

Besides the aforementioned reasons rooted mainly in institutional politics, the absence of a "methodological consciousness" hampered the development of the psychiatric EEG. This is characterized by the piling up of uninterpreted or uninterpretable mountains of data underneath which the original question has been lost. Considering this state of affairs, a widespread resignation about the possibility of gaining knowledge is not surprising. Today, an older generation of high profile researchers who would be able to direct the work potential of the upcoming younger generation into the right channels, based on their own research experience, is desperately missed. Instead, we meet everywhere with an activity that centers around methods and technology thanks to successfully acquired means financed by grants, foundations, and sponsors. The mountains or landfills of data thus created result based on the naïve belief that through primary quantification, i.e., through the mere application of certain signal-analytical procedures that are also used in seismology, for example, scientifically significant insights can be gained. The electroencephalography mutated into an electroencephalometry along with the development of electronic data processing. The fact that patents protect the most prevalent analysis programs should be indication enough for the significant commercial interests involved.

Considering the lack of theoretical guidance, it is no surprise that the non-medical technical support personnel became increasingly important with method-dominated transformations or quantifications. Thus, it was eventually considered normal for research engineers and mathematicians to lead the way in EEG.

However, despite this enormous technological input, who can dispute that the results of these activities are still miserably minute? This faulty development, which is in urgent need of correction, also accounts for the unwillingness of young scientists to do research in the area of clinical electroencephalography. The common misconception that nothing new can be learned from the EEG anyway adds to this problem. Several of the most experienced electroencephalographers have complained about this, for example:

"The trend apparent throughout the world to cut back clinical electroencephalographic units in favor of other neurophysiological investigative techniques is both unjustified and dangerous" (KARBOWSKI, 1990; see also NIEDERMEYER, 1985).

One has to add that the generally observed decline in clinical electroencephalography cannot be reversed by lamentation only. We consider the surgence of newer imaging procedures of the radiologists as an opportunity rather than a disadvantage for the EEG. Since these procedures cover the structural-diagnostic needs of neurology far better than the EEG, it would seem natural to fathom the hitherto idle functional or dynamic information, especially with respect to psychiatry.

In the following sections, we would first like to explain the effects of the lack of methodological consciousness examplified in the discussion about terminology. This will be followed by several chapters in which we gradually develop our framework.

3. 3 TERMINOLOGY

Based on a common consensus, consistent usage of scientific terms is of utmost importance. Compared to the underlying facts, the terms are viewed as less important. Therefore, discussions about the semantics of terms are considered a waste of time. As scientist, one can be interested only in the facts. If one paid enough attention to the facts, the meaning of certain words would become clear by themselves.

In comparison, we consider the terminology of primary importance (e.g., WITTGENSTEIN, 1953). Every act of delimitation happens using symbols or terms. Because no act of delimitation can exist without terms, it is obvious that facts cannot exist without verbal terms. It is not true that the meaning of terms can be deduced from the items they signify. Rather, items can be delimited by the meaning assigned to terms. Therefore, clarifying the scientific terminology must have absolute priority. It is not by chance that discussions about the semantics of terms always become acute when the failure of a science is questioned (KUHN, 1968).

3. 3. 1 "Normal" versus "Abnormal"

BENTE (1961, 1964a) probably saw the problem most clearly when he suggested – half a century ago - the uncritical use of the term "normal" as responsible

"for the paralyzing and unfounded pessimism that has invaded the field of electroencephalography of endogenous psychoses. One cannot start from the superficial and unclear criteria of normality but must be open-minded towards the finer morphology of the EEG" (BENTE, 1961, p. 337-346, transl. from German).

Although many authors before and after BENTE expressed their discomfort with the common practice (DONGIER, 1978; GREENBLATT et al. 1944; HELMCHEN, 1968; KOOI et al. 1964; LAIRY, 1978; LIBERSON, 1944; OBRIST & BUSSE, 1965; STRUVE, 1976; TORRES et al. 1983 etc.), such profound criticism had not the least effect on mainstream research.

"Normal" and "abnormal" are value judgements; thus, they are closely related to a specific reference. "Normal" per se is nonsensical, just as well as "abnormal". In medicine, the term "normal" is applied to discern healthy from ill. Because of the longtime integration of the EEG into neurology, we can assume today that "normal/abnormal" is generally used for the neurology-specific distinction of healthy and ill. The neurological perspective has been adopted as exclusively valid, as evidenced when the neurological criteria for normalcy are applied to study a psychiatric matter. This happens even though different reference points for normalcy are imaginable, such as the ideal type or the statistical average type. If EEGs of psychiatric patients are divided into "normal" and "abnormal" from the beginning

- which until today has been a common practice for clinical routine examinations as well as for clinical studies - then only the "abnormal" EEGs seem noteworthy. The negligible gains of such studies are reflected in the statement that groups of schizophrenics or depressives do not differ or differ only slightly in terms of the EEG - usually because of a higher degree of "non-specific abnormalities". In deploring the unsuccessful search for "disorder-specific" EEG patterns, KUENKEL (1980) emphasized a misguided research strategy. Apparently, the significance of the EEG in psychiatry is being seen as dependent on the degree to which it provides an external validation of the psychopathologically based psychiatric diagnosis. However, "disorder-specific" patterns can be expected only if it were possible to assign specific neurological syndromes to the diagnostic "units" of the psychiatry. As we know today, however, this is explicitly not the case:

"One factor limiting the clinical application of QEEG is the inability to adequately manage the large number of EEG variables, often greater than 100. This is in part because the EEG variables are all interrelated and it is not known which are most useful clinically for detecting abnormalities" (OKEN et al., 1989, p. 1281-1287).

This also makes all prophecies of an objective psychiatric classification through a spectral-analytically quantified EEG implausible (JOHN, 1988; MORIHISIA et al., 1983; MORSTYN et al., 1983; SHAGASS et al., 1984). The formerly widespread consensus that it would be possible, at least in principle, to objectify the DSM-III-classification through calculations with 705 (!) necessarily interdependent variables, calculated without any hypothesis from a one-minute section of a resting EEG, was disproved within few years. Instead of validating clinical diagnoses, we have been reading that "different categories of pathophysiological processes may underlie similar psychiatric manifestations in behavior" (JOHN et al., 1991).

The dichotomy between "normal" and "abnormal" has faded out all those EEG-features that have to be regarded as variations in healthy subjects. However, just those unspecific EEG phenomena might be of importance to the psychiatric patient. Those who like Künkel (1980) who ascribed the terminological disarray to insufficient definition miss the point. This is also true for Gibbs (1982) when he recommended his principle of detailed individual checkpoints that one has to study diligently. He distinguished about 30 specific types of *electroencephalographic normality*; however, simply improving definitions will not do here. Instead, we have to reject value judgements like "normal/abnormal." We are certainly aware of the resistance to such a demand since the search for the diagnostic specificity has the ultimate priority in the medical education. Metaphorically spoken, many psychiatric researchers are still looking in their lab for the "schizococcus." The immensely successful paradigm of infectiology has had far too deep effects on the linear causality-based understanding of medicine and consequently of psychiatry. Far less popular is the idea that for certain disorders, only phenomena that are not specific to this very disorder but nonetheless are of pathognostic significance in the context of certain other, equally unspecific phenomena, can be ascertained.

3. 3. 2 ALLGEMEINVERÄNDERUNG
(General Slowing Down of Frequencies – translated by the author)

Allgemeinveränderung is another term that is limited to the German-speaking countries and hampers the development of the psychiatric EEG. The meaning of the word suggests a general evaluation that encompasses gradations of intensity:

"It is used to describe the curve as a whole" (Jung, 1953, transl. from German).

Hardly any other EEG-related term is equally popular in German-speaking countries. This is probably the result of its undisputable usefulness in evaluating the course of traumatic, inflammatory, or toxic encephalopathies. Although we do not want to engage in any discussion about the expediency or usefulness of the term *Allgemeinveränderung* in neurology and neuro-surgery, we must point out certain inconsistencies. Jung (1953) defined the *slight Allgemeinveränderung* by an alpha rhythm of above-average variability in frequency composition and a certain proportion of theta waves. According to Jung, the "slight *Allgemeinveränderung*" shows *"flowing transitions to the irregular EEG"* and is present in 5 to 10 percent of healthy adults and even more frequently in healthy children between the age of 10 and 14 years. It is our opinion that such a vague definition cannot be satisfactory in a discipline that requires the physician to clarify distinctions. For example, what is the meaning of the slowing of the alpha frequency from 12 Hz to 10 Hz (or a acceleration by 2 Hz) during the course of the illness or a marked discontinuity of the alpha activity with frequent transitions into segments of desynchronized low voltage activity as well as the spreading of the alpha-activity to the anterior brain regions for the user of *Allgemeinveränderung*? Since such statement implies implicitly a pathological change, it is at best misleading to characterize the EEG of healthy children using the term *Allgemeinveränderung*.

Because *Allgemeinveränderung*, at least in its medium degree, connotes a disturbance of the brain function, it further worries us that one also talks about *Allgemeinveränderung* in connection with the effects of psychotropic drugs. Although at first glance very similar, a diffuse theta/delta dysrhythmia in encephalitis certainly represents something completely different from the EEG because of high clozaril dosages. While in the first case, a severe clouding of consciousness might be present, the patient in the latter case will be frequently quite inconspicuous intellectually, a difference often not reflected in the EEG report. This creates additional mysteries for the recipient of such a report.

However, *Allgemeinveränderung* is unsatisfactory not only for semantic and pragmatic reasons. The term also obstructs the gathering of new scientific insights. The implied restriction of *Allgemeinveränderung* to frequency characteristics precludes considering other aspects. This is particularly true in terms of **EEG dynamics,** which is extremely important for the psychiatric EEG. Yet, there has been scant discussion of it thus far. If the terminology allows for the distinction between with or without *Allgemeinveränderung*, markedly disturbed EEG-dynamics would necessarily be classified as without *Allgemeinveränderung*. When *Allgemeinveränderung* and *normal* are equalized, the question about the importance of disturbed dynamics becomes pointless. Therefore, *Allgemeinveränderung* turns out to be a terminological procrustean bed that prevents gaining new insights. The EEG interpreter, who because of generally accepted convention has only the choice between two alternatives, will not dare to seriously consider other possibilities, as a rule.

An additional problem concerns the so-called *variants of normality*. About 10 % of healthy subjects show EEGs with characteristic that are different from the rest. These *variants* are generally regarded as individual types of EEG morpho-dynamics without any clinical relevance. The *variants* could as well be perceived as *state-independent Traits*, indicating a deficit of functional brain maturation and/or vulnerability for the clinical manifestation of psychiatric disturbances. Eventually, the *variants of normality* could be due to an actual pathology and therewith represent a state-dependent phenomenon, i.e., a "*State*" (see Chapters 6 and 7). A valid interpretation requires a repeated recording dependent on changes of the clinical state. However, such investigations are hitherto the exception rather than the rule.

3.3.3 KRAMPFBEREITSCHAFT
(Proneness to Epileptic Seizures)

The question of increased "Krampfbereitschaft" is in tandem with the question about "Allgemeinveränderung," the question most frequently asked by physicians in German-speaking countries. In psychiatry, this question presents itself for all patients treated with psychotropic medication. It is also of particular importance during the withdrawal phase of addiction patients. Under these conditions, clinical experience alone may suggest a higher seizure risk. The physician wants to know from the EEG interpreter whether the risk in a particular case is considered to be higher than expected based on general experience with comparable patients. Another question of interest for the physician is whether the degree of risk has changed in the course of the treatment. Although there is no empirical basis for answering this question, it seems difficult to rectify the general assumption among physicians that the risk of seizure can be deduced from the distinctiveness or even the presence of paroxysmal potentials in the EEG. Unfortunately, some textbooks also contribute to the confusion. Consider the following:

"*They (the paroxysmal potentials - the author) generally are the expression of an increased seizure risk.*" Furthermore, " *such potentials are proof of an increased seizure risk, yet under no circumstance of a manifest seizure disorder*" (KUENKEL, 1980, transl. from German).

We emphatically reject the claim that it is possible to predict an increased seizure risk from an EEG. An EEG- report containing the formulation "seizure risk" is likely to startle the physician in charge. Therefore, the physician might be prone to administer an antconvulsive drug prophylaxis, which is often superfluous and may imply a risk by itself. On the other hand, a real existing seizure risk is generally independent of hypersynchronic potentials in an interval-EEG.

Nevertheless, the prevailing opinion is that paroxysmal potentials in the resting EEG indicate the probability of epileptic seizures to such a degree to justify the use of prophylactic and therapeutic measures. It should be indisputable that a plain nexus between EEG features and epileptic seizures does not exist. This holds notwithstanding the undisputable fact that the EEGs of epileptics in the intervals between seizures show significantly more frequent paroxysmal potentials compared to those of non-epileptics.

Van Donselaar et al. (1992) assessed the cumulative risk of another seizure occring within two years in 81% of the cases with proof of paroxysmal potentials in the interval EEG, as compared to 12 % in cases in which this proof did not exist.

If we examine the historic roots of "*Krampfbereitschaft*" (proneness to epileptic seizures), we again encounter Jung (1950). Although he correlated the seizure risk in epileptics with the degree of *Allgemeinveränderung* rather than with the distinctiveness of paroxysmal potentials, he introduced the solely EEG-based diagnosis of "*latent seizures*" reserved exclusively for healthy persons. As criteria, he used the proof of dysrhythmia in connection with sharp waves. Acceptance of "*latent seizure*" implies the abolishment of the distinction between the logically incommensurable levels of clinical and physiological phenomena. This is manifested in the opinion that it is possible to express the phenomenon of pathological behavior (the epileptic seizure) by a physiological phenomenon (such as sharp waves, spikes etc.) or that the one is a reflection of the other. Such a violation of the logical premises, of course, has practical consequences. Those who equate paroxysmal potentials with latent seizures or increased seizure risk will also justify anti-epileptic medication based solely on the EEG findings. Despite numerous solid arguments to the contrary, this irrational practice is still applied even in university institutions. To our knowledge, there is no empirical proof for a regular interdependence between the risk of seizures and the proof or distinctiveness of paroxysmal potentials. Instead, MILLER & BLUME (1993, p. 128-132) stated:

"*The lack of a significant relationship between tonic-clonic seizures and number and length of epileptiform bursts suggest that EEG is not a reliable forecaster of tonic-clonic seizures in patients with primary generalized epilepsy.*" Furthermore, "*epileptiform bursts occurring only on activation by sleep, photic stimulation or hyperventilation lack prognostic significance....*"

Severals authors also excluded such correlations for patients undergoing drug rehabilitation (KOUFEN & BECKER, 1980; MATISON, 1983; SCHMICKLAY et al., 1989; TYNER et al., 1989; van SWEDEN, 1984; WIKLER & ESSIG, 1970).

The indication for therapeutic anti-convulsive medication has a rational-empirical basis only when an epileptic seizure can be extrapolated from the case history.
Our criticism is certainly not directed at the prophylactic prescription of anti-convulsants after brain lesions or during drug rehabilitation treatment. However, in these cases, the prescription for prophylactic treatment should be independent of the EEG record.

Whether the EEG allows the prognosis of focal-symptomatic seizures after cerebral trauma is at the least doubtful (COURJON, 1970). The sharp high-amplitude waves usually observed under the influence of neuroleptics indicate at best a slightly increased seizure risk. In contrast, the seizure risk in high-frequency spikes and occasionally polyspike patterns is somewhat higher.

The lack of a regular connection between paroxysmal activity and seizure risk even in clinically established epilepsy is evidenced most clearly by the fact that for at least half of these patients, the seizure-interval EEG, even in the case of repeated recordings, does not show any paroxysmal potentials. DESAI et al. (1988) have replicated this finding, which is hardly new, about 20 years ago. Two thirds of 100 randomly selected epilepsy patients did not show any seizure-interval paroxysmal potentials. This seems to confirm HOPKIN'S & SCRAMBLER'S observation (1977, p. 183-186):

"A biometrical test with so many false negatives would never have entered clinical practice."

However, since paroxysmal potentials are considerably more frequent in seizure patients than in healthy persons, we must question the pathognostic significance of these graphoelements. The paroxysmal potentials are generally interpreted as the expression of a tendency of synchronous discharge of distributed neuronal populations. We know from the EEG that these synchronizations have localized accentuations as well as a tendency toward irradiation. Whether this spreading tendency is limited to a specific region or whether a partial or even complete generalization correlated to an epileptic seizure ensues depends on **hypothetical irradiation-restricting mechanisms**. For those mechanisms, no indications exist in the EEG, which could be aligned with the tendency toward synchronization. Therefore, it is impossible to objectify the irradiation-restricting potential that presumably counteracts the excitatory irradiation. However, this is exactly what would be necessary to allow statements about the seizure threshold and thus about the seizure risk from the EEG. A decrease in the seizure frequency may even be accompanied by an increase in paroxysmal activity in the seizure-interval EEG, especially during treatment with carbamazepin. The seizure-controlling effect of the anticonvulsants is reflected in a distinct decrease of the paroxysmal activity only in the primary generalized petit-mal epilepsies (DALBY, 1969; MILLER & BLUME, 1993; MILLICHAP, 1965). In this context, it is remarkable that carbamazapin may induce an increase of paroxysmal activity in every other epileptic. Therewith, the seizure-reduction appears clearly independent of the EEG effect (e.g., JEAVONS, 1972; RODIN et al. 1974; WILKUS et al. 1978).

It would be appropriate to use the terms "paroxysmal potentials", "latent seizures", and "seizure risk" as tantamount only in the case of a one-on-one matching of EEG and clinical seizure phenomena. Since this is not the case, we are obliged to make a logical and clearly defined distinction between these description levels. Exceptions, such as the unequivocal correlation of 3/s-spike-wave patterns along with an observable absence in infants, do not follow this rule.

As with *Allgemeinveränderung*, one can contrast the gain or damage caused by use of the term *Krampfbereitschaft*" (seizure risk). A seizure-prophylactic treatment based solely on the EEG report can even be harmful. On the other hand, one has to expect harm in all false-negative cases (without "seizure risk" in the report) in which necessary therapeutic or prophylactic measures are not taken because there was no proof of paroxysmal potentials: "*persistently normal record is entirely compatible with an increase in the severity of epilepsy*" (STROBOS & KARALLINIS, 1968, p. 622 - 633).

We recognize another detrimental effect of the term *seizure risk* in the unjustified claim of lab capacities because of rationally unfounded "repetitions of recordings." All too often, we are confronted with the demand for short-term control recordings due to the erroneous and stubbornly held opinion that it is possible to objectively detect seizure risks at any time with an EEG. The urgent need to correct assumptions about *seizure risk* is also evidenced in psychiatry with regard to differential diagnoses. A typical question that the EEG clinician asks the physician could be:

Is it possible for a patient with an uncertain epilepsy anamnesis who is currently showing an atypical psychopathological syndrome to actually display an "epileptic equivalent"?

It is understandable that especially colleagues who are still in training and lack experience tend to avoid the responsibility of diagnosing such a serious disease as epilepsy, if possible. Generally, the EEG lab is used for this purpose, with the erroneous expectation of an objective, equipment-backed diagnosis. In an era in which progress in medicine is measured by the degree to which the fallible subject is neglected, it has almost become a matter of civil disobedience to confess adherence to the still valid view that the diagnosis of epilepsy must be based primarily on clinical anamnesis. The contribution of the EEG to the diagnosis of epilepsy will differ from case to case but will never be of decisive importance:

"*The EEG is a limited diagnostic tool for making a positive diagnosis of epilepsia or for resolving unequivocally the differential diagnosis between an epileptic vs. a non-epileptic condition*" (GLOOR, 1977, p. 9 - 21).

This is in line with MATTHEWS (1973), *"Where clinical doubt exists, the EEG will not help."*

A model calculation by Goodin and Aminoff (1984) who took the sensitivity and specificity of the EEG with regard to epilepsy into account showed that the prevalence of epilepsies in the respective population decides whether the EEG will contribute to the diagnosis. The authors based their work on the prevalence of 0.5% found in the general population and on the condition of their own neurological-psychiatric patients. Paroxysmal potentials were found in 4% of seizure-free patients and in 52% of patients with seizures. For a model population of n = 1000 this leads to the frequency distribution presented in Table 1.

		Epilepsy Yes	Epilepsy No	
Paroxysmal Potentials in the Resting EEG	Yes	3	40	Epilepsy prevalence: 0.5%, n=1000
	No	2	955	
	Yes	260	20	Epilepsy prevelance: 50%, n=1000
	No	240	480	

Table 1. Frequency distributions of patients with and without paroxysmal potentials in the resting EEG by the presence or absence of epilepsy. <u>Above</u>: epilepsy prevalence of 0.5%, <u>Below</u>: epilepsy prevalence of 50%. A specificity of 96% and a sensitivity of 52% were assumed for the paroxysmal potentials.

According to the table, 43 carriers of the characteristic are expected with an epilepsy prevalence of 0.5%; 40 of those carriers would be without a seizure disorder, i.e., they would be false-positive. Considering such an unfavorable relation between real-positive people (n = 3, corresponding to 7% of those with the characteristic) and false-positive people (n = 40, corresponding to 93% of the carriers), it would be extremely risky to base the diagnosis on the EEG. However, the diagnostic value of the EEG appears in a different light if we assume a prevalence of 50% of seizure patients - an assumption that seems realistic for the clientele sent to an epilepsy ambulatory for diagnosis. Assuming the same specificity and sensitivity, there would be only 20 (7%) of the patients without seizure disorder, i.e., false-positive cases out of the expected 280 carriers of the characteristic if n=1000. Overall, 260 (93 %) of the carriers would also be epileptics and therefore true-positive. Weighing the usefulness against the risk, the usefulness clearly dominates. The question of primary interest regarding differential-diagnostic significance of paroxysmal potentials in psychiatric patients can therefore be answered through the determination of the epilepsy prevalence in the respective psychiatric population. For our institution, which deals primarily with acute psychiatry, we took the data gathered over a ten-year period between 1981-1991 as basis, considering all patients with an initial diagnosis of epilepsy (ICD 9: 345.0, 345.1, 345.4, 345.5). This resulted in an epilepsy prevalence of 0.39%. When we considered only epileptics with primarily psychiatric symptoms, the prevalence declined to a mere 0.32%. If we viewed these numbers as representative of an in-patient institution for acute psychiatry, we could conclude that paroxysmal EEG activity is insignificant for the psychiatric differential diagnosis. One must be more concerned that by ignoring the biometric premises, the risk of false-positive diagnoses would be significant. Of course, the premises demonstrated here in the example of the resting EEG are equally true for EEGs recorded under provocative methods as well as for the long-term EEG record from the moving patient who carries a cassette. The usefulness of the EEG is then always indisputable when the paroxysmal activity can actually relate to observable epileptic behavior with sufficient certainty. This means that examination intending to confirm or exclude psychiatric manifestations of epilepsy makes sense only if it is conducted in close cooperation between the EEG lab, the treating physicians, and the nursing staff. Each case requires an individual examination plan. The prospects of success increase if during the examination, the frequently detectable seizure-triggering circumstances are considered.

In review, the popular, albeit erroneous opinion that EEG allows an evaluation of the seizure risk touches upon psychiatric questions and, therefore, the psychiatric EEG. *Seizure risk* is a term reserved for clinical descriptions. An interpretation of the clinical meaning of paroxysmal graphoelements cannot extend beyond the physiological level of description. Synonyms are "increased neuronal synchronization", "increased brain-electric excitation", or "epileptiform potentials" but never *seizure risk*.

3. 3. 4 One Feature - Many Terms

One striking peculiarity of clinical electroencephalography is the proliferation of terminology. In general, the creation of a new term is justified only if a truly novel or important phenomenon needs to be defined for practical or theoretical purposes. As numerous examples prove, these conditions are fulfilled only very rarely. A clinical electroencephalography, dominated by the production of terms, especially for single graphoelements, leads one to believe that we are dealing with some kind of substitute activity for the required research that is simultaneously unattainable due to lack of suitable concepts.

It is, for instance, difficult to claim that definition and research of gamma-, kappa, lambda-, my-, rho-, pi-, psi-, sigma-, and zeta-waves (for overviews see DUTERTE, 1978; KUGLER, 1981) resulted in an essential expansion of knowledge. This also holds true for a multitude of other features that we do not desire to list here in their entirety. As can be demonstrated with each example, such kind of pseudoresearch regularly develops in phases. The initial description is followed by the creation of a profile of symptoms. Further confirmations follow. Afterwards, however, disappointment sets in. Independent and, compared to earlier methods, superior research shows the total clinical insignificance of the very feature. From then on, it only leaves a footnote as a historical reminiscence. Pars pro toto, we only want to mention here that the 14 and 6/s positive spike pattern was used for at least 30 different clinical syndromes as pathognomonic before it was found that it can be proved in every fourth healthy young man (LONG & JOHNSON, 1968).

A critical evaluation of the facts reveals that, to our dismay, the stock of knowledge upon which clinical electroencephalography is based consists largely of such footnote ballast. While the aforementioned terms can be blamed only for wasted research potential and time lost for meaningful activities, some terms impede the acquisition of knowledge. In addition to those mentioned in the previous chapter, these terms are more or less those that are used as synonyms for the same phenomenon. Among the many examples, we take particular note of the grouped, fronto-central high-amplitude and rhythmic slow waves pertaining to the subalpha-, theta-, and delta-range (*I*ntermittent *B*ilateral /*A*nterior = **IBA**; see below). This salient phenomenon naturally attracted early attention. SMITH (1938) coined the term *"rhythmic theta bursts of drowsiness."* Numerous authors in later years believed that they dealt with a new feature, which had hitherto not been described in literature and therefore required the creation of a new term. Table 2 provides a list of terms that, in our opinion, all refer to the same phenomenon in the adult EEG.

Term	Author
Rhythmic theta bursts of drowsiness	SMITH (1938)
Abnormal slow potential changes above the frontal region	KORNMÜLLER (1942)
Rhythmic slow discharges	COBB (1945)
Equilateral waves with 6 or 3-4 Hz and frontal emphasis	DUENSING (1949)
Runs of bilateral 4-7 c/sec activity	HILL (1952)
Hypnagogic hypersynchrony	KELLAWAY & FOX (1952)
Dysrhythmia	DALY et al. (1953)
Monorhythmic frontal delta	CORDEAU (1959)
Frontal intermittent rhythmical delta activity (FIRDA)	VAN DER DRIFT & MAGNUS (1961)
Frontal midline theta rhythms	CIGANEK (1961)
Paroxysmal slow activity	GIBBS & GIBBS (1964)
Paroxysmal dysrhythmia	HELMCHEN (1968)
Centro-temporal episodic 6/s rhythm	LIPMAN & HUGHES (1969)
Theta- or Delta-parenrhythmia	PENIN (1971)
Anterior 6-7 Hz moderate amplitude activity	KELLAWAY (1979)
Periodic slow wave complexes	KUROIWA & CELESIA (1980)
Generalized bilaterally synchronous slow bursts	SCHAUL et al. (1981a)
Bilateral paroxysmal slow waves	SCHAUL et al. (1981b)
Episodic anterior drowsy theta in adults	JANATI et al. (1986)

Table 2. Synopsis of terms that can be considered synonyms for the phenomenon of **I**ntermittent **B**ilateral **A**nterior (**IBA**): high-amplitude and rhythmic waves of low and high frequency over the anterior regions.

The asymmetrical, generally left-sided variety of this phenomenon, i.e., intermittent left anterior groups of slow rhythmic waves (**ILA**) of low and high frequencies, was not included in Table 2 since asymmetries were always viewed as related exclusively to focal damages. Therefore, the intrinsic relationship between **IBA** and **ILA** was not considered.

Morphologically, the patterns subsumed under **IBA** correspond to the so-called infantile drowsiness patterns, as described by GIBBS & GIBBS (1950). The frequency of those patterns shifts from the delta- to the theta-range with an increasing age.

Another area, where inconsistently applied and partially overlapping terms cause confusion is the **Low-voltage EEG**. The same EEG is described as either *flat*, *of unstable frequency*, or *beta-typical*, depending on the local "school". Whether the arbitrary determination of formal criteria, such as 20 µV as the upper amplitude limit of the *flat EEG* (JUNG, 1953), is of any help remains doubtful. An important but only rarely mentioned characteristic consists of short bursts of posterior alpha-activity observed in the majority of low-voltage EEGs as a reaction to closing the eyes (COBB, 1978; DAVID & DAVIS, 1936; GASTAUT et al., 1960; RÈMOND & LESEVRE, 1957). In this case, one can observe all gradations of easily overlooked single alpha-waves to spindle-shape modulated groups of alpha-activity. Compared to that, a sustained flat EEG remaining absolutely unchanged under all conditions is a rarity. Another phenomenon, which can be used for differentiation is the hyperventilation effect. It has been demonstrated that a certain percentage of Low-voltage EEGs can be "resynchronized" by hyperventilation (GALLAIS et al., 1957; PICARD et al., 1957). The changes, which occur spontaneously with ongoing resting activity, are of great importance. It is an undisputable fact that, for example, the appearance of the EEG during the first recording minute under resting conditions is as a rule very different from the one recorded during the tenth minute, for example. This is ignored by the still prevailing conviction that any abruptly occuring low voltage desynchronisation independent of the recording time represents an *arousal reaction,* as propagated by the activation concept of LINDSLEY (1961). We remind that the *arousal reaction* is defined as a short-lasting low-voltage desychronisation due to an external stimulus (in the sense of an on/off-phenomenon). According to our experience, low-voltage activity in the resting EEG is generally **not** an expression of *arousal*. Furthermore, it seems hardly possible to prove the "arousal" interpretation since suddenly occuring states of anxious tension as subjective phenomena can at best be assumed but not objectified. EEG technicians often try to meet the demand for a comprehensive behavior documentation during the recording time by making notes about observable signs of tension in case of primarily low-voltage activity. Such a note, however, is usually not the result of the observation of behavior but rather a "petitio principii". Since it is considered true that states of psychological tension or excitement are reflected in longer-lasting low-voltage activity, the presence of the latter is used to conclude the presence of the former. However, the physician who assesses the EEG would tend to relate the note to actually observed behavior and therefore feel confident in his/her opinion.

The increase in lower-voltage desynchronized phases along with increasing recording time in the vast majority of patients is also incompatible with the *arousal-* interpretation. The regularly observable, seemingly paradoxical alpha-activation through sensorial stimulation furthermore proves, without any doubt, that we are not dealing with a manifestation of *arousal* but, on the contrary, with a lowered vigilance. Initially desynchronized EEG that shows the alpha-typical organisation only at a later point in time is very rare. Furthermore, we can point to the findings in healthy subjects subjected to longterm sleep deprivation.

All authors agree that after a progressive discontinuous disintegration of the background activity, around the third day of deprivation, a low-voltage EEG occurs that is otherwise also described as norm variant (e.g., RODIN et al., 1962; BENTE, 1969b).

It is a sign of the power of longstanding errors, as few dared to question the equation of low-voltage and arousal EEG, despite all evidence. According to CHATRIAN (1976), anxious tension can explain only some low-voltage EEGs. Before him, ROTH (1961) had already noticed that any relationship between the frequent low-voltage EEGs in post-encephalitic and post-traumatic states on the one hand and anxiety and emotional instability on the other hand was the exception rather than the rule. Most cases offer evidence for lowered vigilance. The typically discontinuous low-voltage EEGs associated with the detoxification period in alcoholics lasting about 2 to 3 weeks also point against the *arousal*-interpretation.

According to the concept of LINDSLEY (1960), the sensorically induced desynchronisation and amplitude decrease go hand in hand with a more or less evident activation of fast beta-activity. In reality, however, we also find a high proportion of fast beta waves in desynchronized low-voltage activity that can unequivocally be related to a subvigil state (BENTE, 1964b; DAVIS et al. 1938; FROST, 1963; KUBICKI et al., 1987). Even spectral analysis could not distinguish desynchronized activity under unquestionable *arousal*, i.e., immediately after opening the eyes on command, from longer lasting subvigil desynchronized activities occurring with closed eyes (DANIEL, 1966; GEGERELLI & PARKER, 1966). Therefore, it is impossible to use beta-activity to distinguish between *arousal* and subvigil activity. The terminological chaos surrounding desynchronized low-voltage activity becomes complete by relating EEGs with increased or dominant beta-proportion in certain cases to the so-called norm variants, "beta-typical EEG" or "frequency-unstable EEG". VOGEL (1970) was right when he pointed out that only a minority of beta-EEGs are genuine, i.e., constitutional variants.

Drawing some preliminary conclusions, we cannot deny that the thesaurus of electroencephalographic knowledge is nothing but an unstructured conglomerate of unconnected individual facts of dubious meaning. As DANDEY & GACHES (1977) remarked, the interpreter bases his assessment of the EEG on a hodgepodge of half-truths, which, for most part, do not satisfy strict empirical or scientific standards. To put it more bluntly, this means that the clinical EEG lacks a rational foundation in psychiatry. However, such a rational foundation would be the condition not only for the integration of all disconnected facts, but also for focused observation. It would eliminate the real reason for the limited intersubjective reliability of visual evaluation that is generally observed and deplored (STRUVE et al., 1975; VOLAVKA et al. 1973b; 1975; WILLIAMS et al. 1985). Contrary to popular opinion, this is not a problem of insufficient standardization of terminology. When a scientific discipline stagnates due to terminological difficulties, the actual problem never reflects the terminology. With some good will to compromise, it could be standardized. The true problem is that the terminological bewilderment results from differing opinion about the essence as well as the possibilities and the limitations of the method. Terminology problems are, as JASPERS (1946) already knew, usually the consequence of the absence of a concept.

"When a science seems to stagnate and, despite the best efforts of many people, does not seem to make any progress, one can notice that the cause for this is often found in a certain traditional way of thinking about things, in a terminology adopted at one time which the masses accepted and followed without further thought and which thinking people only in individual cases and only with great reluctance rejected in a few instances" (v. GOETHE, (1823, p. 123-124, transl. from German by the author).

3. 4 Theoretical Foundations

3. 4. 1 Systems Physiology, Cybernetics and Biorhythms

WEISS (1941) originally coined "System physiology" as opposed to the upcoming doctrine of "microprecise causality" later promulgated especially by HESS (1969). Nowadays, the term is essentially obsolete. The scientific use of "systems" as the guiding idea of the organismic unity of mind and body has its roots in German idealism (SCHELLING, 1977). Though dismissed by the subsequent materialistic-mechanistic alignment of biological research, systemic thinking was kept alive by a minority of outstanding scientists with philosophical background.

    C. BERNARD'S *Milieu de l'interieur* (1878), which inspired CANNON to develop his concept of *homeostasis* (1929) exerted much influence. Merit deserves also UEXKÜLL (1920) with his *Funktionskreis von Wirken und Merken* (functional circle of acting and perceiving, transl. from German), HEAD'S (1923) theoretical construct of *Vigilance*, WIENER'S (1948) *Cybernetics*, BERTALANFFY'S (1970, 1977) *General*

Systems Theory, FOERSTER'S (1985) distinction between *trivial and non-trivial systems*, as well as the distinction between *allopoietic* and *autopoietic* systems by VARELA (1979) and MATURANA (1982). This coarse listing would be incomplete without mentioning authors who were far ahead of their time and went therefore essentially unnoticed down to the present day. Among them are JACKSON (1884, 1959), GOLDSTEIN (1934), SELYE (1952), ASHBY (1962), EIGEN (1975), PRIGOGINE (1969; 1985), PIAGET (1974), and HAKEN (1982).

The central concern of *Systems Philosophy* was to explain how natural machines (including all naturally occurring interactional phenomena, be it about macromolecular structures of chemistry or living organisms) could maintain their structure and identity in spite of permanently changing embedding conditions. A crucial advancement of this endeavour was highlighted by the publication of WIENER'S "*Cybernetics*" published in 1948. The exciting news of cybernetics was that it was applicable to any kind of system, be it simple man-made systems or complex natural ones. Thus, it had the status of a metascience. As such, it was independent of knowledge about the substantial realization of its objects (ASHBY,1985).

Before addressing the EEG from this vantage point, a misunderstanding, near at hand, has to be cleared up. As already stressed, cybernetics can characterize or explain any natural process. Since human beings are natural processes, man-made machines, just as watches or bicycles but also weather and seismic activity, as well as living organisms have to be regarded as natural processes in the same vein.

From a cybernetic point of view, differences between them exist only with respect to their degree of complexity or behavioral predictability. As such, the phenomenon of *life* acquires a special logical category. The classical natural sciences (sensu strictu) are not concerned with the phenomenon of life nor that of mind. The equalization of natural process and life is a categorical fallacy. In other words, the common antinomy of life and death is nothing but a verbal attribution by a human observer. To natural science, the true antinomy is that between "being" and "not-existing". The "being" may be determined either by the actual given environmental conditions or by inward orientation due to its own past history. To be precise, in the latter case, the determination will result from an interaction between actual outward- and historically developed inward information. In the first case, there is only one single system-state. Its dynamics are to be characterized as linear since each disturbance/impact implies a certain predictable effect. V. FOERSTER (1963, 1985) designated such systems as *trivial* and ascribed them to the *First Order Cybernetics*.

In contrast, systems characterized by a permanent interaction with their environment, implying non-linear system dynamics and unpredictability, were designated as *non-trivial* and ascribed to the *Second Order Cybernetics*. Unpredictable systems should not be designated as "indeterminated" but rather "chaotic determinated" (SCHUSTER, 1994). Chaotic determination is the degree of the system's complexity. It can be quantitatively expressed by means of certain algorithms (e.g., GRASSBERGER-PROCACCIA algorithm: Correlation dimension D2 or LYAPUNOV'S exponent).

An intriguing example of chaotic determination delivers meteorology, which allows only short- or middle-term weather forecast, at best. The Spontaneous Resting EEG represents another example. Each single stimulus or interaction with its surrounding changes the system. Therefore, it is impossible to stimulate the same system, or EEG, twice. This resembles the proposition of the ancient greek philosopher HERACLIT according to whom one never may enter the same river twice. The unpredictability of complex, non-linear, non-trivial processes refers to both the physiological level of function and the psychological level of performance/experiencing. Because we are dealing here with categorically different domains, the one cannot be deduced from the other. Consequently it is of utmost importance to always make clear whether experimentally obtained data refer to the domain of function (exact physiological measurement) or to the domain of performance (assessment by qualitative psychological methods). The common practice of reducing the one to the other equals a trivialization of a non-trivial system. The deleterious effects of this epistemological fallacy become especially obvious with certain popular interpretations of modern neurosciences (KURZWEIL, 1999; 2009).

Though WIENER'S cybernetics reinforced systemic thinking across a broad front, it lost its initial effect as a metascience within a few decades, particularly within medicine and psychology. Instead of working out the profound heterogeneity between trivial systems and non-trivial living organisms, mainstream science was in contrast essentially engaged with emphasizing the homogeneity between them, i. e., trivializing non-trivial research topics like the EEG.

Neurobiologists increasingly considered themselves as "brain physicists", implicitely admitting their incompetence concerning the phenomena of the living and of the mind. The progredient disappearance of "Biology" in favour to an affirmative use of "Life Sciences" seems to reflect a discomfort with this modern self-conception.

The conception of the Second Order Cybernetics, elaborated by the Biological Computer Laboratory (BCL, Urbana/Ill) 1958-1975 under the direction of Heinz v.

FOERSTER, promised a true progress that was hardly acknowledged up to that point. This truly epochal achievement was the result of an inspired multi-disciplinary research activity. The staff comprised such illustrious scientists as WIENER; Mc CULLOCH; ROSENBLUETH; ASHBY; GUENTHER; LOEFFGREN and MATURANA to name a few.

This deficiency will remain unchanged as long as Life and Subject are being excluded from research as "wissenschaftliche Tatsachen" (in the sense of L. FLECK, 1935; "scientific facts", transl. from German).

First tentative attempts towards a systems theory-based organismic physiology date back to the 1970s (e.g. DRISCHEL 1973; HASSENSTEIN, 1973; RENSINGER, 1973; SELBACH, 1974). The failure of such efforts may be ascribed to an inability to break away from the prevailing pretendedly atheoretical empirism.

3. 4. 2 The Spontaneous Resting EEG (SR-EEG) as a non-stationary process

Viewing the **SR-EEG** as a time function with a certain order (*Verlaufsgestalt* in German) takes for granted a certain hierarchical order of Cerebral Global Function (**CGF**), as postulated by JACKSON (1884) long ago and later on modified by HEAD (1923). However, BENTE initiated the development of a **psychophysiological or psychiatric EEG** by conceiving **SR-EEG** as an indicator of **CGF** (Ulrich, 2012). The visuo-morphological patterns, which occur along with the recording of the **SR-EEG,** are qualitative phenomena of our empirical reality. The distinction *requires* the "tool" of human pattern-perception (*Gestaltwahrnehmung*). This "tool" is to be regarded as scientifically legitimate (LORENZ, 1959) and indispensable for defining naturally occurring patterns. With respect to the spatio-temporally distinguishable patterns, BENTE (1961, 1973a, b) coined the term "*höhere Strukturmerkmale*" (higher structural characteristics, translated from German). He regarded these characteristics as products of an ontogenic maturational process (GIBBS & GIBBS, 1964). Constitutive for them were certain so-called *formative Tendenzen* ("formative tendencies", transl. from German), i.e., changes in **amplitude, synchronisation, frequency,** and **topographical differentiation**. From the viewpoint of systems theory, the *formative tendencies* are to be regarded as partial processes of the "brain-electric mass activity".

Apart from the "higher structural characteristics", the **SR-EEGs** may be visually distinguished with regard to their overall dynamics. Three different predilection types may be discerned with one view by means of a so-called chronospectrograms (see Fig. 45, 46, 47). Thereby a certain number of FFT spectra calculated from consecutive 2s epochs of a **SR-EEG** (in the following examples, 300 2s epochs correspond to a 10 min record) were arranged behind one another and displaced laterally. If one tried, as it is common, to distinguish the three EEGs quantitatively by averaging the 300 spectral power values, the obvious qualitative differences would be missed due to eliminating the dynamic information.

The interaction between a system and its environment goes along with a deflection of functional parameters of the system. This leads to an instable, indetermined disequilibrium state, which brings about a counter-regulation in favour of the pre-existing (more) stable equilibrium state. It is generally disregarded that an exact equilibrium can never be achieved principally. Considering this fact, it may be claimed that systems are permanently oscillating about their default equilibrium states without ever reaching it. Therefore, any regulatory deflection has to be regarded as overcompensation. Each overcompensation causes a counterregulation into the opposite direction and so on and so forth. Since the "set value" ("Sollwert" in German) is only achievable by approximation, the resulting time function will never be periodical but only *quasi-periodical*. Obviously, *quasi-periodicity* of a process is the precondition of its continuity. Exact reaching of the set value would mean a standstill or an idle state, tantamount to "death" in the case of a living organism. In view of the succession of "waves", which amounts to the process of the Spontaneous Resting EEG, each single "wave" can be regarded as an overcompensation of the previous one. Any visuo-morphologically discernible change of the EEG-patterning (corresponding to BENTE'S, 1963, *höhere Strukturmerkmale*, "higher structural characteristics", transl. from German) indicates a change in regulation with regard to the hierarchical organization of the system. A physiological example thereof is the spindle-like patterning of the posteriorly accentuated Alpha rhythm, which is typically observed among alert healthy subjects and matched to stage A1. The spindle-like appearance results from reasonable higher alpha-frequencies associated with lower amplitudes both at the beginning and at the end of alpha formations. This kind of patterning indicates a stepwise regulatory mechanism. Within the first half of the spindle (the so-called *squeezing on*), frequency slows down increasingly as a reflection of a transitory negative feedback mechanism, whereas the amplitudes increase by means of concurrent positive feedback. Within the the second half of the spindle, the regulatory mechanisms reverse their direction (the so-called *squeezing off*). Anteriorization of the Alpha rhythm, which indicates subvigil Stages A2-A3, accompanies a falling apart of the Alpha-spindles. With stage A3 only the first half, if at all, resembles the well-ordered symmetrical Alpha-spindles of stage A1. Increased transitions into low voltage desynchronized activity with predominance of rapid ("subvigil") Beta activity, which is typical for an undisturbed recording from min 4-6 and coordinated to stage B1 (ROTH, 1961), indicates another type of regulation. The same holds for the patterns that were coordinated to the remaining stages of lowered EEG-vigilance, including those of sleep.

From this vantage point, it is inherently consistent to interpret pathological EEG patterns, for instance those observed with epilepsy, in the same way. In contrast to the patterns coordinated to physiological vigilance regulation, epileptiform patterns indicate pathological or maladaptive types of vigilance regulation. The well-known association between epileptic seizures and spontaneous or induced changes of the EEG-vigilance level supports this interpretation.

Special attention should be paid to BENTE'S (1964, 1981) additional characterization of the **SR-EEG** as a process with cyclic order reflecting differentiation and goodness of adaptive behavior.

If we define health as the maintenance of a dynamic equilibrium within certain limits (v. BERTALANNFY, 1970, 1977), we need adequate parameters. Since the opposition of healthy and sick is reserved for living systems characterized by high complexity, only variables representing the highest organizational level possible will have to be considered.

The micro-detail anlyses of modern biology, which result in cascades of chemical reactions are tracing down to the molecular level. It needs not to be stressed that this kind of information does not provide us with knowledge about the highly integrated functional mechanisms that are needed for our purpose.

"*Life*" belongs to the logical category of metaphysics. It is not a topic of the natural sciences. A holistic top-down- or a meristic bottom-up-strategy will not tell us anything about its essence. Physics and chemistry place boundary conditions, thus leaving this "essence" undefined. From a thermodynamical point of view, there is no difference between the flame of a candle and a living system. Every now and then we are concerned with a dynamic equilibrium, albeit only living systems are "seeking" a higher states of order. WEISS (1969, 1970, 1978, see also ULRICH, 1997), who introduced the term *system* into biology, specified certain determinants that characterize living systems without explaining their very "essence". Thus, living systems may spontaneously change their states of order by means of a hierarchically organized sequence, which depends on the actually realized transactional relation with the environment (WEISS, 1969, 1970, 1978, see also ULRICH, 1997). GOODWIN (1994) summarized these determinants using *dynamic organization,* which is compatible with our systemic notion of the Spontaneous Resting EEG as a macroindicator of cerebral global function (3.4.4). As already mentioned, the transitions between different states of the system are reflected by the visuo-morphologically defined wave patterns of *EEG-vi*gilance both spontaneously and due to environmental stimulation. So called "Alpha-blocking" consists of a very short lasting attenuation or even complete disappearance of Alpha waves due to an acoustical stimulus or opening of the closed eyes. It goes without saying that the prerequisite of Alpha blocking is a preexisting Alpha-rhythm. This so-called *arousal-effect* has to be interpreted as a passing desynchronization without a specific behavioral meaning. The *arousal effect* has to be distinguished from longer lasting low voltage desynchronized activity occurring without any sensorial stimulation. In case of pre-existing activity of this kind, sensorial stimulation will be followed by an activation of synchronized Alpha-activity, indicating EEG-vigilance stage A. Accordingly, it has to be concluded that the pre-existent desynchronized low voltage activity represents decreased EEG-vigilance corresponding to subvigil stage B rather than a state of *prolonged arousal*. Thus, this kind of Alpha-activation is by no means "paradoxical", as it is commonly termed. It necessarily follows from the fact that all stimulations of the system affect an increase in EEG-vigilance, with its duration being dependent on the effect of the stimulation.

Therewith, we meet the challenge of a quantitative evaluation of the continuously changing macroindicator of cerebral global function, i.e., the **SR-EEG**. This first step of the task consists of a visuo-morphological demarcation of the spatio-temporal wave patterns representing the cyclic order of the process. Subsequently a quantitative reconstruction of the qualitative information is required, both as a time course profile and as mean-values across the total recording time.

3. 4. 3 EEG AND VIGILANCE

LAIRY & DELL (1957) took the first step towards a theoretically founded electroencephalography. HEAD'S (1923) construct of *vigilance* played a decisive role in their work. LAIRY & DELL considered the electroencephalographic pattern dynamics as an expression of the Cerebral Global Function (**CGF**) as well as of the maturity state. The global functional state (*état fonctionnel global*) has been considered the equivalent of HEAD'S vigilance. The authors emphasize certain passages of HEAD'S original work, which clearly indicate that this term did not stand for psychological facts, such as a behavioral state or a behavioral disposition. *Vigilance* had "*une signification trés générale.*" The equation with alertness or wakefulness was erroneous, although tempting because of the word stem. *Vigilance* would be indicated by the spontaneously occuring spatio-temporal patterns, which were discernible in the EEG under the so-called resting conditions as well as by the dynamics of transition between these patterns. The distinction between waking and sleeping conditions, therefore, seems to be of subordinate importance. BENTE (1961, 1964a, 1964b, 1979, 1981, 1984) adopted this approach and demonstrated its heuristic fertility in an article published exclusively in the French language. BENTE explained, a certain order of succession dominates the pharmacogenous and pathological *Form- und Funktionswandel* (morphological and functional change in the brain's electrical activity). The respective order represents a modification of the physiological process of falling asleep or waking up. This clearly rejects the common practice of the arbitrarily isolating analysis of features that ignores the morphological context.

"*Since the EEG is a complex structure of a variety of features, all attempts to consider or measure the individual features without regard to its structural relationships harbor the risk of wrong conclusions that might have grave consequences*" (BENTE, 1961, p. 337 - 346; transl. from German).

To Bente, a profound knowledge of the brain-electrical patterns regularly observable during the transition from wakefulness to sleep was prerequisite for a psychophysiological or psychiatric electroencephalography (BENTE, 1981, 1984). Referring to LAIRY & DELL (1957), BENTE postulated a correspondence of this sequence with a decrease/increase in differentiation and availability of environment-related behavior. BENTE viewed the crucial information as residing in the spontaneous vigilance dynamics. Therefore, the EEG taken under resting conditions (sitting comfortably, eyes closed, undisturbed in a quiet darkened room) was of central importance to him.

To him, the sleeping EEG as well as the EEG under defined cognitive load were only interesting methodological supplements. BENTE called the EEG-patterns at the center of interest, that is, complex structures of grapho-elements in a certain arrangement varying in time and topography, "higher structural characteristics" (*höhere Strukturmerkmale* in German). The appropriate instrument for their delineation would be primarily visual gestalt perception (see also 3.4.2).

Dating back to the beginnings of electroencephalography, LOOMIS et al. (1937) classified the time course of the Spontaneous Resting EEG beginning with full alertness up to deep sleep into stages (stage A to E; Fig. 1 above). Later, the DEMENT & KLEITMAN'S (1957) classification (Fig. 1, below) in which the focal point of interest shifted to the sleep (sleep stages II to IV as well as REM stage) gained wide-spread acceptance.

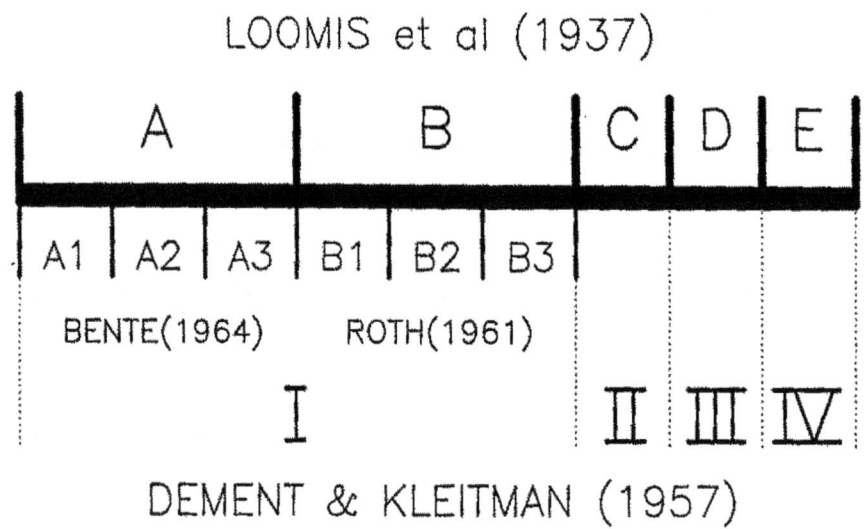

Figure 1. Synopsis of commonly used visuo-morphologically defined classifications of the EEG-stages occuring between relaxed wakefulness and deep sleep.

The latter staging was inspired by the assumption that sleep may be physiologically better discerned into stages than wakefulness. Nevertheless, through the introduction of a certain framework of conditions, the EEG of wakefulness can be equally well defined, a fact that motivated LIBERSON (1944) to propagate his *functional electroencephalography*. With healthy adults, the **SR-EEG** shows characteristic changes in accordance with the recording representing the physiological dynamics (**PM**). The initial stage A is generally maintained for about 4-6 Minutes (see Fig. 2, 3). Thereafter, transitions into stage B patterns may be observed, followed by recurrences to A-stages. Along with recording time, a current trend indicates a decrease in stage A patterns and an increase towards mid and late B stages (B2, B3). Eventually, a short-lasting Stage C may be reached.

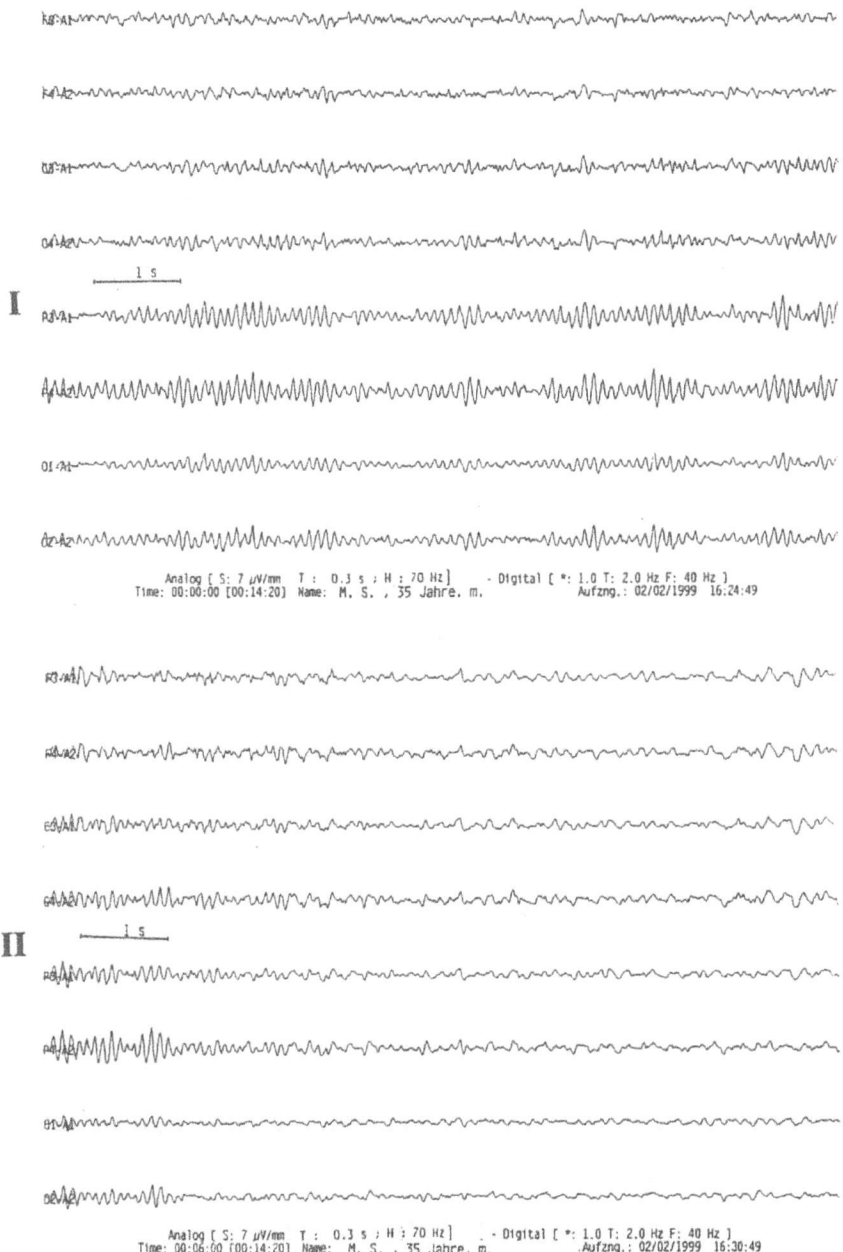

Figure 2. At the beginning of the SR-EEG (min 1-5), a continuous and spindle-like modulated Alpha rhythm of about 9-10/s prevails (I); thereafter (min 6-10), transitions into segments of low-voltage desynchronized activity increase, corresponding to stage B1 with increasingly interspersed Theta-waves (stage B2, B3).

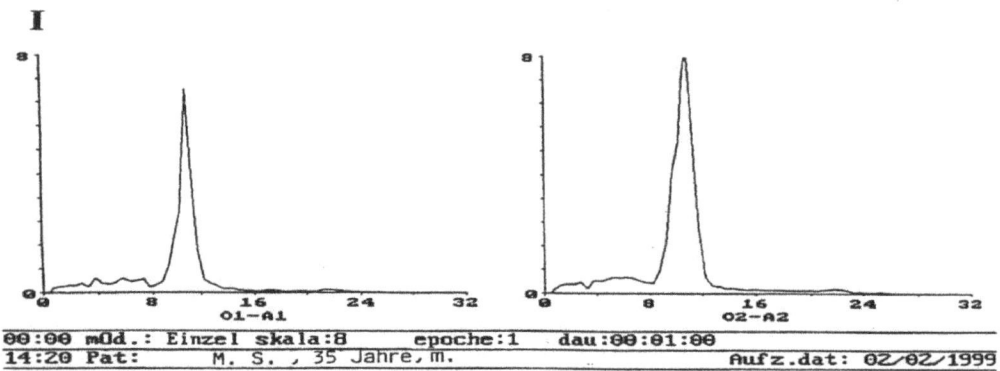

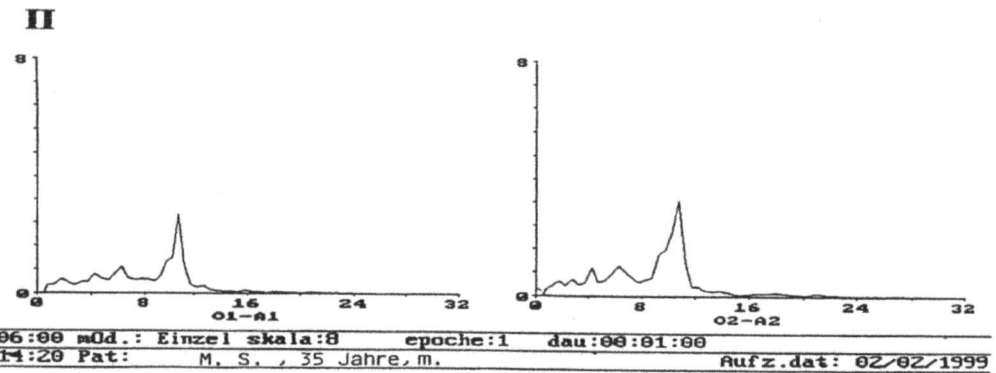

Figure 3. The FFT-spectrogramms, calculated for the 1st and the 6th minute (leads O1-A1, left side and O2-A2, right side) confirm the pronounced decrease in Alpha-activity together with an increase in Theta-waves occurring between min 1-5 and min 6-10.

Illustrations 5-23 show the subvigil intermediary stages, which can be observed during wakefulness (these have been subdivided by BENTE (1964b) and ROTH (1961)) as well as at the sleep onset and during light-sleep stages. The International 10-20 System for the electrode placement in Fig.4 is intended for orientation purposes. In comparison to the stage A1 with its characteristic posterior accentuation of the basic rhythm (Figs. 5, 6), an anteriorization occurs during the transition to stage A2 (Figs. 7, 9) accompanied by

- a moderate increase in voltage
- a moderate increase in continuity (stability of course)

- a moderate decrease in frequency, more obvious in the anterior than in the posterior
- a moderate increase in synchrony
- a moderate anteriorization of the alpha-activity in the mid and frontal regions (ear reference!)

The degree of anteriorization was originally related to the EEG taken against ipsilateral ear reference (BENTE, 1964b). We retain this convention. As the following curve examples demonstrate, frequently a more or less distinct discrepancy between the reference and the source derivation exists with regard to the anteriorization. In the reference derivation, the anteriorization is considerably more pronounced in the majority of cases than in the source derivation. The opposite is hardly ever noted. We also frequently find a distinct anteriorization with reference recording and an equally distinct posteriorization with source recording. Such peculiarities indicate high within-subject stability. Furthermore, the existing, distinct between-subject variability leads to the conclusion that the phenomenon of alpha-anteriorization resists the unequivocal neuroanatomical correspondence, i.e., it ignores brain lobe boundaries. While in most cases of anteriorization, we are dealing with an ear electrode generated *temporalization* (TIIHONEN et al. 1991; LU et al. 1992), in some other cases, the anteriorization actually is more of a frontalization.

The fully developed stage A2 (Fig. 9) accentuates all these tendencies. The criterion for the delineation with respect to stage A1 is the degree of anteriorization with an anterior alpha-amplitude of about the same magnitude as the posterior.

THE THEORETICAL INTERPRETATION OF ELECTROENCEPHALOGRAPHY (EEG)

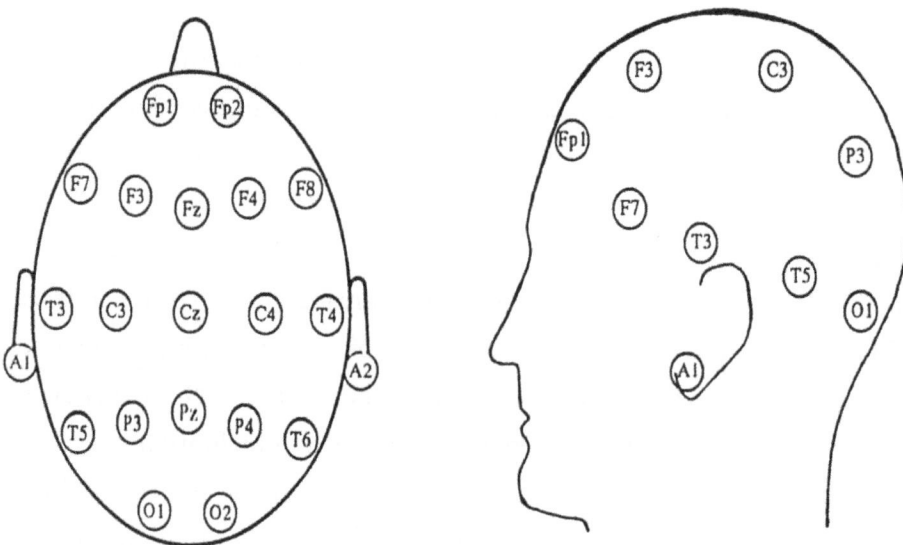

Figure 4. Placement of electrodes according to the International 10-20 System.

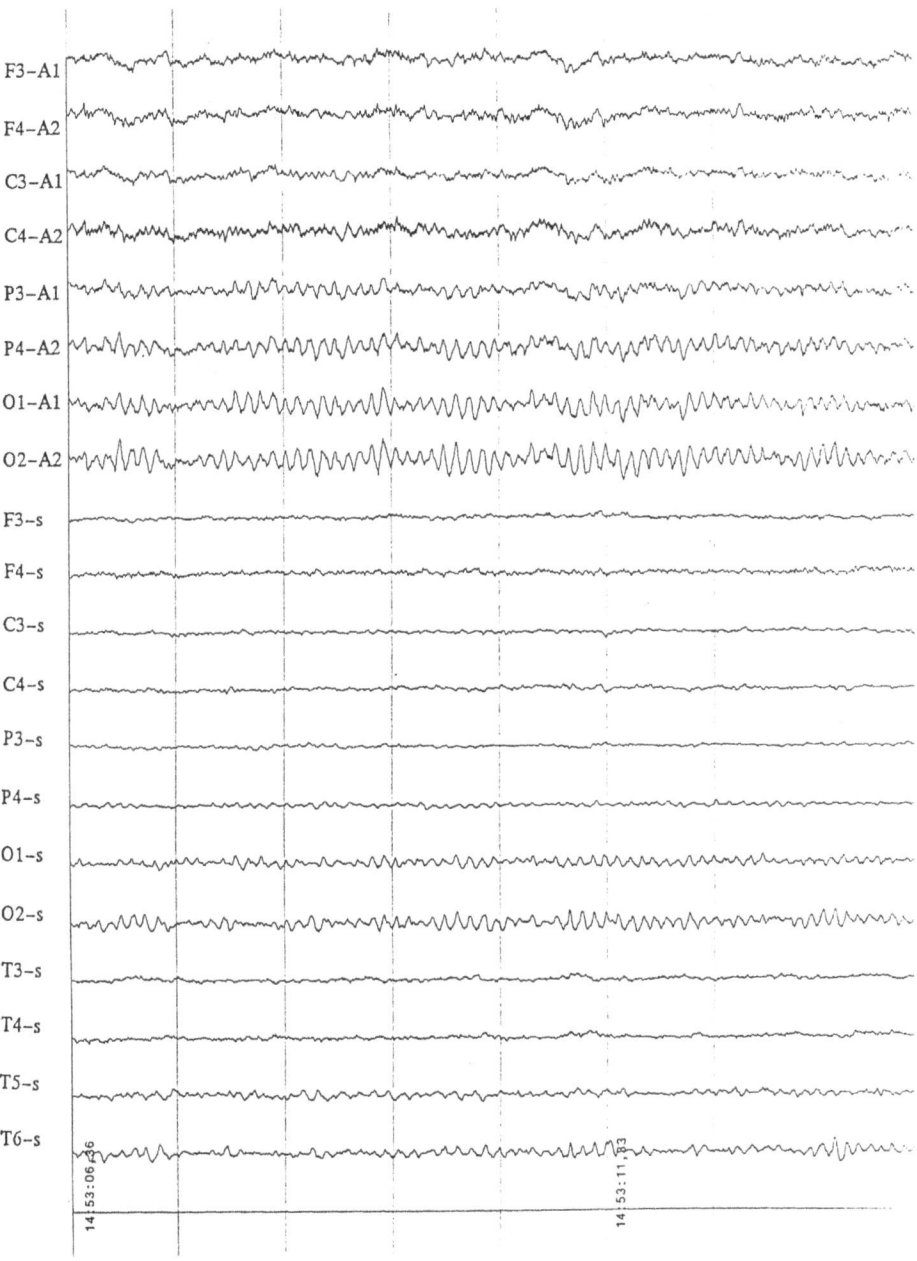

Figure 5. Stage A1: 8.5/s-alpha-activity with a distinct posterior accentuation (the following curve examples – fig. 5-23 with identical electrode montages).

THE THEORETICAL INTERPRETATION OF ELECTROENCEPHALOGRAPHY (EEG)

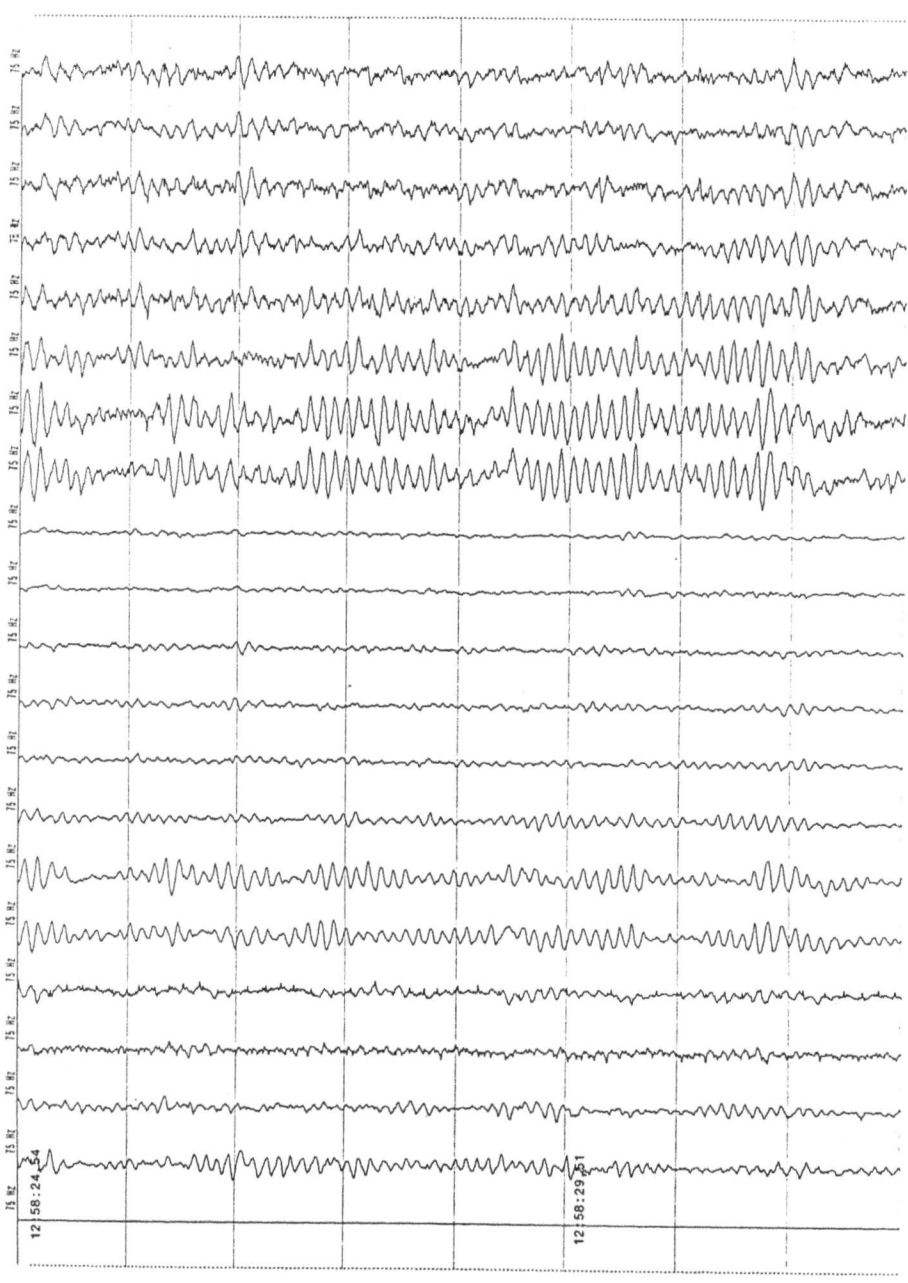

Figure 6. Stage A1: Slightly spindle-like modulated 9/s alpha-activity with posterior maximum. An alpha-rhythm can also be distinguished above the frontal and mid regions but at significantly lower amplitudes compared to the above the posterior regions

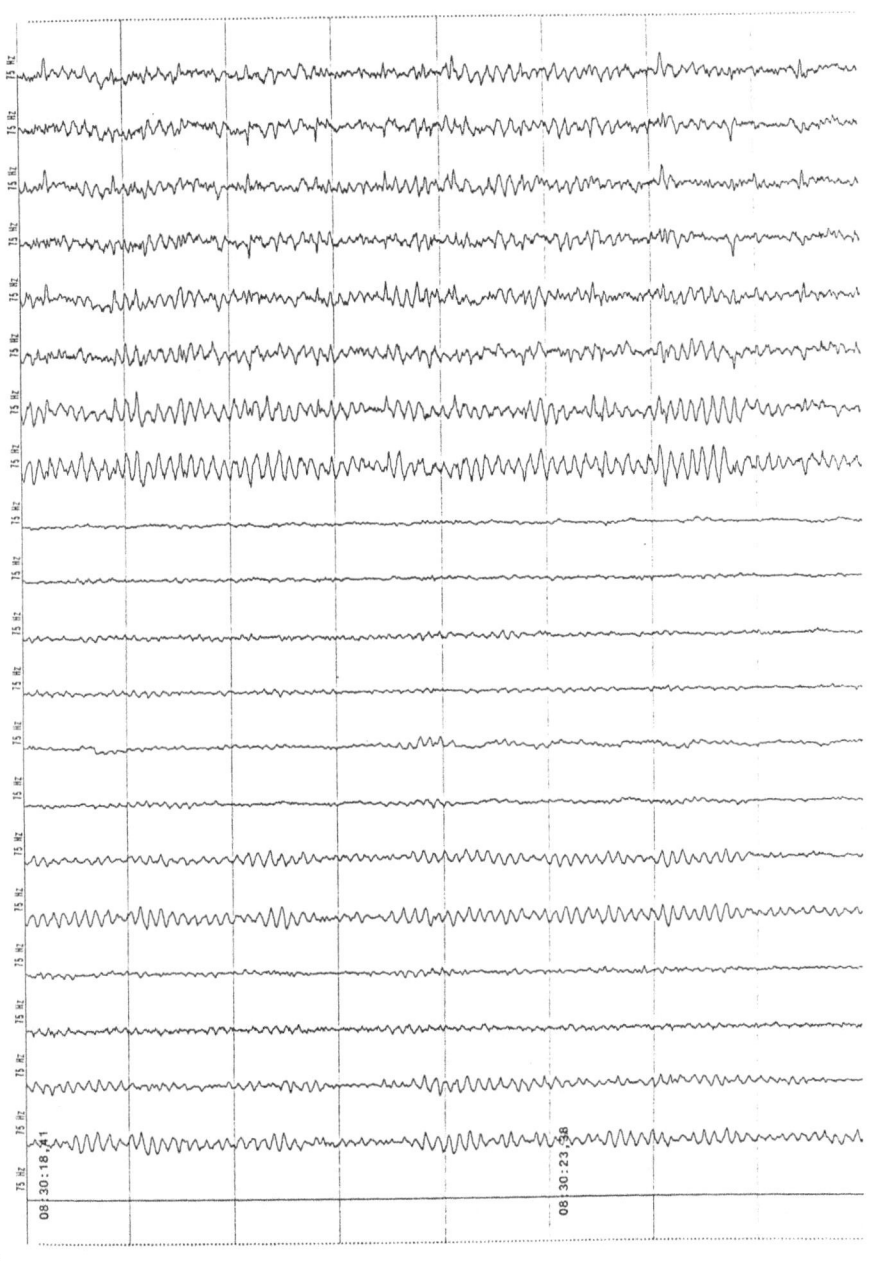

Figure 7. Stage A1 > A2: 9.5/s alpha-activity with posterior accentuation during the first 3 seconds spreads to the front in the 5th second, corresponding to a stage A2.

THE THEORETICAL INTERPRETATION OF ELECTROENCEPHALOGRAPHY (EEG)

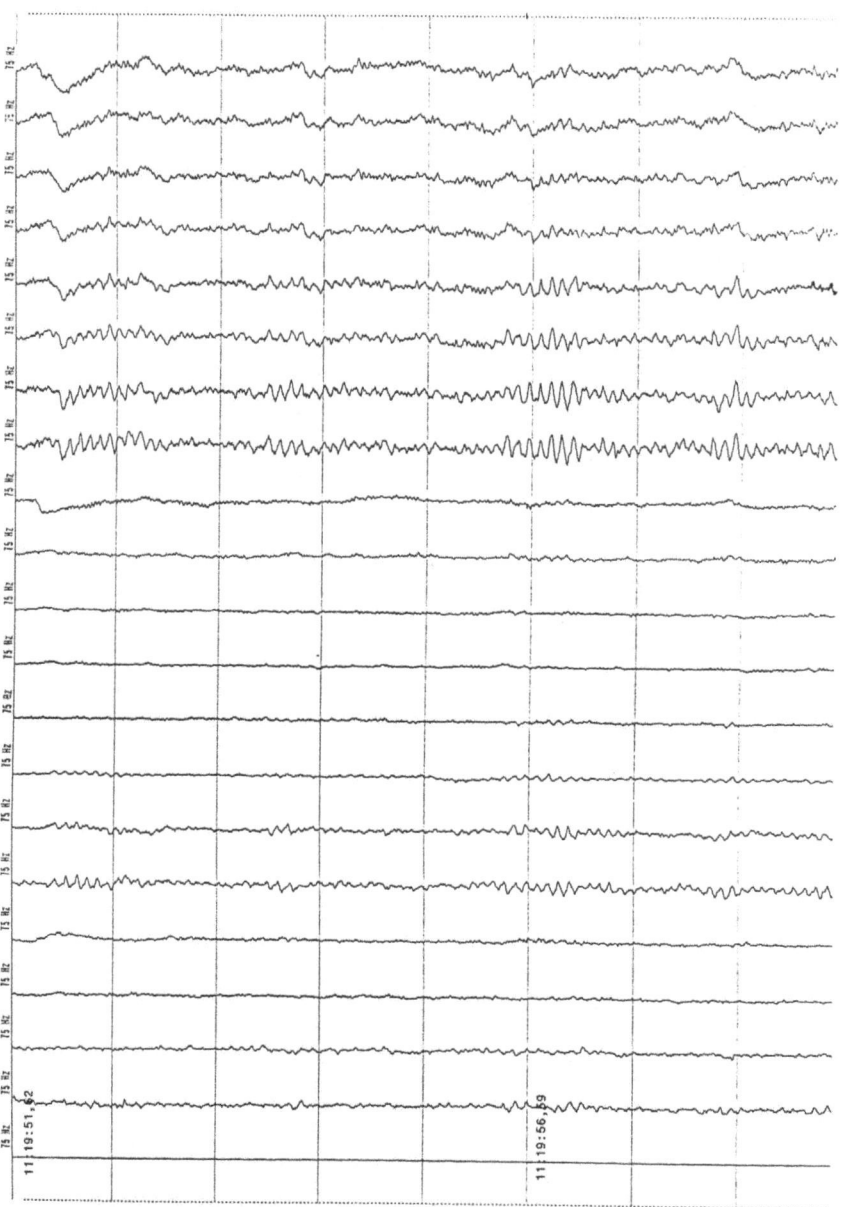

Figure 8. Stage A1 > B1: Discontinuous and posterior-accentuated alpha-rhythm at 9.5/s with transitions into short (1s) desynchronized segments of low voltage corresponding to a stage B1.

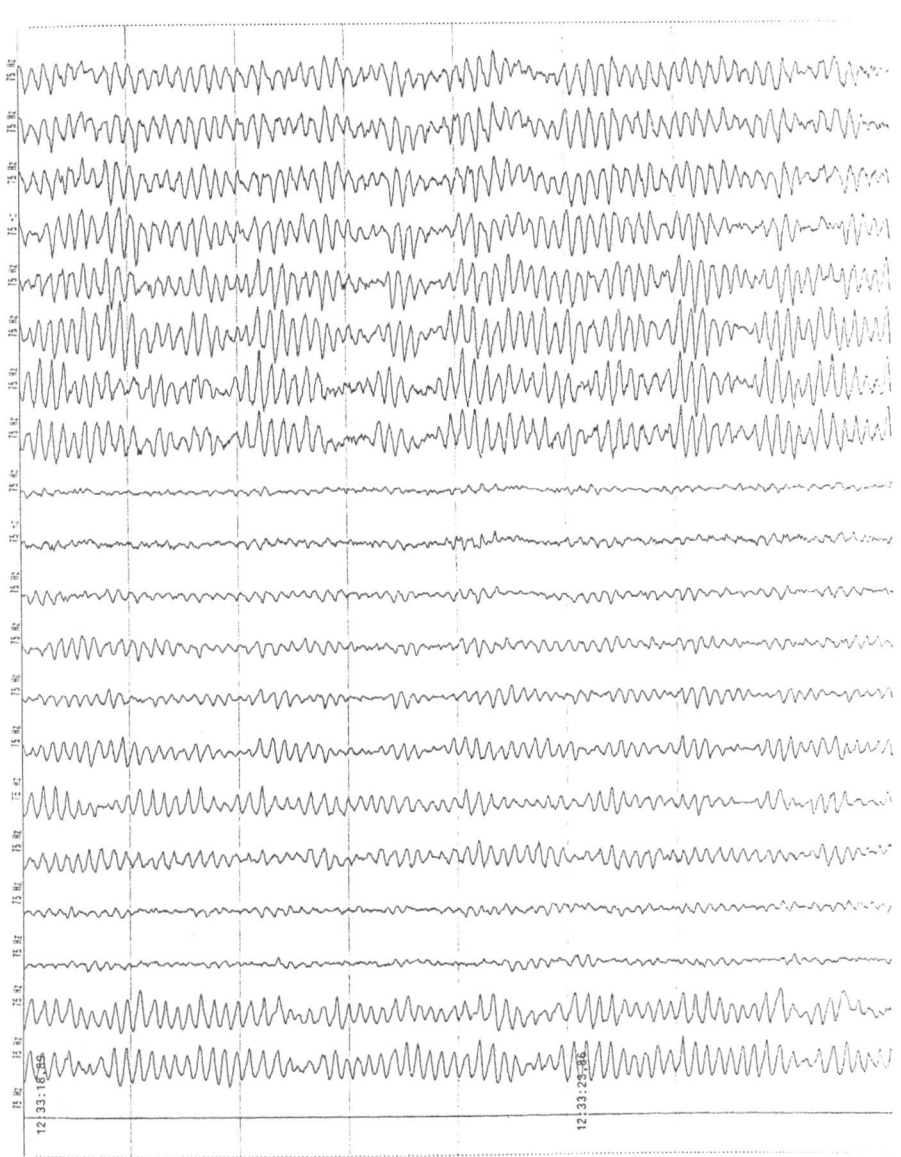

Figure 9. Stage A2: Consistently anteriorized, relatively monomorphous alpha-activity with an anterior-posterior frequency dissociation of about 1.5 Hz (posterior: 9.5/s, anterior: 8/s) exceeding the physiomorphic range. While the anterior-posterior amplitude relation is almost balanced in the reference derivation, the anteriorization in the source derivations appears to be relatively smaller.

THE THEORETICAL INTERPRETATION OF ELECTROENCEPHALOGRAPHY (EEG)

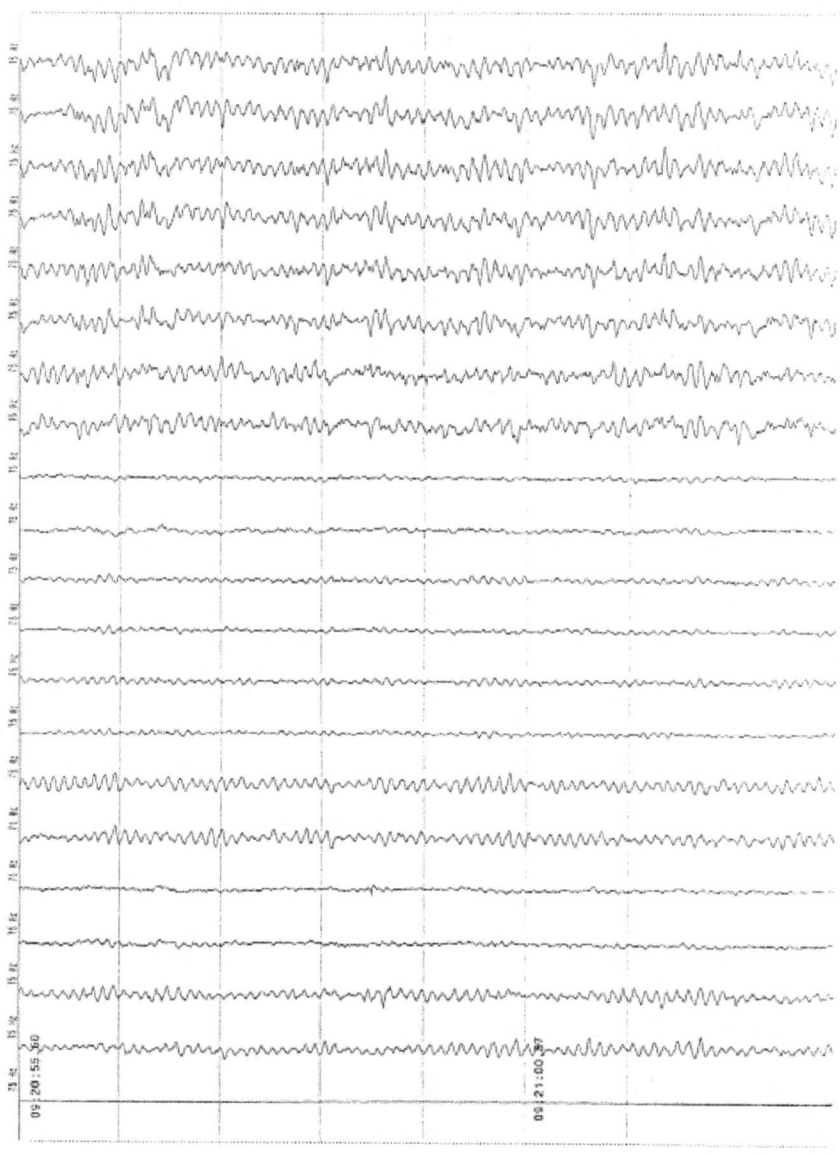

Figure 10. Stage A2/A3: slightly anteriorized 9/s alpha-activity from the beginning. The source-derivations, on the other hand, shows a continuous alpha-dominance of posterior amplitudes.

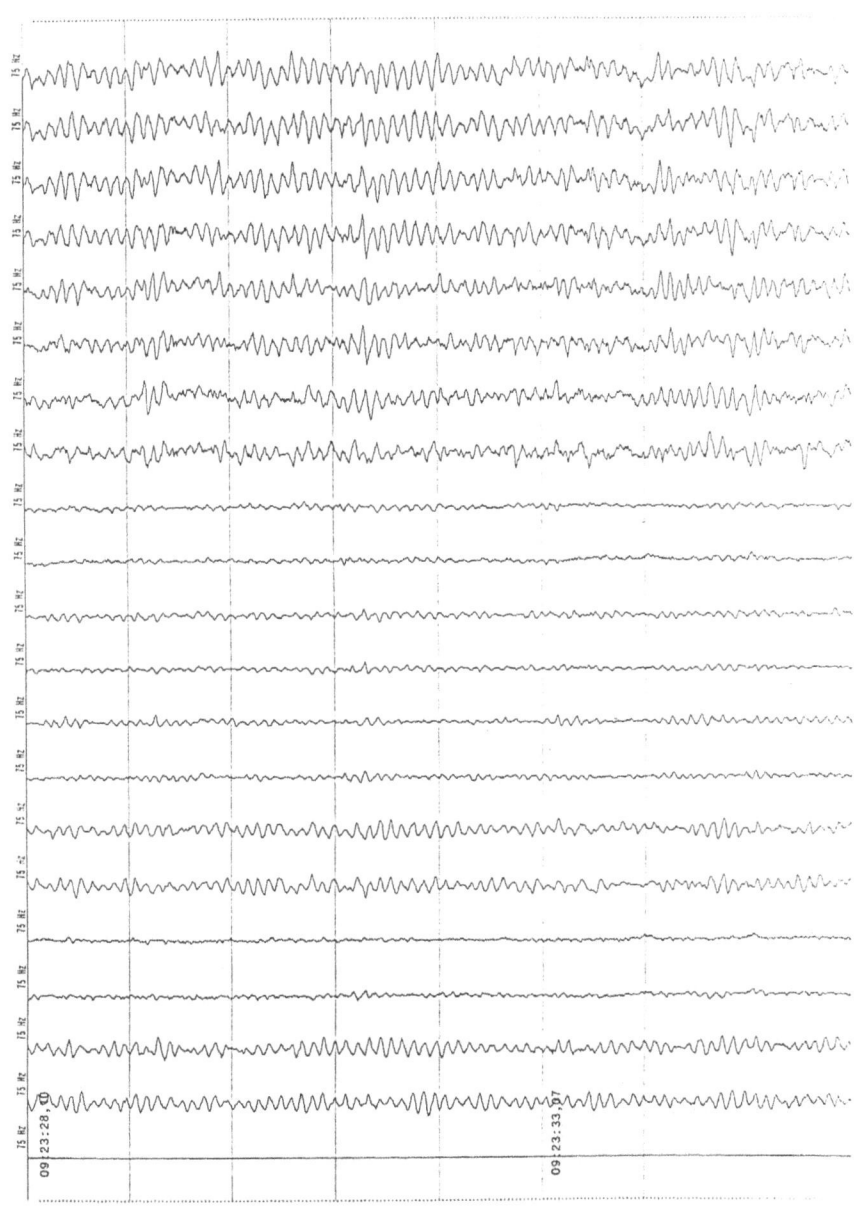

Figure 11. Stage A3 > A2: Obvious anterior amplitude dominance of a 9/s alpha-activity from the 1st to 6th second (not in the source derivations!), followed by a transitional A2 stage.

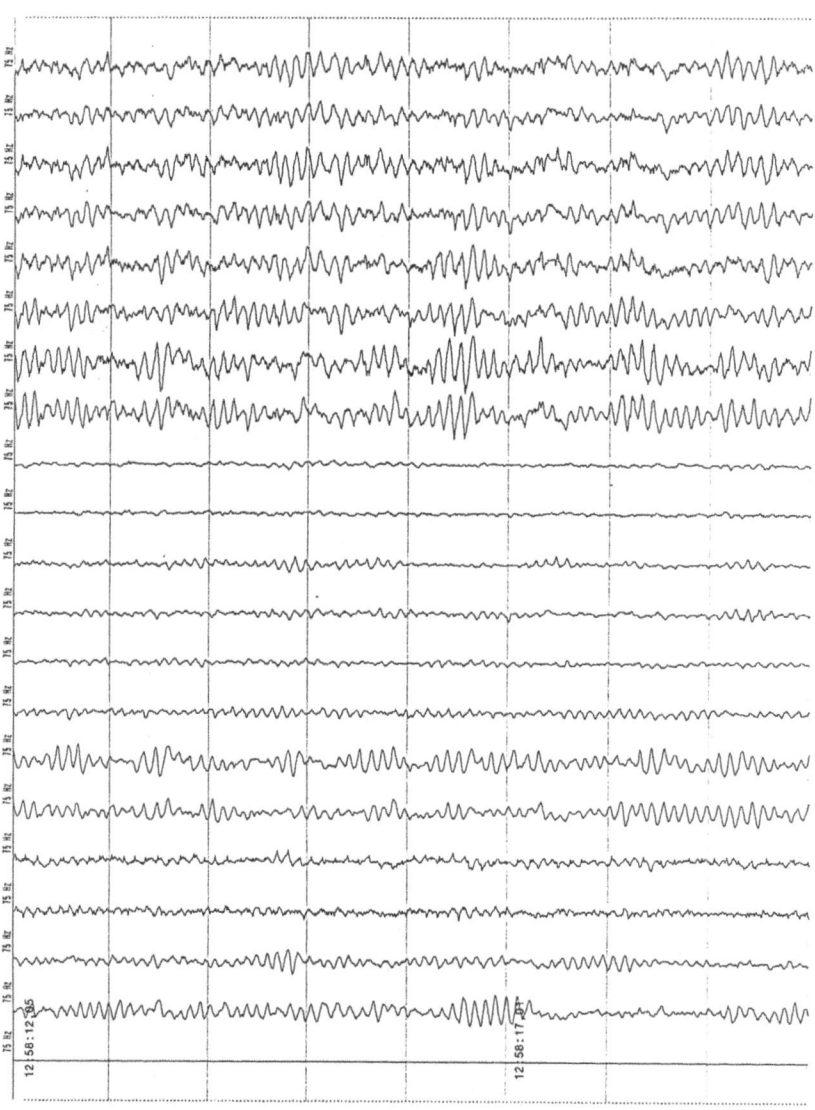

Figure 12. Stage A1 > A2 > A3: A clearly posterior-accentuated 10/s alpha-activity (A1) spreads in the 2nd and 3rd second to anterior (left-emphasized) with a temporary passing of stage A3 in the transition from the 3rd to the 4th second. Between the 5th and 7th second, there is again a posterior-accentuated alpha-activity corresponding to a stage A1, followed by another anterior increase in the 8th second (stage A2). The source derivations reflect the topographic changes only vaguely.

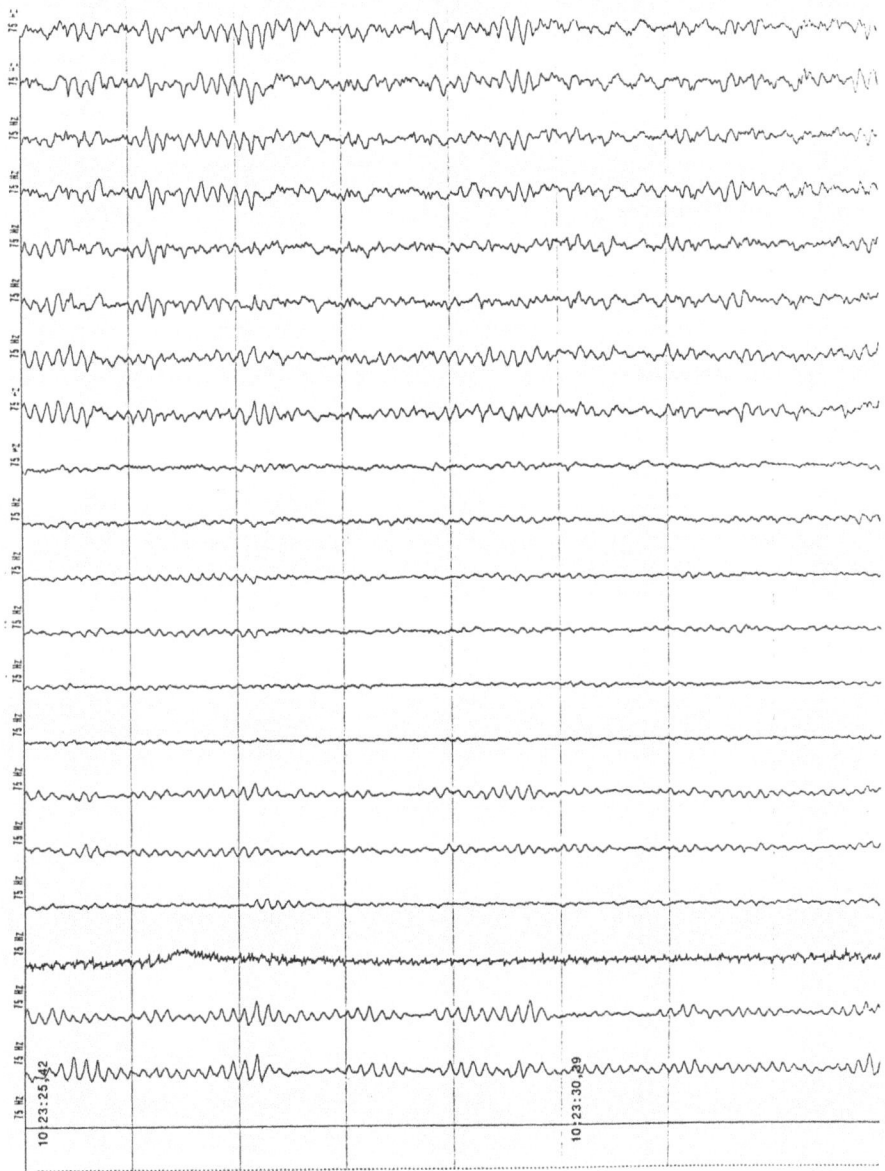

Figure 13. Stage A2 > A3 > B1 > B2: The progressive anteriorization with a 9/s alpha-activity (A2-A3) in the first two seconds is followed by the transition to a short lower-voltage desynchronized stage, corresponding to a stage B1. An anterior-accentuated alpha-activity in the 5th second is followed temporarily by an irregular theta-activity in the 6th to 8th second (B2).

THE THEORETICAL INTERPRETATION OF ELECTROENCEPHALOGRAPHY (EEG)

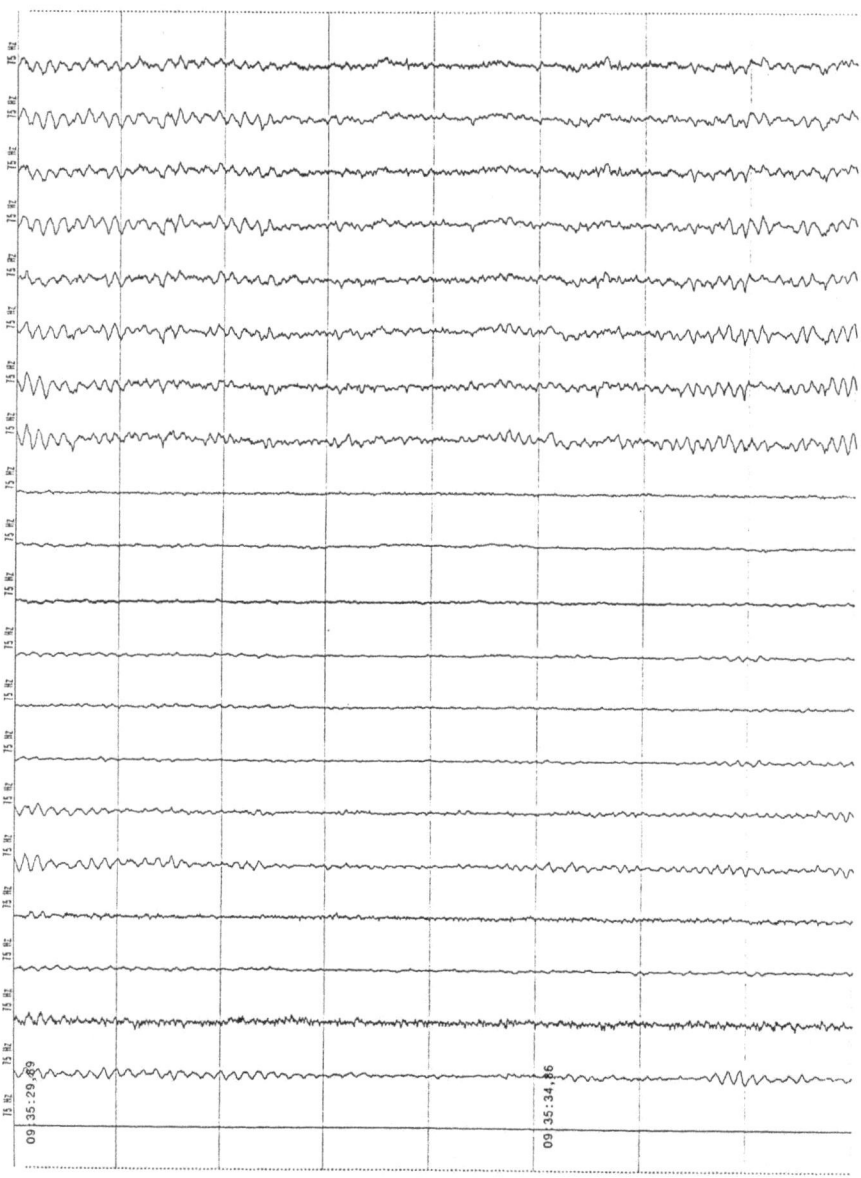

Figure 14. Stage A2 > A3 > B1 > A1: Increasing anteriorization of an 8/s alpha-activity from the 1st to 3rd second (A2, A3), followed by a low-voltage desynchronized stage of activity (B1). In the final two seconds, the restitution of a posterior-dominated 9/s alpha-rhythm occurs.

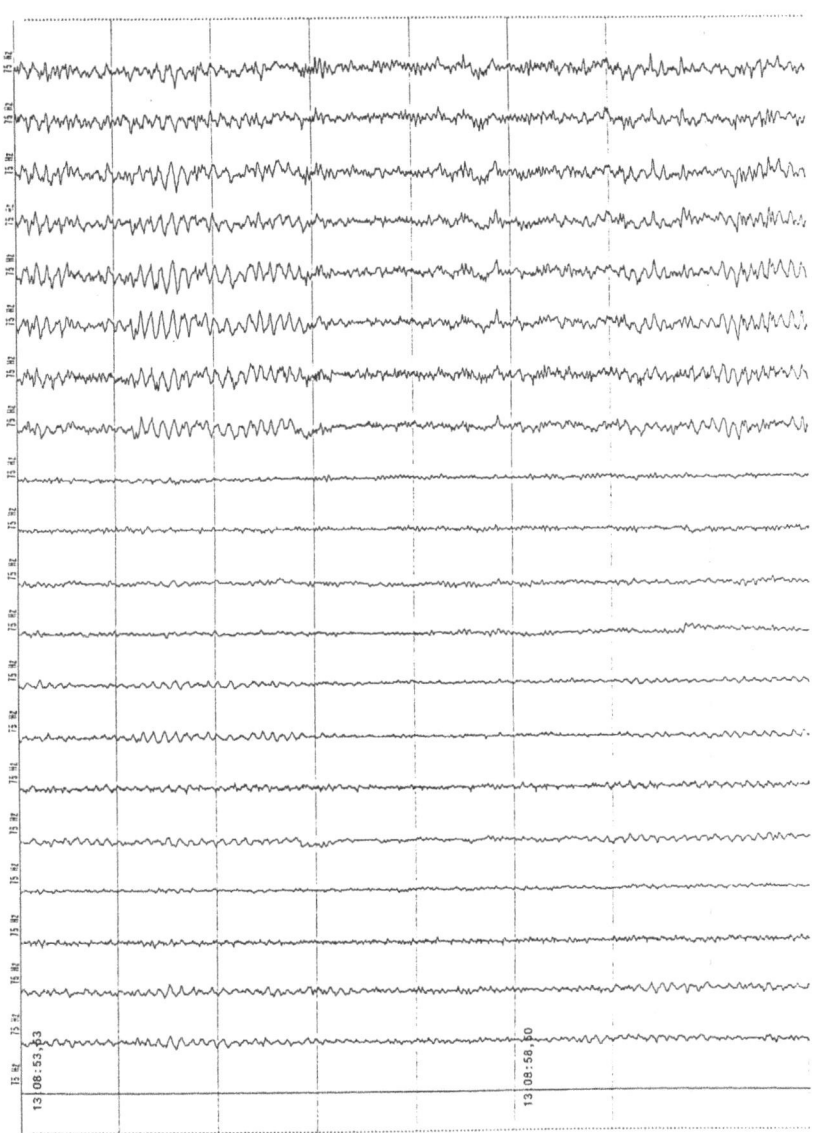

Figure 15. Stage A2 > B1: A moderately anteriorized 9/s alpha-activity switches abruptly in the 4th second to a low-voltage and desynchronized stage with predominant *subvigil* beta-activity of approximately 20/s. In the 7th and 8th second, a posterior-accentuated 9.5/s alpha-activity recurs.

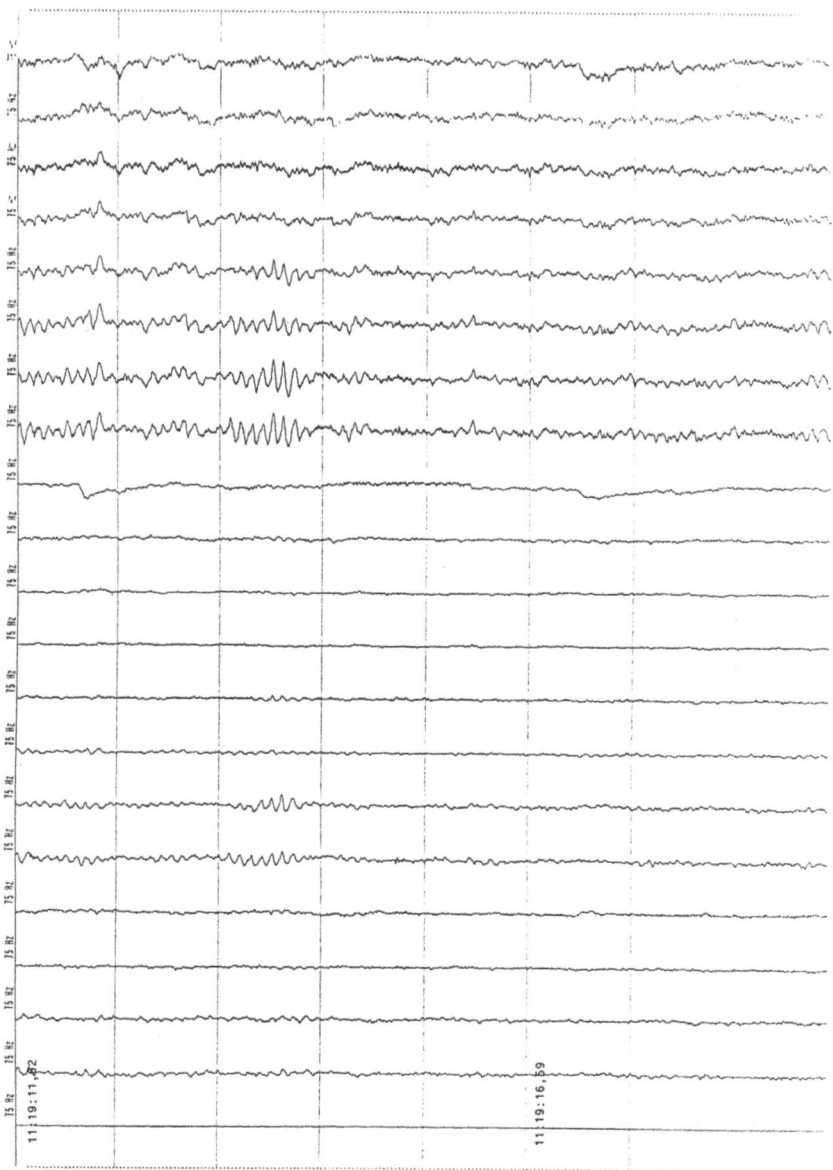

Figure 16. Stage A1 > B1/B2: Abrupt transition of a posterior 9/s alpha-activity (A1), without intermediary mid and late A-stages, into a low-voltage desynchronized activity with interspersed irregular theta-waves (B1/B2).

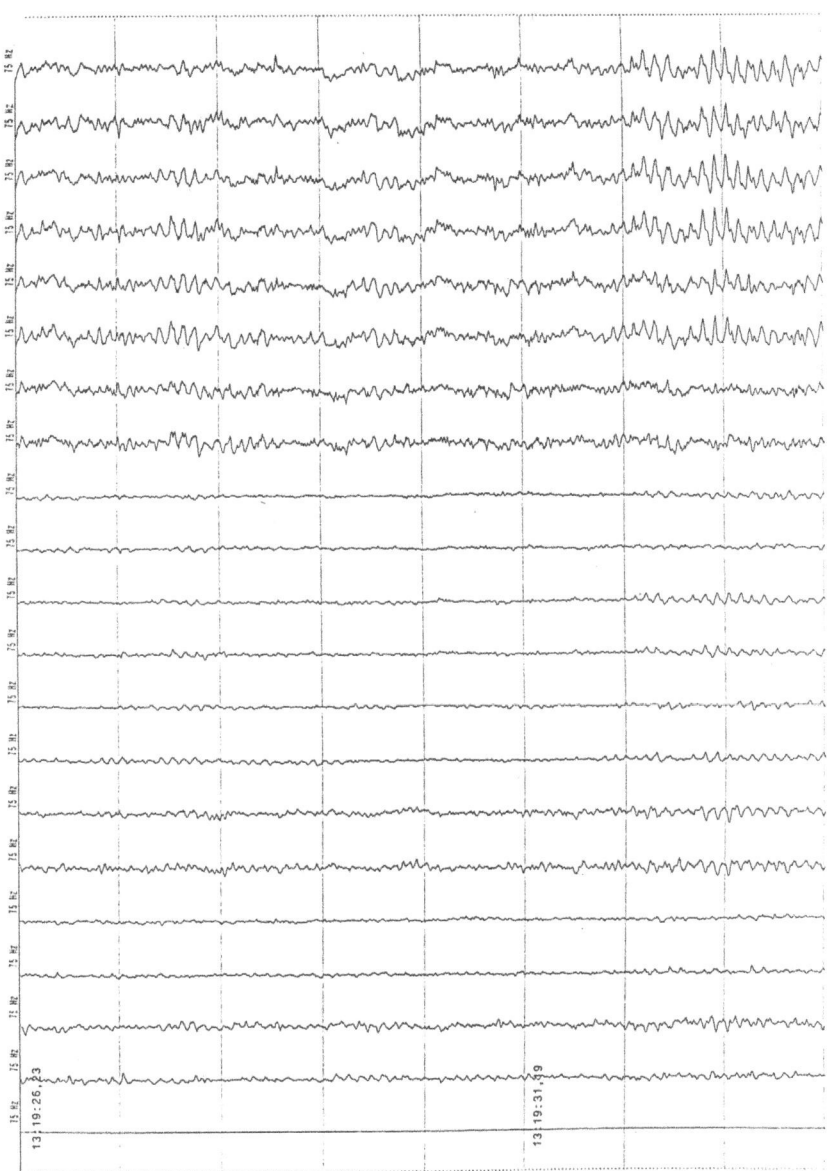

Figure 17. Stage B1/B2 > A3: After a desynchronized phase of activity with interspersed irregular theta-waves (B1-B2), an abrupt transition to a clearly anteriorized 9/s activity corresponding to a stage A3 occurs in the 7th second. This anteriorization can also be seen in the source derivations.

THE THEORETICAL INTERPRETATION OF ELECTROENCEPHALOGRAPHY (EEG)

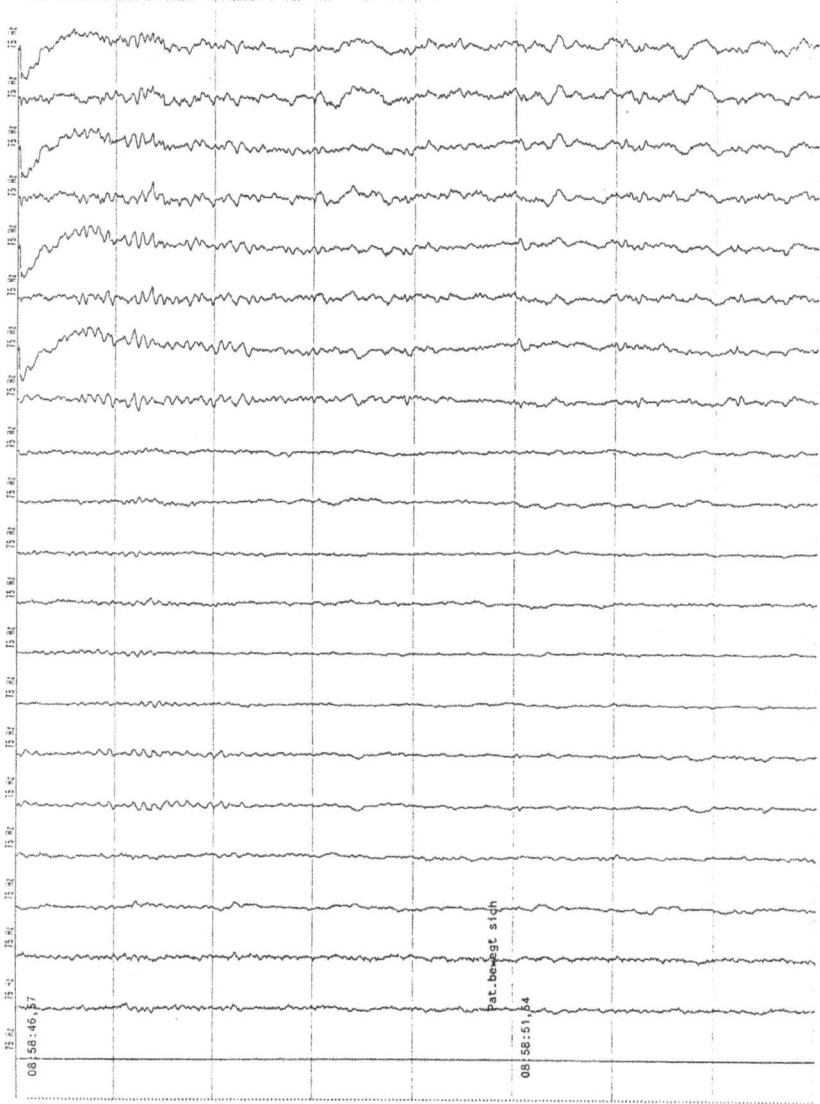

Figure 18. Stage A2 > B1 > B2 > B3: A moderately anteriorized 9/s alpha-activity (A2) changes in the 3rd second to a desynchronized stage (B1) into which theta (B2) and anterior-accentuated delta-waves (B3) are interspersed from the 3rd second.

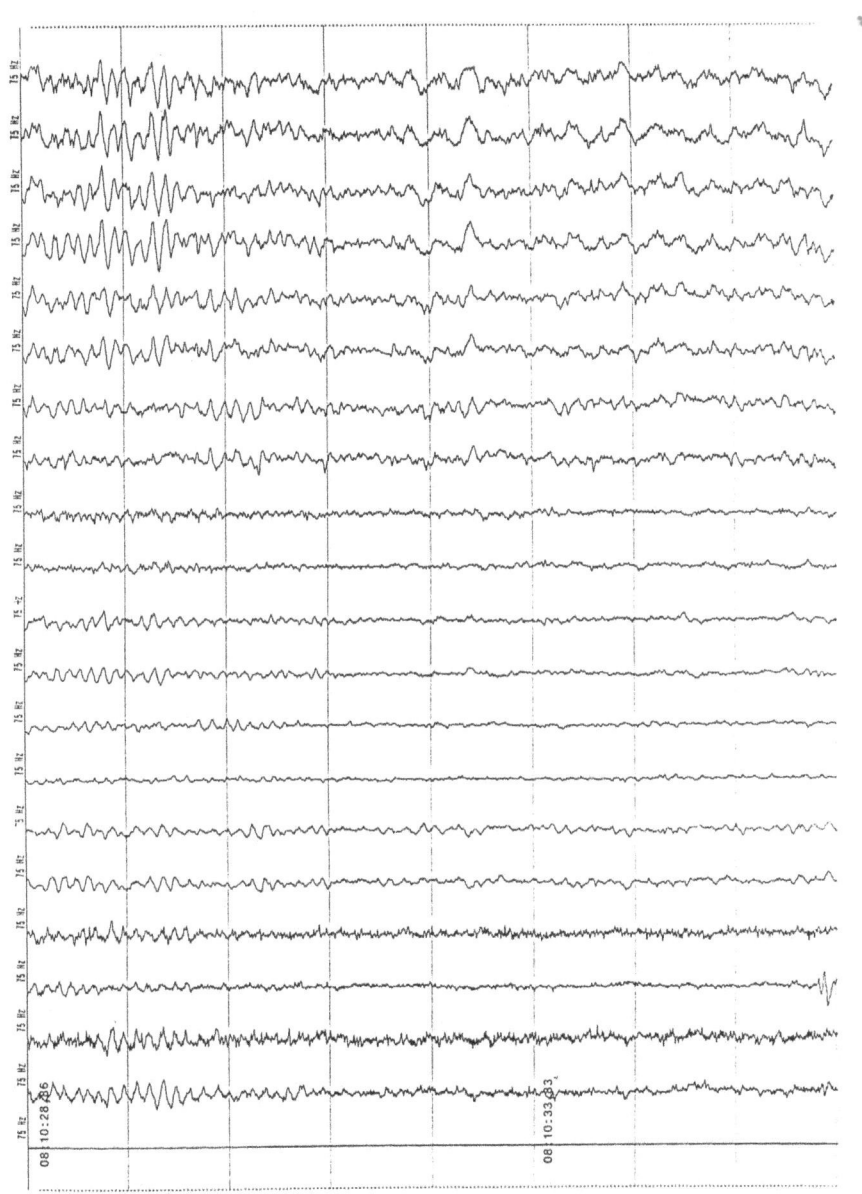

Figure 19. Stage A3 > B1 > B3: A relatively slow anterior-accentuated 7-8/s activity (A3) changes in the 3rd to 4th second via a temporary stage of desynchronized activity (B1) into an anterior-accentuated irregular delta-activity (B3).

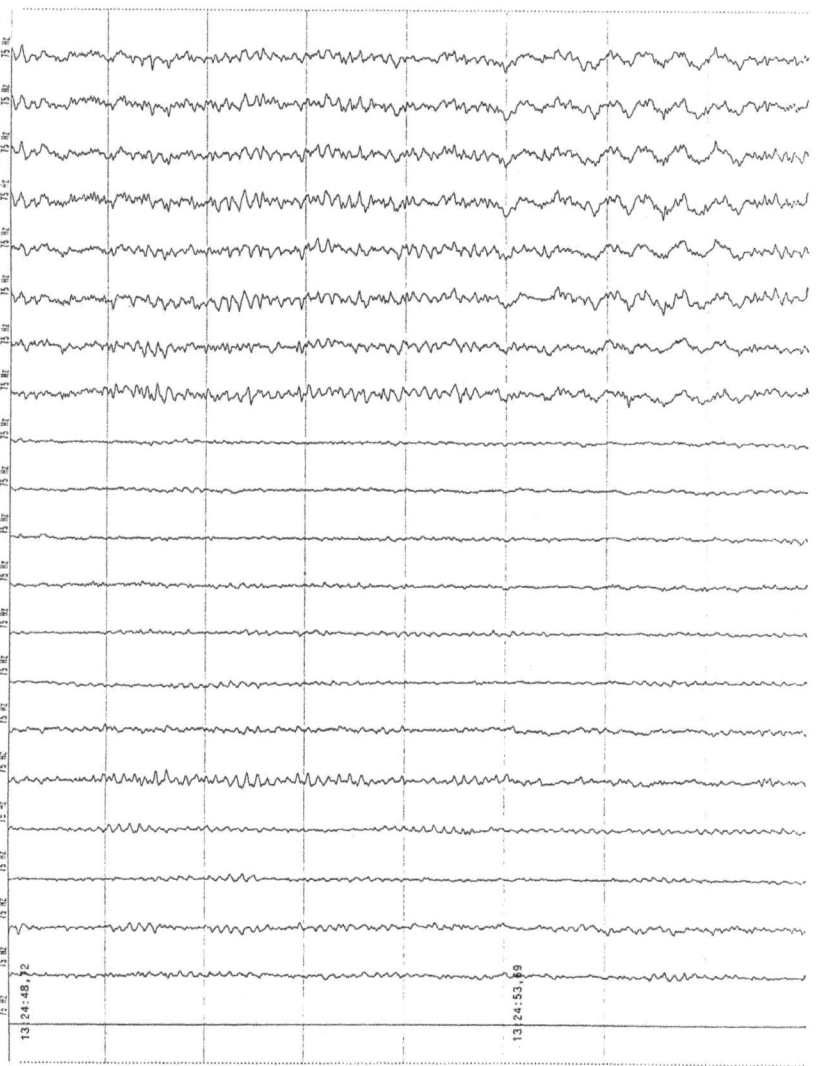

Figure 20. Stage A2 > B1 > B3: A medium degree anteriorized 9/s alpha-activity (A2) changes in the 6th second into an anterior-accentuated 2-3/s delta-activity (B3). These dynamics cannot be observed in the source derivations.

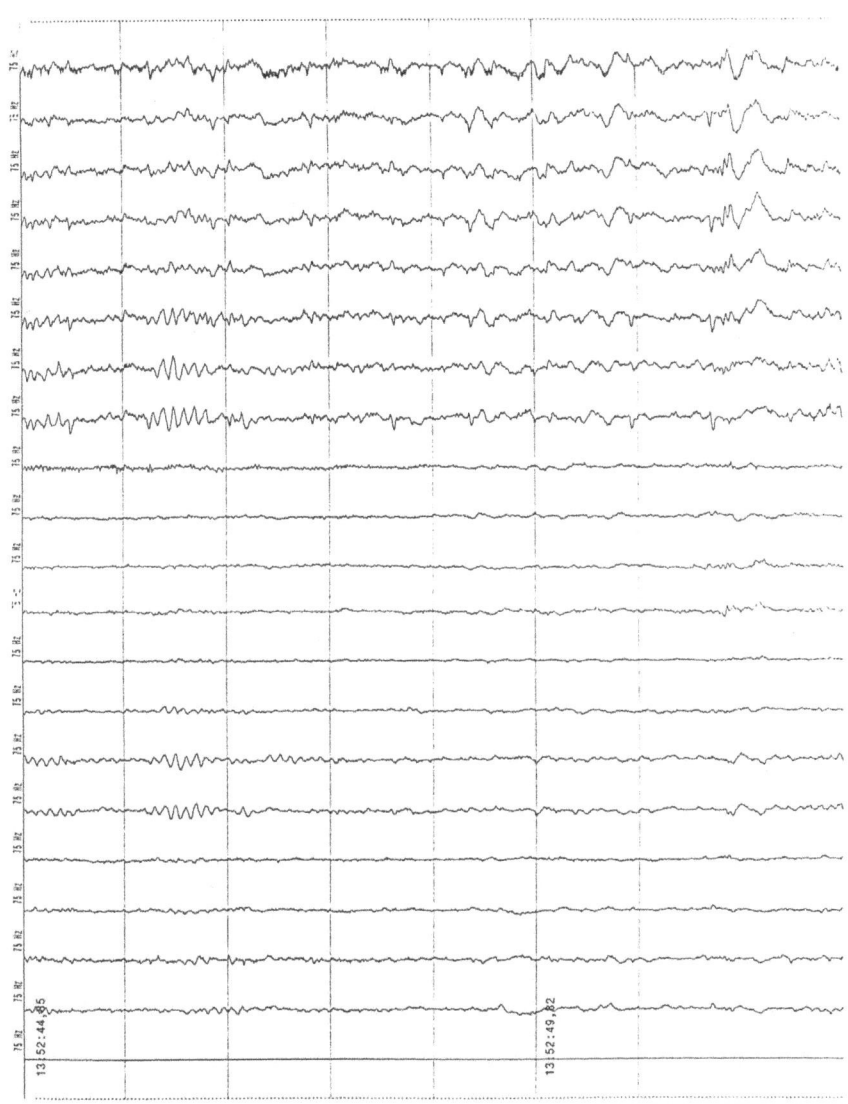

Figure 21. Stage A1 > B1/B2 > B3 > C: A posterior 10/s alpha-activity changes in the 3rd second into a desynchronized activity, corresponding to a stage B1-B2. In the 5th and 6th second, anterior-accentuated irregular delta-waves (B3) take prevalence with a transition into an atypical K-complex, i.e., 14/s beta-activity occurs simultaneously with a so-called vertex potential (C).

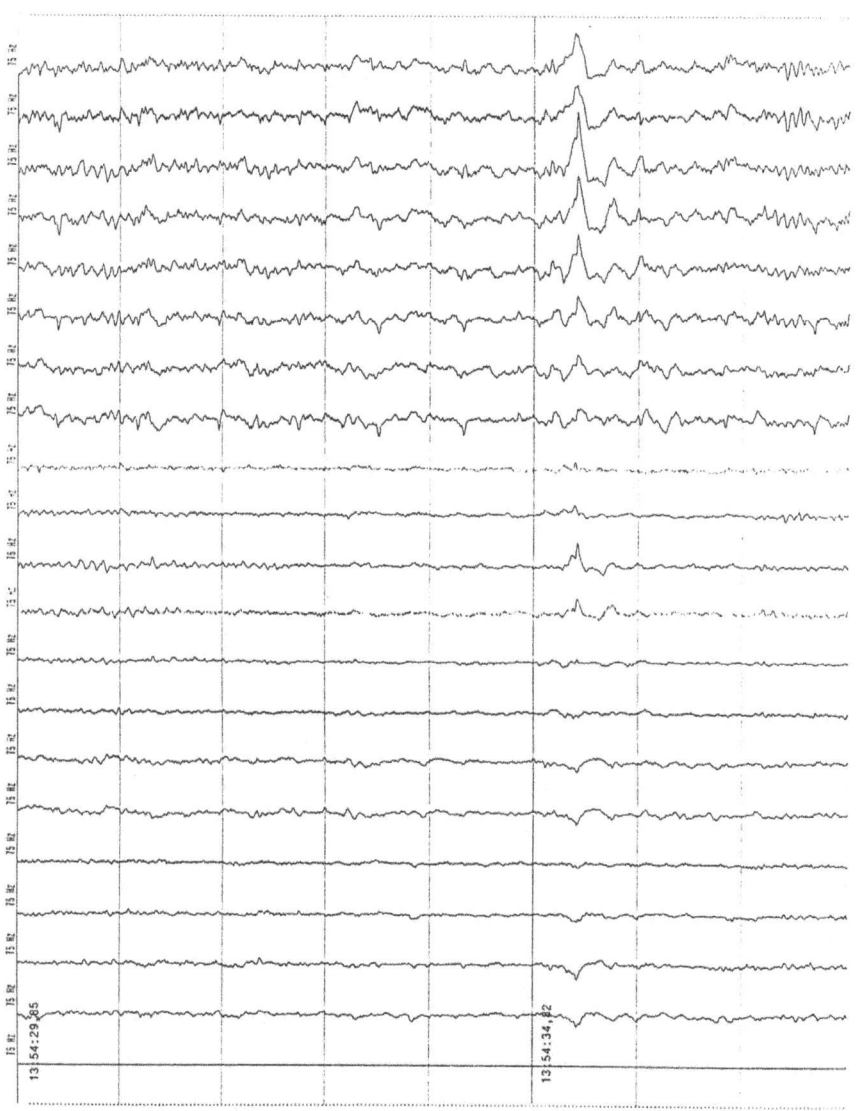

Figure 22. Stage B1 > B2/B3 > C: From a desynchronized activity in the 2nd and 3rd second, (B1) develops in the 4th and 5th second through interspersing with irregular theta- and delta-waves at stage B2/B3, followed by a stage C (K-complex, 14/s beta-spindle) from the 6th to 8th second.

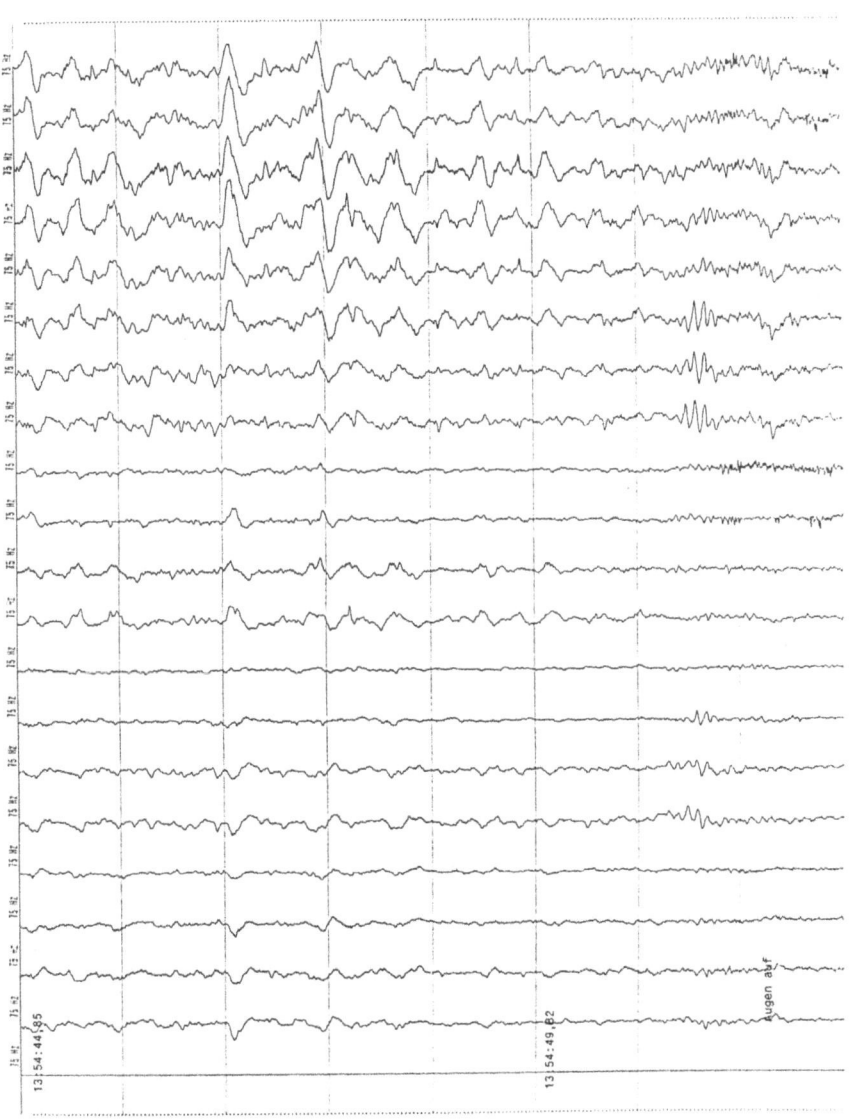

Figure 23. Stage C: During the first 6 seconds, anterior-accentuated 2-3/s delta-waves prevail in connection with sharp, likewise anterior-accentuated waves (so-called vertex potentials) and a touch of 14/s beta-waves. In the 7th second, a posterior 10/s alpha-activity reappears together with anterior beta-activity of approximately 14/s.

In stage A3, a shift of the amplitude maximum from the posterior regions to the frontal regions occurs (Figs. 10, 11, 12). The transition to stage B1 is marked by a discontinuous dissolution of the increasingly shorter spindle-like modulated anterior alpha-activities (Figs. 13, 14, 15). Stage B1 shows a desynchronized low-voltage activity (Figs. 14, 15). The interspersing with rapid (*subvigil*) 20-30/s beta-waves is facultative. In stage B2, irregular theta-waves of relatively low-voltage occur (Figs.16, 17, 18), in stage B3, high-voltage 3-4/s delta-waves, typically with accentuation above the frontal and mid regions (Fig. 18, 19, 20, 21), can be observed. The appearance of 12-14/s spindles finally marks the transition to stage C (Fig. 21, 22, 23, stage II according to DEMENT & KLEITMAN, 1957). The transition to deep sleep takes place (stage D and E or III and IV) with the dissolution of the spindles and the evolution of irregular high-amplitude 1-3/s delta-waves. In younger healthy persons, an increase of epochs corresponding to early B-stages can be observed from about the 5th minute of the recording. Late B-stages can be expected after about 10 minutes. Reaching stage C (or stage II) under the described conditions is not common. Until today, there is a disagreement about which pattern exactly marks the beginning of sleep. Many authors consider the lower-voltage desynchronized activity, corresponding to our stage B1 as the beginning of sleep. This empirically unsupported assumption can be traced back to LOOMIS et al. (1937). Much more evidence links the beginning of sleep with stage C or stage II. As we will explain in more detail, we are not faced with a sharp boundary but with a wide transitional zone. The answer to the question of which kind of staging conforms better to our matter clearly favors the assumption of LOOMIS et al., since it allows a considerably better differentiation of the EEG recorded in a state of wakefulness.

Whereas the delineation of these stages in subjects with prevalent alpha-rhythm is without problems, the low-voltage or flat EEGs with only sporadically detectable alpha-rhythm or only singular alpha-waves have been discutable. Some claimed that such EEGs, which were also termed *norm-variant*, defy any staging. Research done by VOGEL (1970) that seemed to prove an autosomally dominant hereditary line of the characteristic low-voltage supported this opinion, which we reject. VOGEL classified the decidedly rare category of EEGs without any rhythmic alpha-activity in conjunction with the much more frequent EEGs, showing a temporary alpha-rhythm as a reaction to the closing of the eyelids which has the same appearance as the conventional activation of the alpha-rhythm under hyperventilation. If we accepted the accuracy of the genetic basis of VOGEL'S claims, we would confronted with the question of what exactly is hereditary. It does not seem very plausible to us that there could exist a certain hereditary predisposition for a characteristic that is so crucially dependent on the recording conditions, like the amplitude of cortical potential variations. Much more plausible is the assumption that a certain regulation characteristics, as reflected for instance in dynamic lability (**DL**), is hereditary. In practically every EEG with dominating desynchronized low-voltage activity, a more or less temporary posterior alpha-rhythm can be provoked during the closure of the eyes that has to be preceded by a short phase with open eyes. Therefore, since the close-the-eyes open-the-eyes maneuver acts as a stimulus, the alpha-rhythm provoked this way can only be the manifestation of a temporary rise of the vigilance level. Therefore, we consider it obvious to associate a desynchronized low-voltage activity with a subvigil stage B1. This means that we must assume that in a minority of people, because of their constitution and possibly genetics, desynchronized low-voltage activity, corresponding to a stage B1, prevails under the usual conditions for relaxation instead of an alpha-rhythm, corresponding to a stage A.

In the literature, we find that for this kind of patterning of the resting EEG observed with wakeful subjects, terms such as "*états subvigile*" (SOUCACHET, 1952), *transitional stages* (SIMON & EMMONS, 1956) or *subvigile Intermediär-Stadien* (BENTE, 1964b). These morphologically clearly distinguishable stages (see also Figs. 8 to 26) have generally received little attention. This might be responsible for the fact that they have been considered as mere transitional phenomena attributable neither to a waking nor a sleeping stage. This made them appear to be some kind of negligible biological disturbing variance. This profound misunderstanding until today hampered the development of a psychophysiologically oriented electroencephalography, as written, for example, in a handbook article entitled "EEG and Dynamic Psychological States":

"At this point, however, it might be mentioned that some attempts at least have been made to describe EEG patterns related to stages of vigilance. BENTE (1964) subdivides into 7 stages the original A and B stages of LOOMIS et al. (1938)..." and further: *"..we propose to limit the discussion of vigilance to those states that LINDSLEY associates with some degree of efficient behavior, considering that this "vigilance" appears to be only an absolutely dispensible, superfluous name for alertness, vigility, wakefulness, attention, etc.."* (DONGIER, 1977).

Based on this misunderstanding, a deeply lowered *vigilance* is equated to somnolence. Especially in pathological somnolence, it is obvious that we are dealing with a relatively clearly delineated phenomenon or neurological symptom with a certain etiopathogenesis. Therefore, *somnolence* belongs to a different logical category than the theoretical ordering term *vigilance,* which is related to the global functional level. Defined this way, *vigilance* obviously cannot be equated with "arousal" or "activation." Such misunderstandings have become almost common knowledge, as evidenced by the title of a monography, "The EEG of Drowsiness" (SANTAMARIA & CHIAPPA, 1987). Despite their attempt at comprehensiveness, no reference to LAIRY & DELL or BENTE or even HEAD can be found. However, with regard to the title of their work, the authors' claim, "*The literature is largely quiet on this subject.*" Their statement, "*the analysis of sequencing drowsy stages has only scratched the surface of what we feel may be an interesting area*", cannot fool us about the fact that the authors have no EEG-conception that includes or supersedes the partial aspect of "drowsiness." Contrary to HEAD'S original conception (see above), "vigilance" is today used almost exclusively in relation to behavior, like in the sense of "sustained attention" (MACKWORTH, 1948).

The heuristic potential inherent in **SR-EEG** has been rather hypothetical. The following outline of a theoretical framework aimed at a clinical utilization refers to early fundamental publications by BENTE (1961, 1963, 1964a). Since all of them were written in German, their content has essentially remained unknown in English literature. Our theoretical framework may at present be sketched as folllows:

- **SR-EEG** reflects the integrated mass activity of cortical neurons.

- The dynamics of the SR-EEG may be specified as a synergetic, non-linear process. Since its time-course dependent spatio-temporal characteristics (i.e., its *Verlaufsgestalt*) are governed by a certain lawfulness one cannot assume an underlying stochastic random process – for instance conceived as kind of an attendant phenomenon of neurotransmitter chemistry.

- **SR-EEG** is the macroindicator of the organizational level of Cerebral GlobalFunction (**CGF**), which reflects the interaction of brain-endowed living systems with their environment (*Umwelt*).

- **CGF** is a time-function exhibiting spontaneous cyclic dynamics observed in the spontaneous EEG under resting conditions. The quality of the respective *Verlaufsgestalt* is grosso modo correlated with the intensity of wakefulness/sleepiness assessed introspectively between the full alertness and falling asleep. With regard to scientific requirements, such stronger or weaker, sometimes even paradoxical negative correlations are insufficient.

- The spontaneous cyclic dynamics of the EEG consists of a more or less regular sequence of visually distinguishable wave-patterns which are to be corellated with certain central-nervous states of order, the so-called *intermediary vigilance stages* according to BENTE (1964a; 1964b).

- Such a time-dependent order of EEG-patterning can be proven with about 90% of a basic population of healthy adult people.

- Dynamics and proportioning of the EEG-vigilance stages represent the psychophysiological relevant information of the **SR-EEG.**

- With a minority of about 10% of healthy adults, spontaneous cyclic dynamics may only be recognized with low markedness. Without additional information, whether one deals with a constitution-bound pecularity (*trait*) that points to a deficient functional maturity of the brain, possibly indicating a disposition (vulnerability or diathesis) for the manifestation of certain psychiatric disorders, remains unsettled. From the viewpoint of pattern morphology, subjects with reduced or missing spontaneous cyclic dynamics can be coordinated either with Dynamic Lability (**DL**) or Dynamic Rigidity (**DR**). Proportionally, the so-called norm-variant of the low-voltage (**DL**) prevails by far.

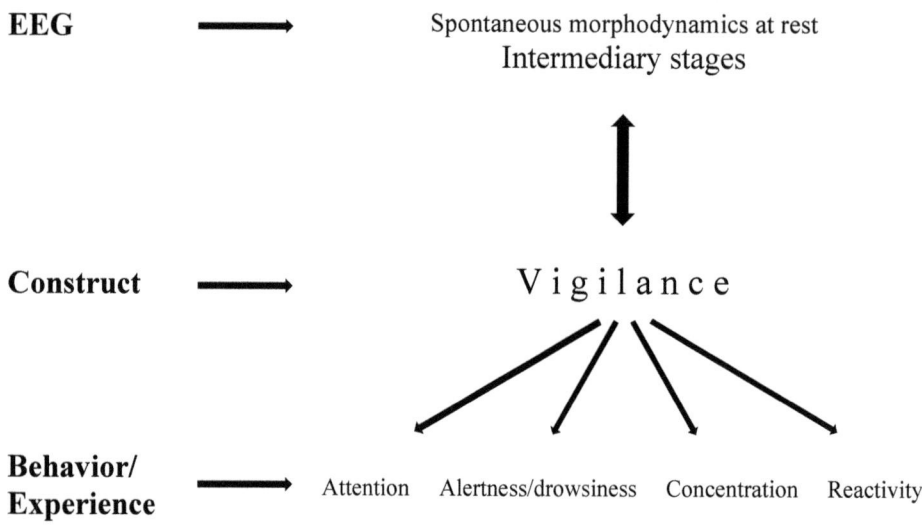

Figure 24. *Vigilance* as theoretical construct.

Several attempts to distinguish between *vigilance* (HEAD, 1923) as a term describing the functional state of a biological system and *vigilance* as a term describing behavior/experience (PETERS, 1976; BENTE, 1977; ULRICH & GSCHWILM, 1988) were modestly received at best. Regardless of the EEG or behavior/experience, *vigilance* is used without making any discrimination. Inevitably, this leads to paradoxes. It has been claimed, for instance, that it could be methodically more advantageous to determine the vigilance level through electroencephalography rather than through self-assessment (MATOUSEK, 1984). The critical question of whether psychological data can be expressed by physiological data or vice versa will still be discussed in detail (see Chapters 3.4.7; 3.4.8). Even the widely used definition of *vigilance* as a readiness of the organism to react adequately to a stimulus (KOELLA, 1984) does not address the essence. "Readiness" is the designation of an attribute by the observer who is focused on the interaction of an organism with its environment rather than an operational characteristic of the organism! "Adequate" is a subjective value judgement. Thus, KOELLA'S definition is adequate for living as well as dead systems. Thus, what should keep us from defining "automobilance" as the readiness of the automobile to react to a specific stimulus, such as pushing the accelerator with an adequate acceleration? According to this definition, an older car could be assigned a lower "automobilance" than a new car. In a less convoluted way, one could say that the old car does not function as well, just as a living organism with lower vigilance does not function as well. That leaves us with the question of why HEAD nonetheless saw the need for a new term. HEAD'S writings indicate clearly that he derived his theoretical construct of *vigilance* from the observation of living systems and only wanted them to be associated with those. He explicitly equated "vigilance" with "vital activity." Different from dead machines, living organisms do not possess an initial state of functional rest. They change their functional state permanently in a cyclic process without even being required to fulfill a certain performance. In order to meet this decisive distinction between living and dead systems, HEAD introduced the concept of *vigilance*. In other words, the necessity of *vigilance* is derived from the impossibility of a one-on-one relation of phenomena described by "brain language" (EEG or brain physiology) with phenomena described by "mind-language" (experiencing or psychology). Relating these two logically incommensurable domains of description can only be substantiated by means of the theoretical construct of *vigilance*. As a theoretical construct, "vigilance" is independent from these domains. Of course, *vigilance* as a technical term for the functionality of living systems cannot be subdivided into "local vigilances" (KOELLA, 1984). Otherwise one would have to assign each of the cooperatively acting neuronal assemblies its own vigilance. *Vigilance* can exist only in its entirety or not at all, just like an arch as a self-supporting edifice.

3.4.4 THE IMPORTANCE OF THE SR-EEG AS A MACROINDICATOR OF CEREBRAL GLOBAL FUNCTION (CGF)

As mentioned in the preceding chapter, the concept of a psychophysiological electroencephalography can be traced back to LAIRY & DELL (1957) as well as BENTE (1964b). This conception is consistent with the findings – not necessarily the conceptions - of recent brain research. Accordingly, the EEG is the result of a network of cooperative neural elements, which are coherent across the entire derivation area. The sensitivity and reactivity of each single neuron depend on the state of excitation of all other neurons (LOPES DA SILVA, 1991). This leads to an "integrated wholeness" (CREUTZFELDT, 1975) within which neuro-anatomical delineations are for the most part blurred. The EEG appears as the manifestation of the *Global Function* (STORM VAN LEEUWEN, 1978).

Therefore, the **SR-EEG** was repeatedly denoted as the **macroindicator of the brain's bioelectric mass activity** (BENTE, 1963; CREUTZFELDT, 1975; FREEMAN, 1975; STORM VAN LEEUWEN, 1978).

Expedited by the rapid developments of the theory of non-linear systems or synergetics, this holistic view increasingly complements the meristic or elementaristic paradigm of columnar cortical organization, which is based on an imagined additive mosaic of elements that can be functionally isolated. Findings according to which the cortico-cortical or horizontal connectivity is considerably more pronounced than thalamo-cortical or vertical connectivity play an important role with this modified approach (BASAR, 1980).

According to non-linear systems theory, the EEG belongs to the class of cooperative or synergetic self-organizing processes that inevitably occur in systems with uniform, non-linear, interactive elements (HAKEN, 1982; ROTH, 1981; AN DER HEIDEN, 1985). One talks about self-organization when a spontaneous formation of structures can be observed. "Spontaneous" means that a new structure was not imposed by external forces but originated because of the specific characteristics of the components involved. A spontaneous repetition of similar structures, such as activity patterns, is called a self-organizing process of cyclic order. This is exactly what happens in the EEG. Insofar as each state of the system is involved in the creation of the following one, the system can also be considered internal state-determined. This cycle is a highly complex process with a wide intra- and interindividual range of variation regarding the proportioning and the dynamics of the course of the subvigil stages. We must consider it less a system of rigid rules and more an ordering system, which allows relating a multitude of individual phenomena in a certain way.

From the perspective of the so-called chaos theory, the cyclically repeated activity patterns can also be regarded as dynamic attractors (see 7.4). According to recent findings, the EEG is most probably a *deterministic chaos* (SCHUSTER, 1994), i. e., a deterministic process the course of which cannot be predicted despite the knowledge of the relevant parameters.

The global functional state of the system, i.e., its vigilance, is evidenced in its cyclic dynamics. A modification of the functional order, as under resting conditions, in German pointedly termed "Funktionswandel" (CONRAD, 1947) or *functional change* in English, can occur under physiological, pharmacological, as well as pathological conditions. The ultimate physiological condition of a *functional change* is sleep with a very specific cyclic order. A *pathological functional change* of lesser degree usually manifests itself in a change of proportioning and temporal sequencing of those patterns that constitute the subvigil intermediary stages. This can mean increased dynamic rigidity as well as lability (see below). However, a *pathomorphical functional change* of a lesser degree can also manifest itself in the intermittent occurrence of certain morphological variations of subvigil patterns without interfering with the cycle dynamics. In the case of more pronounced *pathomorphical functional changes*, as in diffuse dysrhythmia, a delineation of stages - and thus an evaluation of the dynamics - is no longer possible.

3. 4. 5 EEG AND MATURATION: GENERAL POINTS OF VIEW

Since structure and dynamics of brain-electrical activity are the product of a maturation process, each assessment of the actually given level as well as of the dynamics of *vigilance* requires the complementary specification with regard to the associated *ontogenetic maturation level*. The theoretical constructs of *vigilance* and *maturation* belong to different but complementary time grids; they are related to each other in the manner of orthogonal coordinates.

Equally complementary are onto- and phylogenesis, emanation and evolution, homeostasis and homeorrhesis (WADDINGTON, 1966), synchronic and diachronic equilibration (PIAGET, 1983), as well as simply the "state" and "trait" aspects.

As a theoretical construct, *maturation* is just as inaccessible for direct observation as *vigilance*. It also can be conceived by specific empirical indicators only.

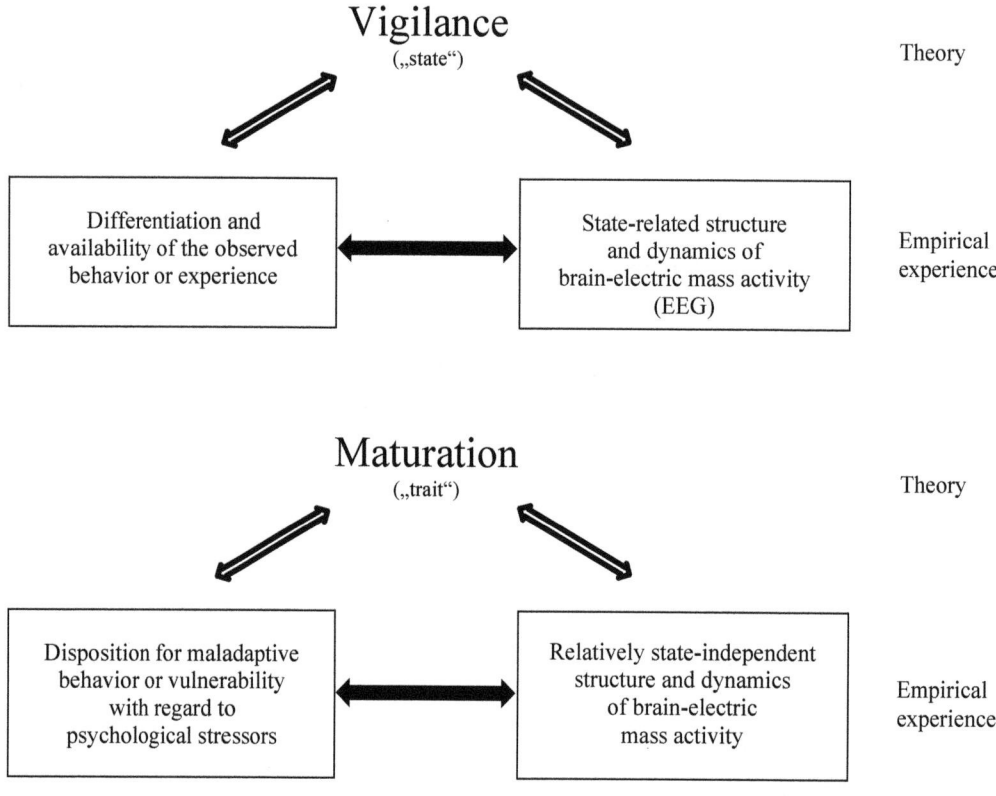

Figure 25. The significance of the theoretical constructs of *vigilance* and *maturation* for hypothesis-based empirical research.

While the electroencephalographic vigilance indicators find their immediate behavioral correlates in the differentiation and availability of the observed behavior or inner experiencing, we can only postulate a correspondence with maladaptive behavior patterns for the electroencephalographic immaturity indicators. However, since a disposition need not necessarily be realized under favorable circumstances, one has to expect inconsistent results and probably significant only when calculating group statistics.

3. 4. 6   EEG and Maturation : Individual Indicators

While thus far we were exclusively occupied with the **state-related** varying phenomena, i.e., the indicators of EEG-vigilance, we now want to focus on the **state-unrelated**, i.e., constitution-related phenomena. As with the former, here, too, we must answer two questions first:

- Which patterns can be considered indicators of immaturity, with which explanation?

- Which correlations can be established for these patterns at the description level of behavior/perception?

It seems plausible to assume that in adults, all those EEG-phenomena point towards a brain-functional immaturity characteristic for certain "normal" maturation phases in healthy infants and adolescents. The attempt to arrive at systematics of EEG immaturity indicators assumes an intense familiarization with the ontogenesis of the EEG.

For the EEG, too, the progression from the undifferentiated to the differentiated, and its maintenance, is considered a general biological principal of maturation. In the EEG of the new-born with a relatively low-voltage 1/2-2/s-activity - with superseding 10-30/s waves - no order of any kind is recognizable. A very coarse distinction is possible between the waking-EEG and the sleeping-EEG. Only after a period of 6 months can we talk about a subvigil intermediary stage in the form of groups and sequences of a rhythmic 2-4/s activity. We must remember that the interindividual variability of the speed of maturation differs widely even within the normal range. Instead of discussing the ontogenesis of the EEG by means of the common chronological ordering of isolated features, we prefer a cursory sketch of the general developmental principles that allow to preserve a coherent overview.

In the first 10 years of life, development is determined by *formative tendencies* that result in steady increase of amplitude and synchronization, with frequency showing a topographical accentuation towards the posterior regions.

THE THEORETICAL INTERPRETATION OF ELECTROENCEPHALOGRAPHY (EEG)

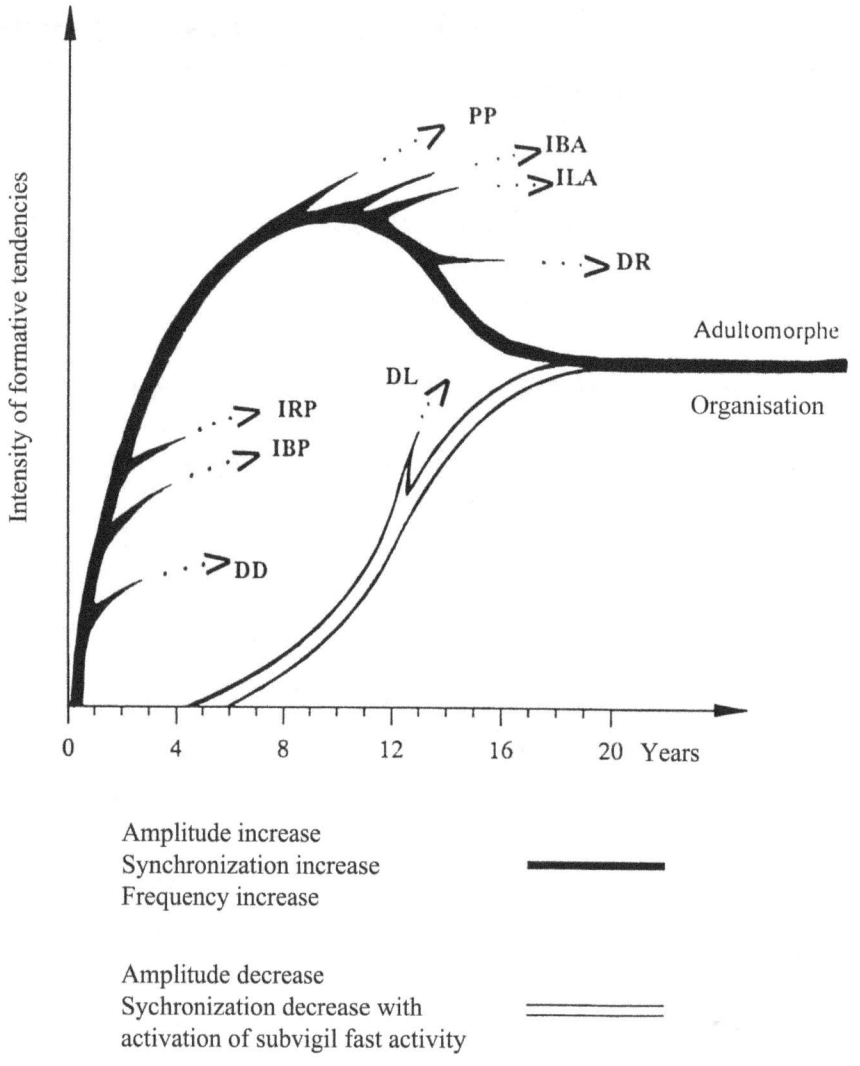

Figure 26. Ontogenesis of the EEG. Ideal course and possible deviations.

To the degree that the amount of irregular diffuse slow activity is pushed back, and a more rhythmic and fast acitivity becomes dominant. A lateral difference also exists approximately around the 3rd to 4th year, when a passing intermittent right-posterior accentuation of irregular slow waves (EEG-OLOFFSON, 1971) corresponding to a topographical heterogeneity of the maturation process is found. Around the 9th year, the alpha-activity becomes posteriorly accentuated. The EEG differs from the adultomorph only because of a more or less high amount of interspersed slow waves. That the development is by no means completed at this point is evidenced especially during the transition from wakefulness to sleep. Groups and sequences of rhythmic high-amplitude, frontally-acccentuated waves with a frequency of 6-7/s (in infants from 3-5/s), mark this transition from childhood until puberty and even beyond that point.

This relatively uniform pattern represents the infantile and juvenile equivalent to the 6 intermediary stages distinguishable in the adult EEG, i.e., the patterns A1, A2, A3, B1, B2, and B3. Formally, this infantile drowsiness pattern corresponds to the phenomena, subsumed by us in the adult EEG under **IBA**. The often observed persistence of these patterns into early adulthood or even beyond can be retraced to an exaggerated and unrestrained effect of the formative synchronization tendencies associated with infancy. This is confirmed particularly by the fluent transition observed both in children and adults, with rhythmic to dysrhythmic paroxysmal activity explained by a different degree of synchronization. The increase in synchronization is also evidenced in the degree of coherence between the frequencies and phases of different regions. An interesting, up to now hardly noticed, partial aspect here is the one of interhemispheral coordination.

DD	Diffuse dysrhythmia because of prevailing irregular slow waves
IRP/IBP	Intermittent right- or bilateral posterior-accentuated irregular (but also rhythmic) theta- and delta-waves
PP	Paroxysmal (epileptiform) potentials
ILA/IBA	Intermittent left or bilateral anterior-accentuated rhythmic theta- or delta-groups
DR	Dynamic rigidity
DL	Dynamic lability

Table 3. Relatively persistent EEG-features (traits) as indicators of a functional cerebral maturation deficit.

While the development of certain synchrony over the central region can be observed after only 4 weeks, a bilateral harmonizing of the posterior regions is occuring only during the 3rd to 4th year of age. The two temporal regions remain independent of each other the longest (WERNER et al., 1977). Around the 4th year of age, the *formative tendency* of "active desynchronization" as an expression of a lowered vigilance level is added to the picture. The maturation of the underlying mechanism, which is the basis of the adult B1-stage, continues until about the 14th year of age. The mature morphodynamics of the adult EEG, which results from the functional integration of the mentioned developmental tendencies, takes additional 4-5 years.

The EEG indicators of functional immaturity, as exhibited in Table 3, can be regarded as deviations, disproportionings, or deficient integrations of the developmental trajectories modelled in Fig. 26.

They may also be observed in combinations. Only **DR, DL**, and **DD** are mutually exclusive. Problems of delineation arise between **ILA/IBA** and **PP**, since both of these phenomena, which are due to exaggerated synchronization, show flowing transitions (see above). A close morpho-genetic relationship between **DD** and **IBP** or **IRP** can also be assumed. According to our model (Fig. 26), these are degradation levels of an ontogenetically early deficit.

As pointed out earlier and restated here, most of the phenomena listed as immaturation indicators, i.e. **DR, DL, ILA/IBA**, and **DD,** can also manifest themselves as state-dependent with cerebral affections, thus indicating a *pathological gestalt change* of the EEG.

Now we want to address the second basic question of this chapter, the question regarding the clinical and psychological significance of our supposed immaturity indicators. A common misunderstanding among laymen is to equate brain-functional immaturity with delayed intellectual development. According to popular opinion, which can be traced back to the pioneers of the EEG, there exists no EEG-correlate for intellectual or mental impairment (f. i., OSTOW, 1950; GIBBS et al., 1960). LA VECK & DE LA CRUZ (1963) who examined a large number of mentally defective people found a "normal" EEG in 34% of them. "Normal" EEGs were even not infrequent in the most severe cases of idiocy. The most frequently observed deviation from the norm was the diffuse dysrhythmia (**DD**). We admit that we have our reservations about such statements, since they are based on the neurological norm concept criticized by us as inappropriate for psychiatric questions. For us, whether correlates of feeblemindedness might be proved by subtle morphodynamic analysis EEG - where we think foremost of our immaturity indicators - is an equally unanswered but interesting question. We do not want to go as far as to expect that it might be possible to diagnose a deficiency of intelligence from the EEG. Here, too, the principle applies that a one-on-one association of EEG and behavior/experience cannot be assumed. After all, we must remember that the features of Table 3 can also be observed in absolutely healthy and intelligent persons. However, studies with healthy persons that could provide the desperately needed empirical foundation for the developmental-biological aspect in psychiatric research are extremely rare. However, the first noteworthy study, which remained without consequences, was performed by DAVIS & DAVIS (1936). The authors divided healthy probands into those with rather continuous and regular and those with rather discontinuous and irregular activity. Since these features could be largely reproduced in repeated recordings, the authors assumed that they were constitutional and possibly hereditary. From this, they derived the following question that could also be considered as a research program:

"If one is dealing with hereditary patterns and types, with what mental or neurological features and tendencies may particular cortical electrograms be related?"

Without mention or in ignorance of this suggestion that never found any resonance, VAN PRAAG (1990) complained, more than half a century after DAVIS & DAVIS, about researchers who had neglected to also consider the physiological correlate of certain personality structures, *biological underpinnings* as he called ,when searching for the pathophysiological correlates of psychiatric diseases.

He stated that knowing it is indispensible to know these correlates because a specific personality structure provides the disposition for certain psychiatric diseases. If we continued to pursue this highly plausible suggestion, we could formulate the hypothesis that samples of remitted psychiatric patients differ from samples of healthy persons with regard to the distribution of our listed immaturation indicators. Such a differentiation or characterization of remitted psychiatric patients, thus far not even considered, opens up the possibility of arriving at developmental-biological groupings that could be, beyond the common diagnostic classifications, clinically meaningful, for instance, for therapy planning and with respect to prognosis

In our developmental-biological model of immaturation indicators (Fig. 26, Table 3), diffuse dysrhythmia (**DD,** Figs. 27, 28) appears to be the characteristic (*trait*) that is associated with the earliest developmental stage. This is the manifestation of impeded processes tending towards an increase in synchronization and frequency acceleration. The importance of **DD** as an indicator of brain-electrical immaturity was noticed early on (LENNOX et al., 1940; HILL & WATERSON, 1942; HILL, 1952; LIBERSON, 1956; PICARD et al., 1956; COHN, 1958, 1961; GASTAUT et al., 1960; WISSFELD & KAINDL, 1961; HARRISON et al., 1968).

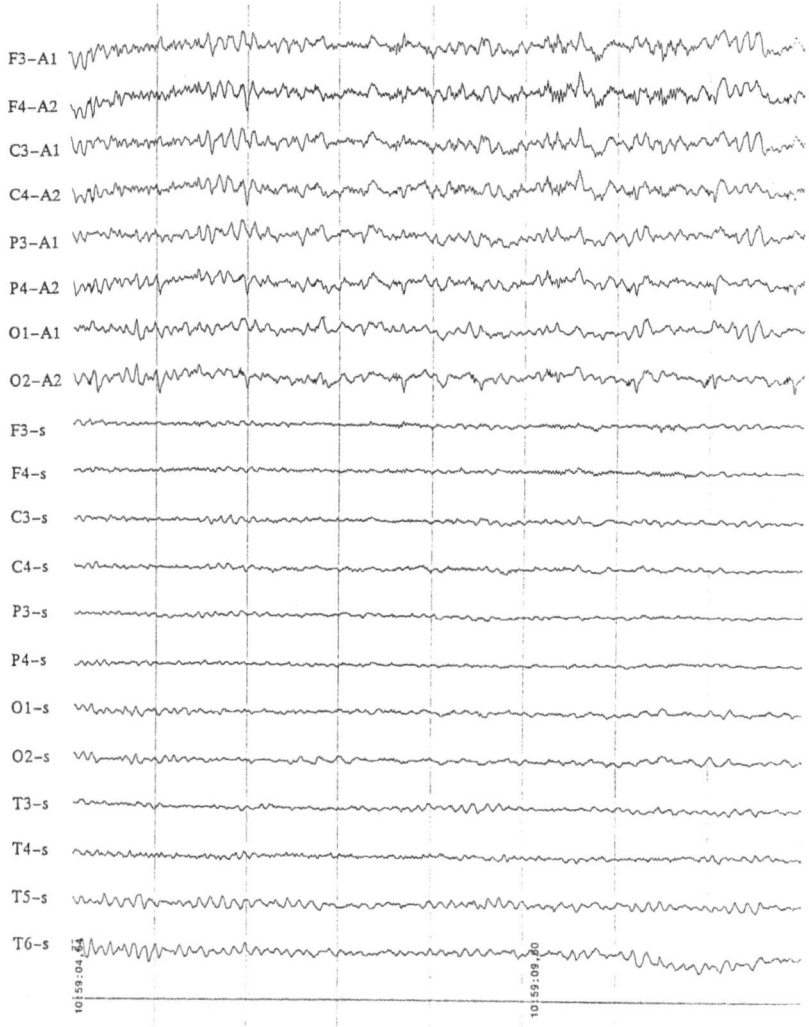

Figure 27. Slightly diffuse dysrhythmia (**DD**) with occipital accentuation in patient with hebephrenia interpreted as constitutional since it was recorded in a medication-free state (K. A., 20 y., m., EEG-nr. 1201/92). (Figs. 27-37 identical derivation schema).

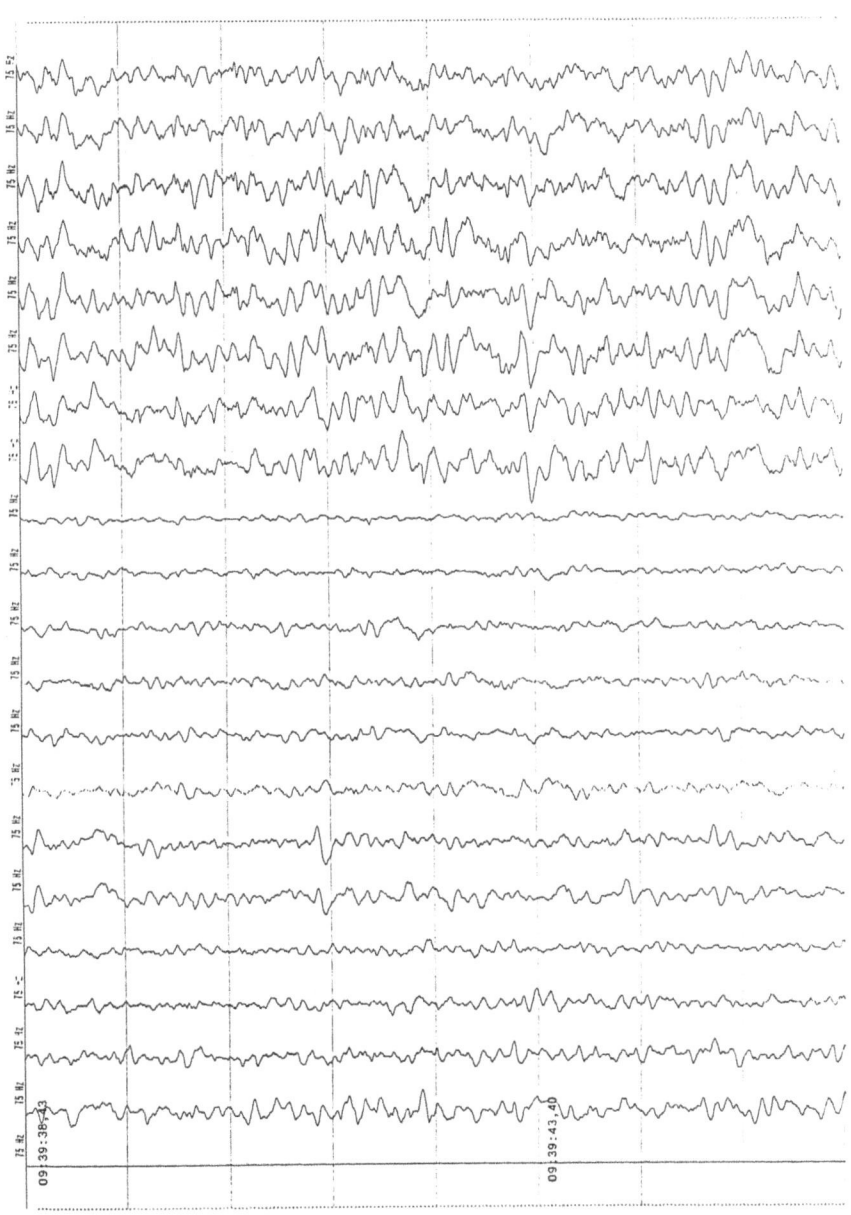

Figure 28. Pronounced diffuse dysrhythmia (**DD**) with intermittent right-posterior accentuation (**IRP**) in a patient with personality disorder interpreted as constitutional since it was recorded in medication-free state (J. E., 24 y., m., EEG-nr. 444/93).

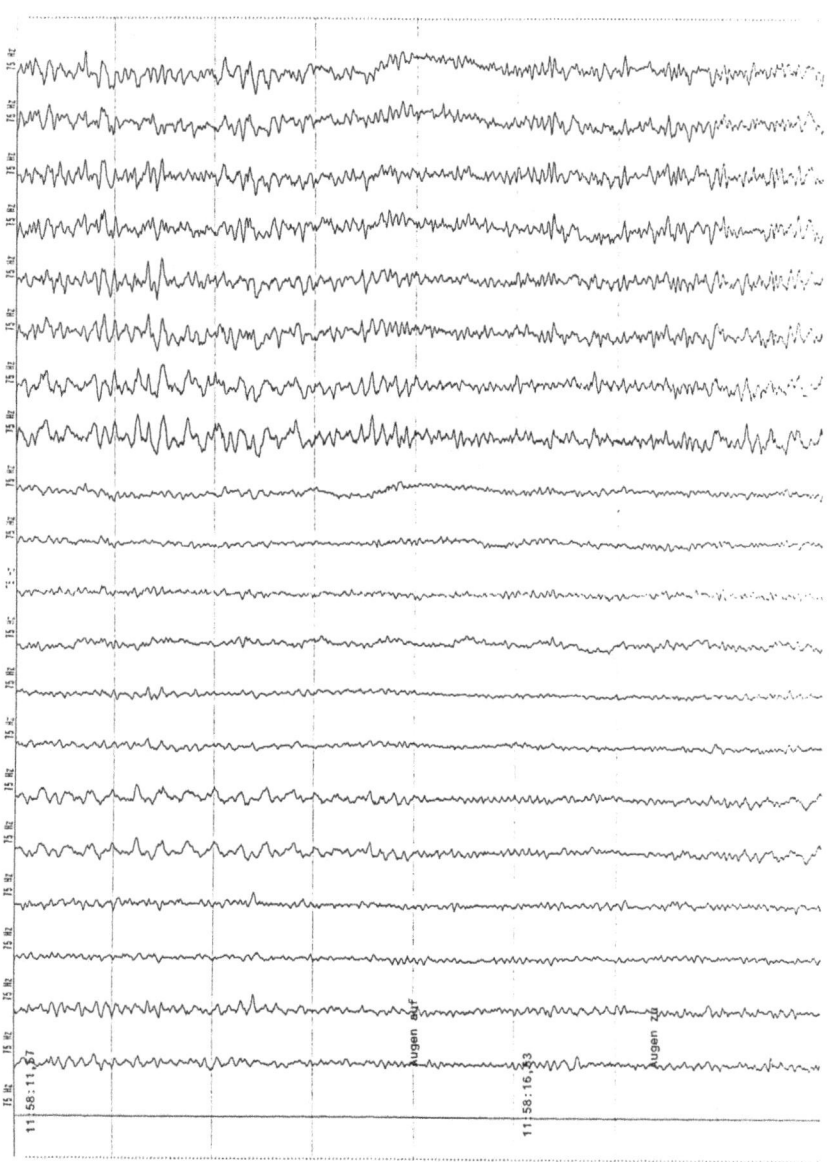

Figure 29. Intermittent bilateral posterior groups and sequences of a 3-5/s activity (**IBP**) in patient with anxiety neurosis (10 mg/d diazepam). Picture of a so-called posterior theta-variant interpreted as constitutional (K. K., 32 y., f., EEG-nr. 666/93).

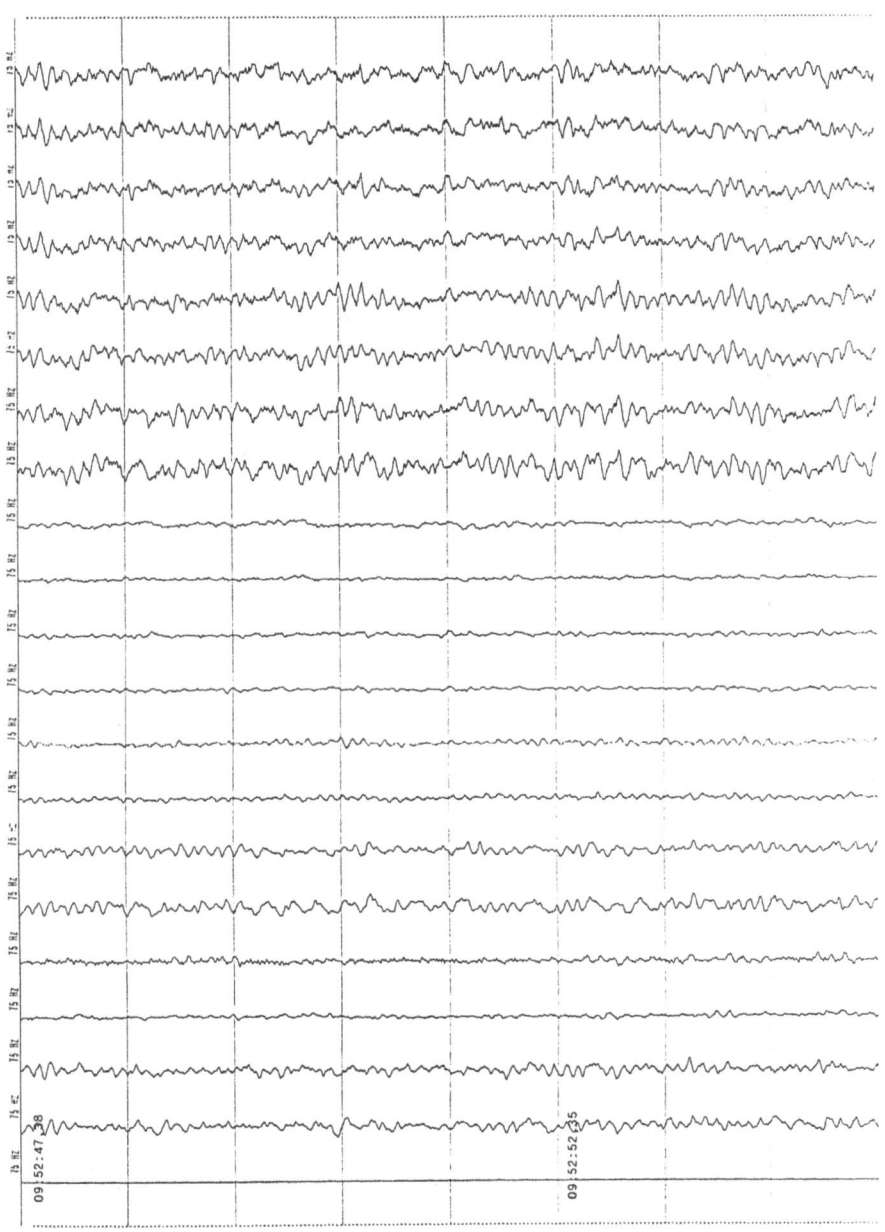

Figure 30. Intermittent right-posterior (occipital) groups and sequences of irregular slow waves (**IRP**) in a patient with schizophrenic psychosis under 300 mg perazine (J. P., 22 y., m., EEG-nr. 387/92).

THE THEORETICAL INTERPRETATION OF ELECTROENCEPHALOGRAPHY (EEG)

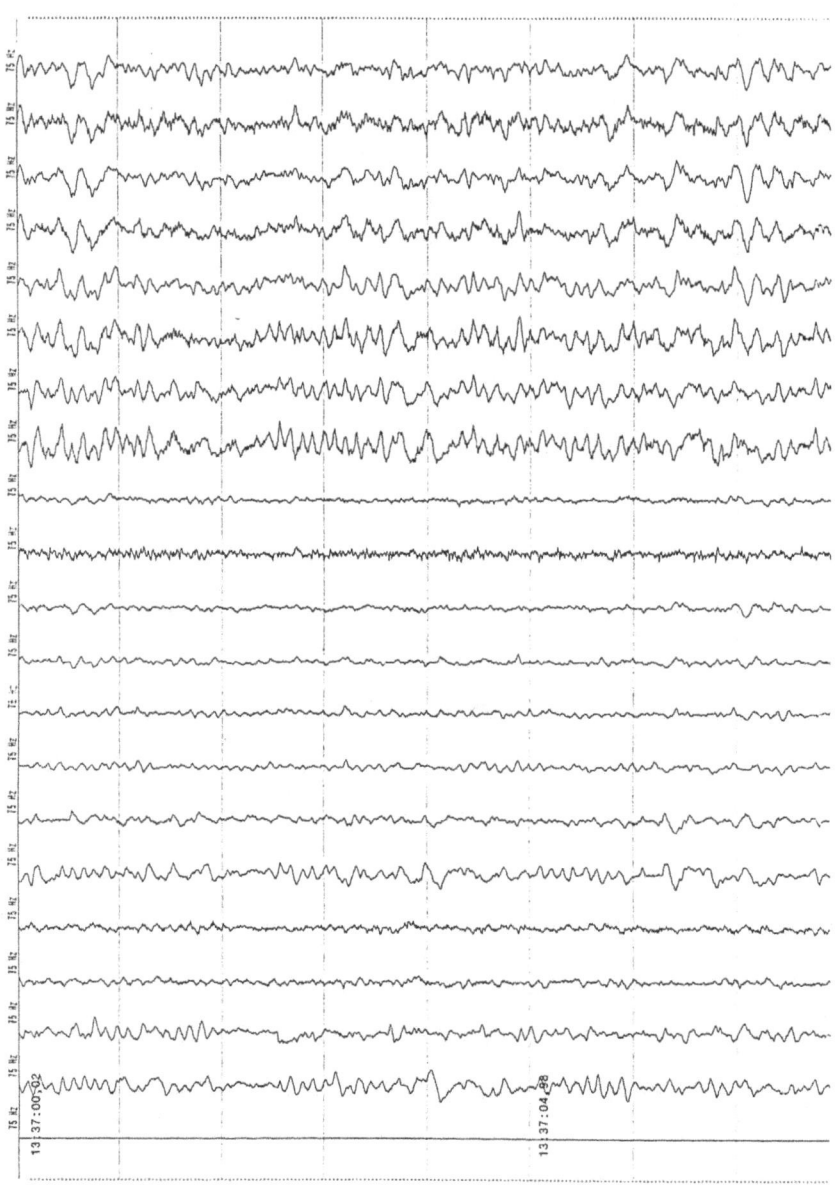

Figure 31. Intermittent right-posterior (occipital and temporo-posterior) accentuated singular and grouped irregular slow waves (**IRP**) in patient with schizo-affective psychosis under 150 mg/d perazine and 100 mg/d clomipramine (K. A., 47 y., f., EEG-nr. 606/93).

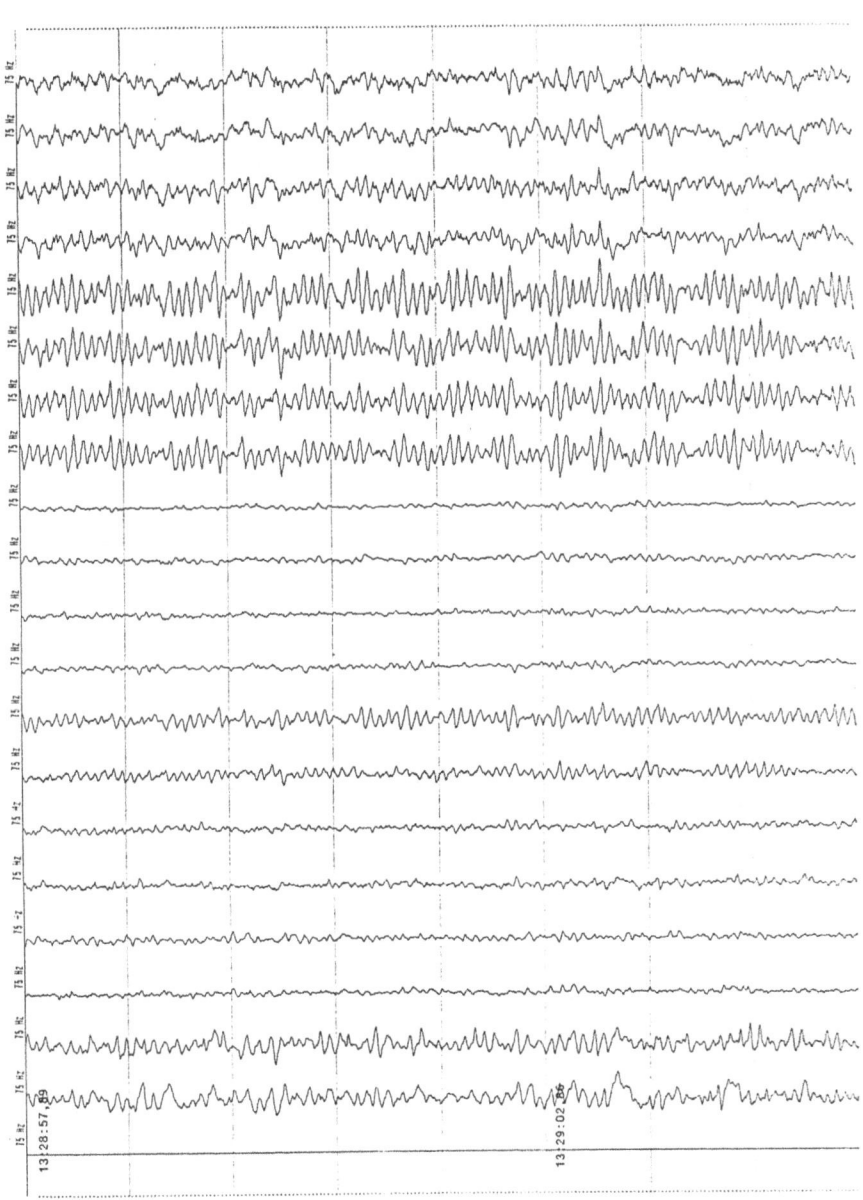

Figure 32. Intermittent right-posterior (only temporo-posterior) accentuated singular and grouped irregular slow waves, partially also resembling sharp- and slow-wave complexes (**IRP**) in patient with schizophrenia simplex under 15 mg/d haldol (A. S., 34 y., m., EEG-nr. 303/93).

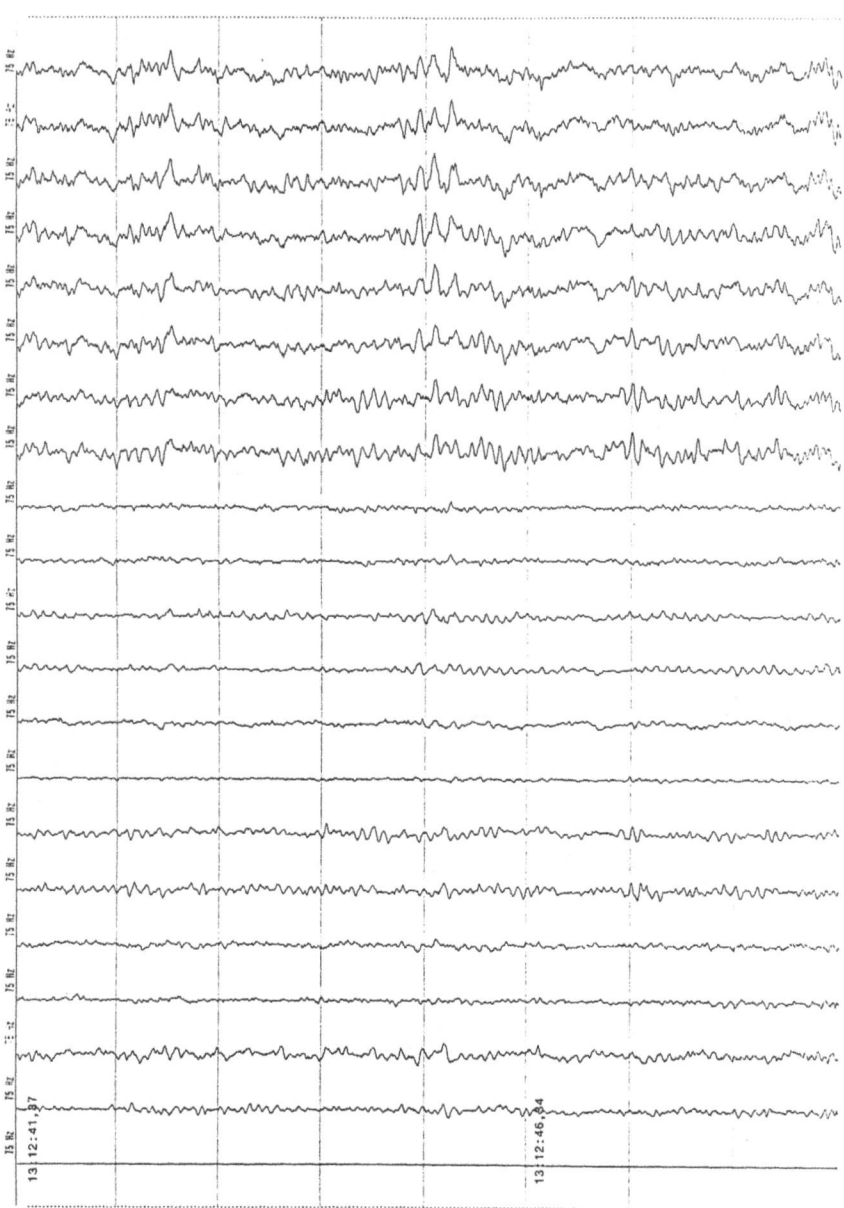

Figure 33. Intermittent left-posterior (only temporo-posterior) accentuated irregular slow waves (**ILP**) in a patient with personality disorder, medication-free (N.N., 22 y., m., EEG-nr. 1001/3).

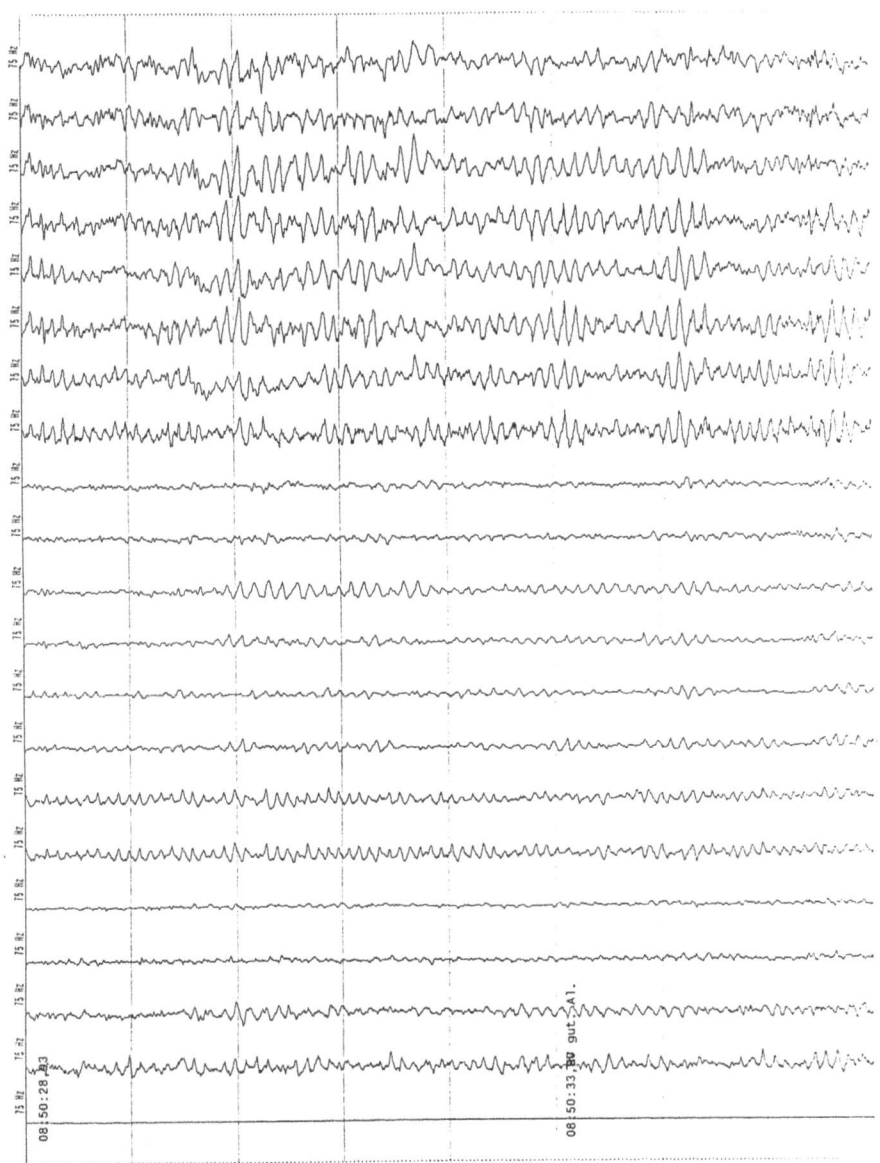

Figure 34. Dominating 10/s-activity with intermittently left-anterior (fronto-central) accentuated groups of rhythmic and high-amplitude 7/s waves (**ILA**) interpreted as constitutional since it was recorded in a medication-free patient with anxiety neurosis (I. S., 42 y., f., EEG-nr. 707/93).

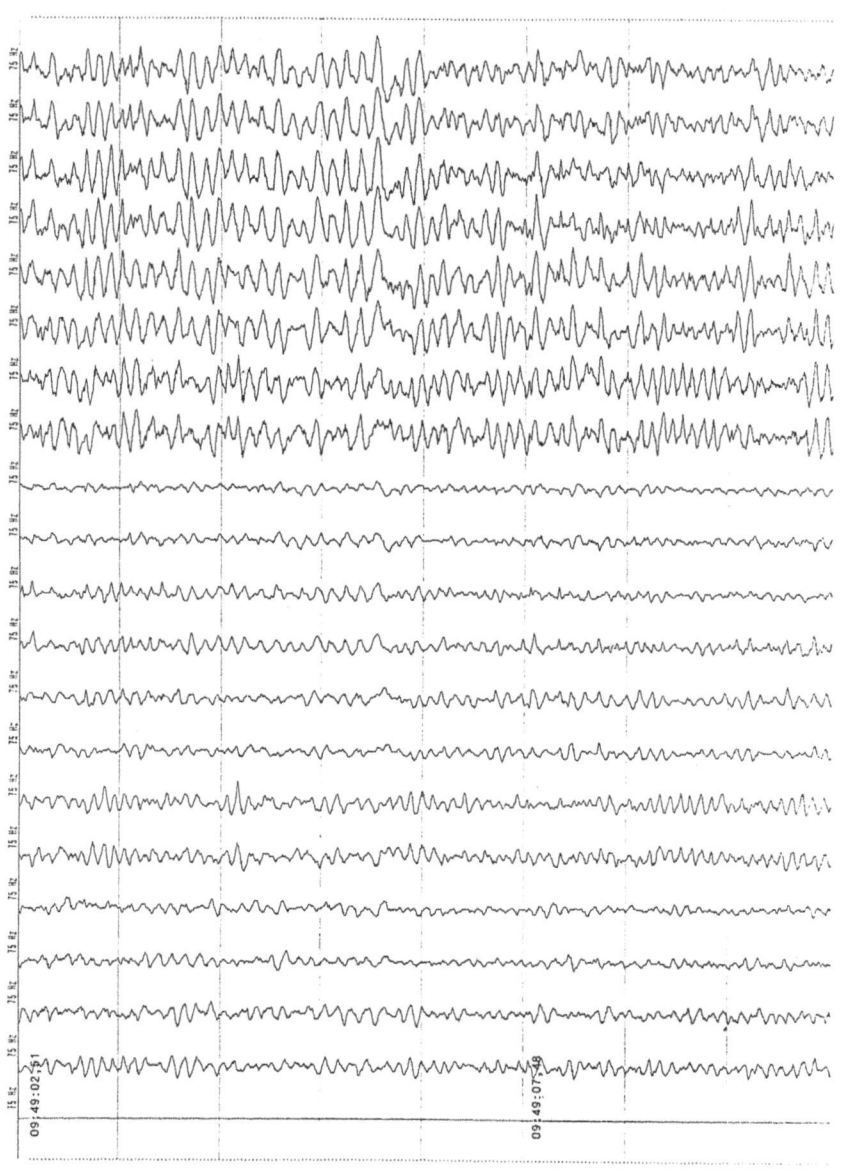

Figure 35. Posteriorly accentuated background activity of approximately 10/s with anterior accentuation in groups and sequences of bilateral symmetrical higher-amplitude 6-7/s waves (**IBA**) interpreted as constitutional since recorded in a medication-free patient with personality disorder (O. P., 23 y., m., EEG-nr. 813/93).

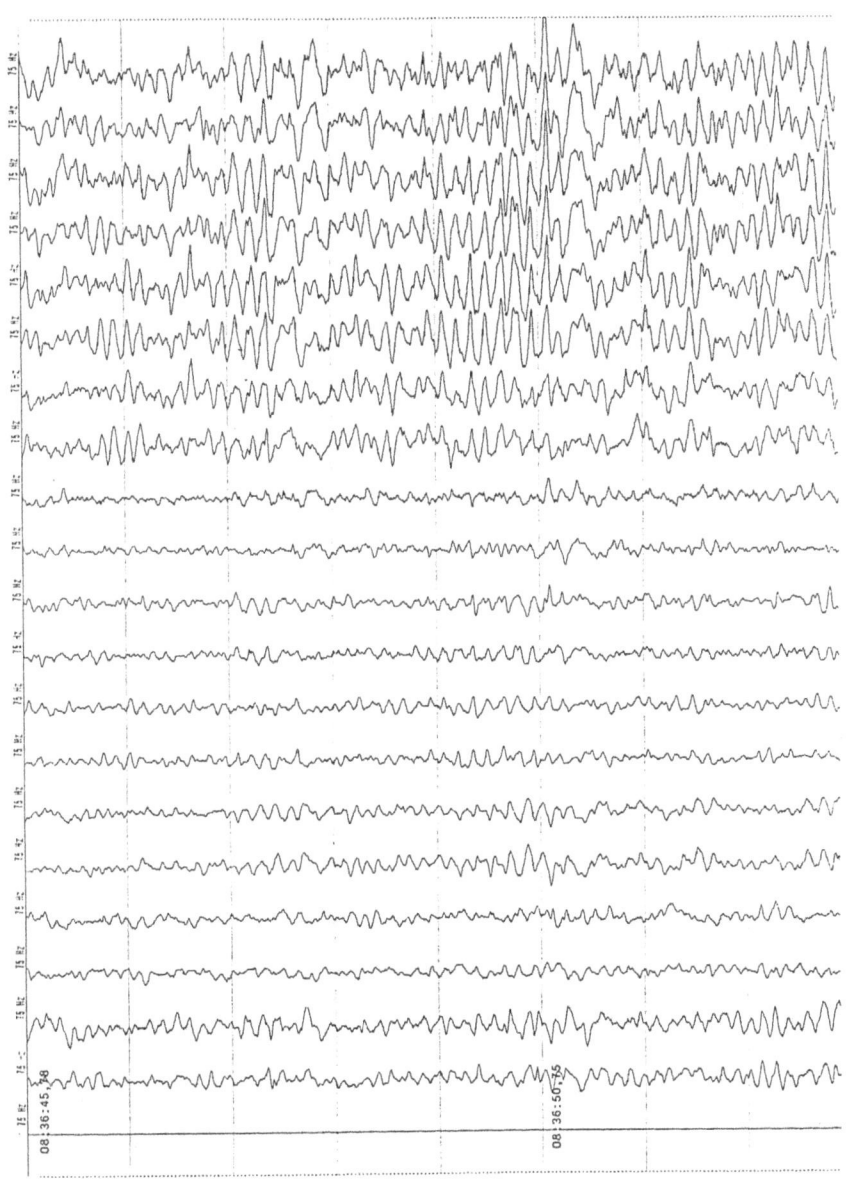

Figure 36. Predominant is a higher frequency, anteriorized and somewhat slow 7-8/s-activity; moderate dysrhythmia due to diffuse interspersed irregular slow activity; intermittent anterior-accentuated bilateral symmetrical high amplitude groups of rhythmic waves that often assume hypersynchronic characteristics; recorded in a patient with chronic schizophrenia under 40 mg/d dipiperone (K. S., 54 y., m., EEG-nr. 111/93).

THE THEORETICAL INTERPRETATION OF ELECTROENCEPHALOGRAPHY (EEG)

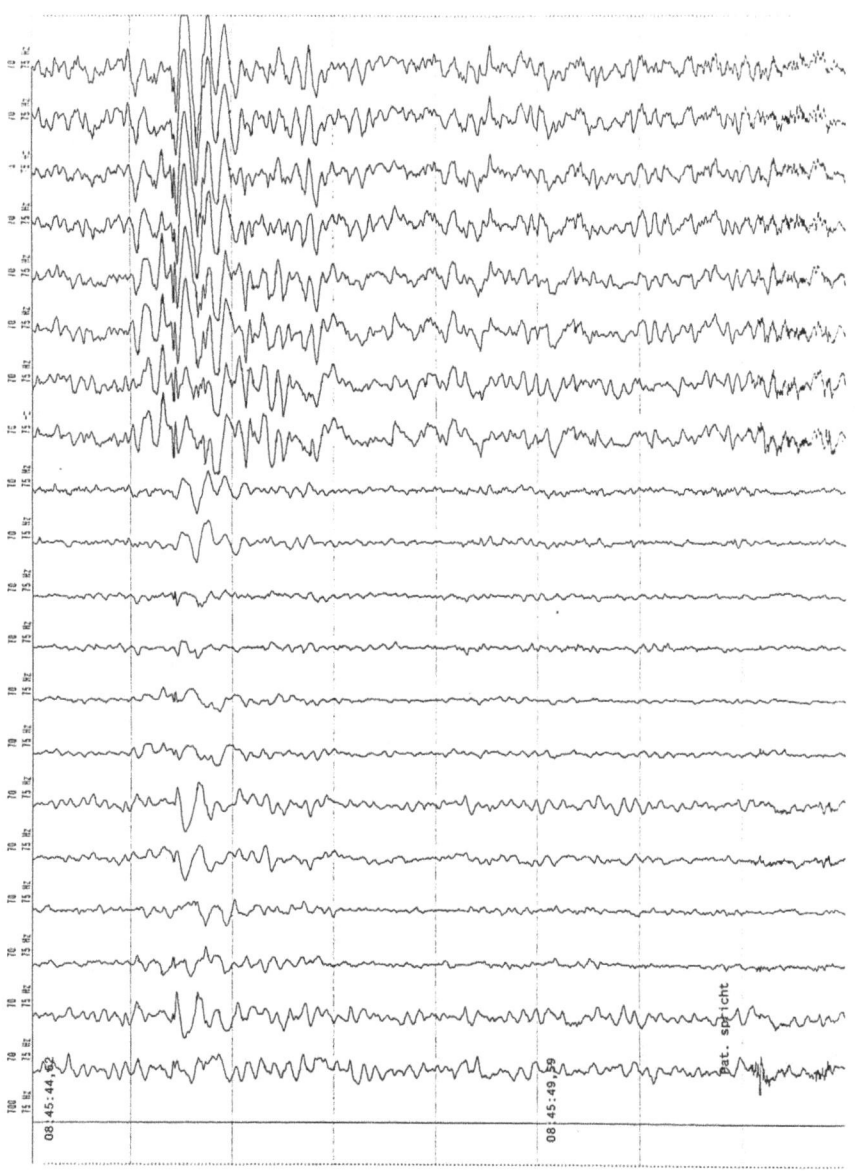

Figure 37. Paroxysmal-dysrhythmic formation with Sharp-and Slow- wave complexes (PP) interpreted as constitutional since recorded in a medication-free patient with disturbed impulse control (K. K., 28 y., m., EEG-nr. 1303/93).

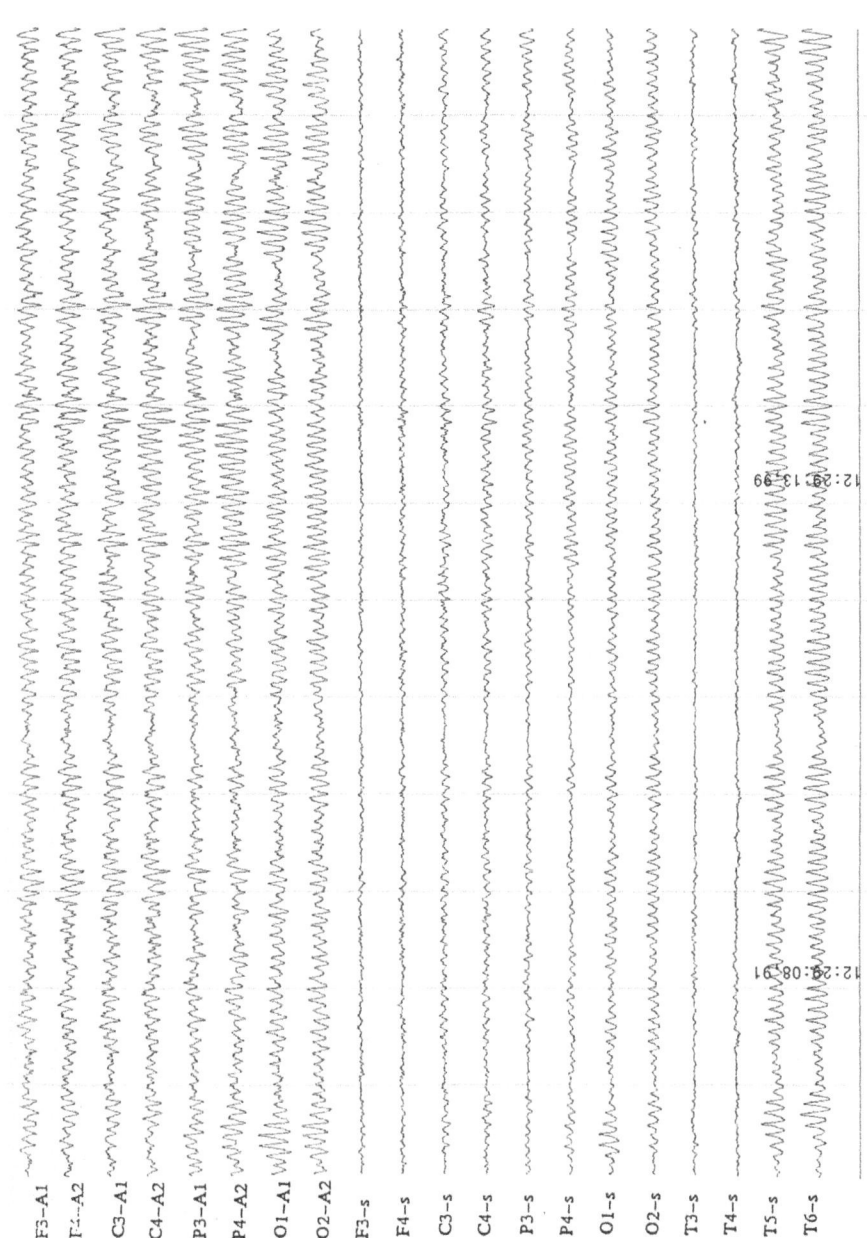

Figure 38. Monomorphic 9/s activity with continuous anterior spreading (DR); interpreted as constitutional since recorded in a medication-free patient with a compulsive disorder (C.A., 39 J., m., EEG-Nr. 64/93); Fig.39-40 with the same derivation.

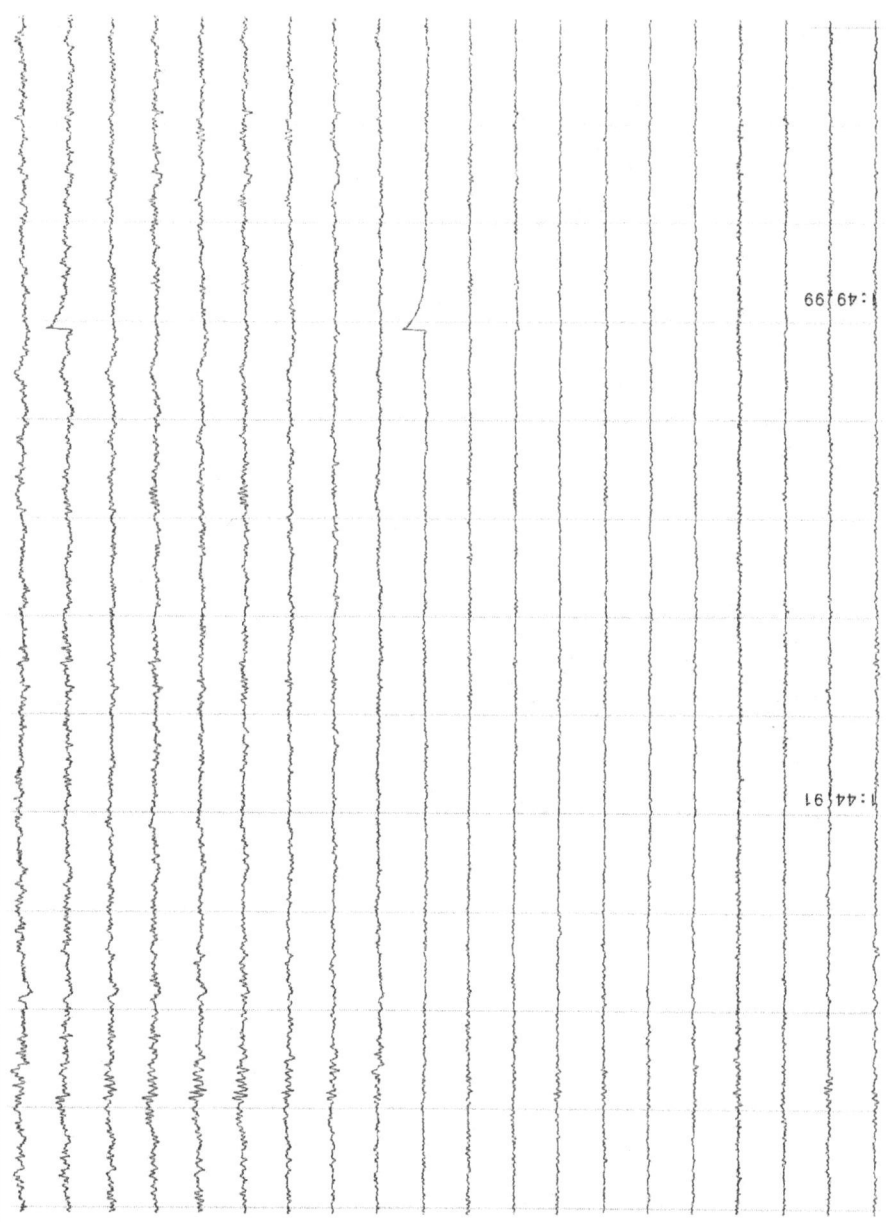

Figure 39. 12-13/s activity appears only in short groups typically for 1-2 s after closing the eyelid. Dominating is a low-voltage desynchronized activity corresponding to a subvigil stage B1 (DL) interpreted as constitutional since recorded in a medication-free patient with asthenic personality (R. F., 28 y., m., EEG-nr. 87/93). Identical derivation scheme as with Fig. 38.

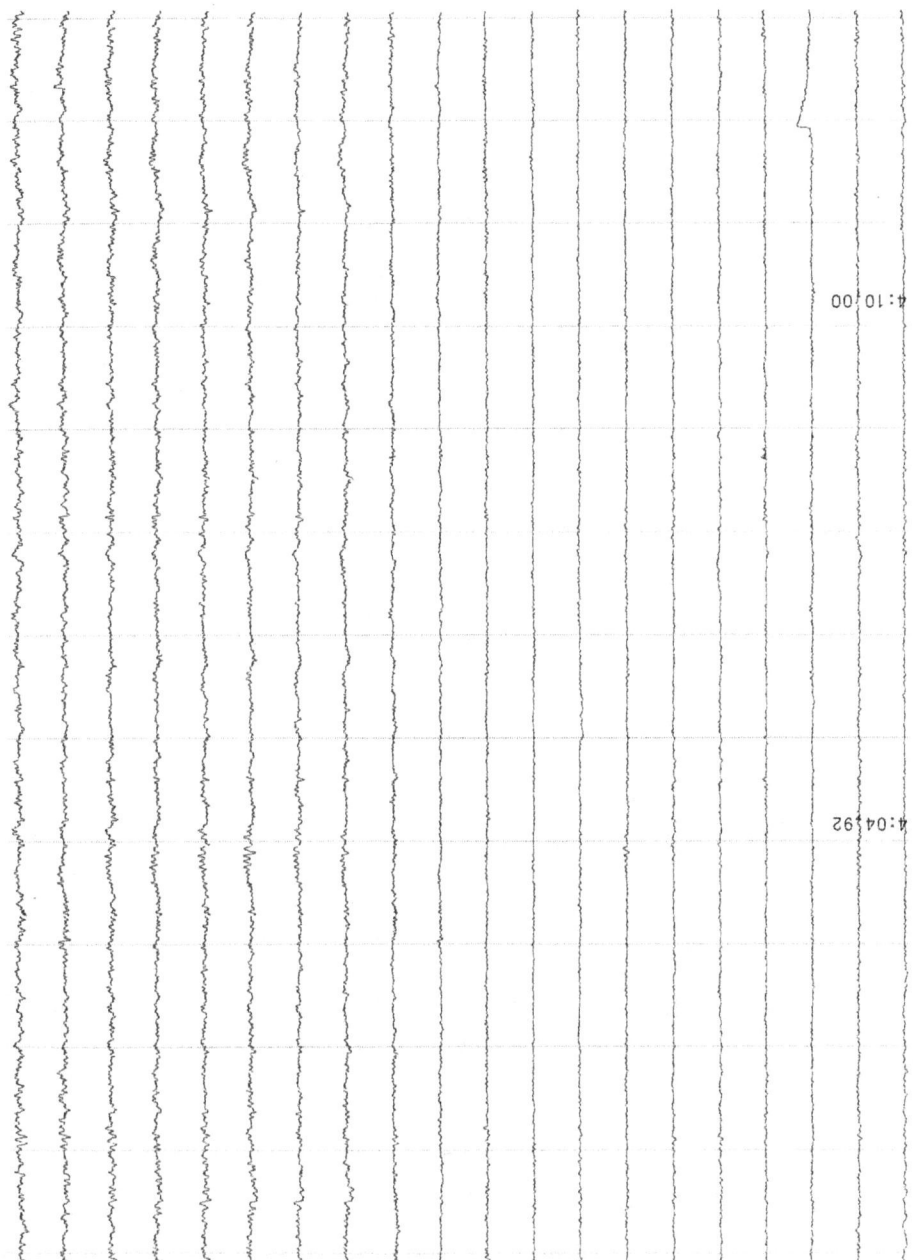

Figure 40. Similar appearance as in Fig. 39, this time in patient with a chronic schizophrenia under 4 mg/d pimozide; for historical reasons, the DL may also be called a schizophrenia-typical "choppy activity" (P. S., 34 y., f., EEG-nr. 999/93). Identical derivation schema as in Figs. 38, 39.

HILL (1952) stated a prevalence of 0.7% ("theta dominant record") in the average healthy population. He found Theta dominance much more frequently in adolescents with behavioral disorders. Because of the frequency of **DD** in patients with genuine epilepsy as well as their primary relatives, it is being considered a possible hereditary feature, predisposing for epilepsy and related psychiatric disorders (LENNOX & GIBBS, 1940; LENNOX et al., 1940).

We consider the mostly intermittently appearing groups and sequences of slow irregular waves confined to the posterior derivation regions - be it the bilateral symmetrical (intermittent bilateral posterior = **IBP**; Fig. 29), the asymmetric, usually right-accentuated (intermittent right posterior = **IRP**, Figs. 30, 31, 32), or the rare left-accentuated (intermittent left posterior = **ILP**; Fig. 33) variant - as a developmental-biological form of degradation of the **DD**. A sufficient number of studies have reported **DD**-correlated behaviour and personality disorders (AIRD & GASTAUT, 1959; BERGES et al., 1966COHN & NARDINI, 1958; GASTAUT et al., 1957; HEINTEL, 1975; HILL, 1952; JURKO & COLLE, 1982; KASPAR & KICK, 1987; KUHLO et al., 1969; MÜLLER-KÜPPERS & VOGEL, 1965; NEUNDÖRFER, 1970; PETERSEN & SÖRBYE, 1962; SCHEULER et al., 1988; ULRICH & BOHN, 1988; ULRICH & OTTO, 1984a, 1984b; WENDLAND & FENZEL, 1992; ZANGMEISTER & BUSHART, 1977).

The area of behavioral correlates considered typical ranges, from bland adjustment problems and habitual violence to delusional syndromes of atypical appearance. The often confirmed findings that the posterior-accentuated irregular 2.5-4.5/s activity that is considered developmentaly-typical in infants shows a right-accentuation until the age of six support a powerful argument for the acceptance of **IBP** and **IRP** (or also **ILP**) as immaturation indicators. This proves that the maturation process that leads to the adult morph posterior-accentuated alpha-background rhythm occurs asymmetrically. Obviously, the left-posterior regions mature faster in these cases in comparison to the right-posterior ones.

The findings obtained from children provide another argument for the interpretation of the **IBP-/IRP (ILP)**-phenomena, observed in adults as immaturation. COHN et al. (1958) found a slow posterior activity in 17% of psychologically inconspicuous children between the ages of 6 and 12 and in 62% of children of the same age group with behaviour disorders. Previous studies have confirmed a much higher prevalence of this feature in children with behaviour disorders compared to children without this disorder (f. i. SILVERMAN, 1958; KELLAWAY, 1958). This prevalence decreases with increasing age towards the end of the maturation process and finally remains constant. Because of the relative age-relatedness, proving this phenomenon in adults and children or adolescents is very different. Thus, it is only in adults that we are allowed to consider **IBP/IRP** (**ILP**) as immaturation indicators in the more concrete sense. During childhood and adolescence, the phenomenon permits only the assumption of a delay in maturation because of its potential reversibility. An evaluation of the possible clinical significance of **IBP/IRP** (**ILP**) requires prevalence comparisons between normal samples of behaviorally inconspicuous persons on the one hand and samples of psychologically disturbed persons on the other hand. A study indicated that about 0.12 or 0.24% of healthy candidates for a pilot career were the carriers of the feature (VOGEL & FUJIYA, 1969) compared to 5-7% of psychiatric inpatients under the treatment (COHN & NARDINI, 1958; KASPAR & KICK, 1987; ULRICH & BOHN, 1988; ULRICH & OTTO, 1984a; 1984b). As with all other immaturation indicators, the genesis of this phenomenon seems to be independent of the nature of the influences that hamper the development.

In Fig. 26, we tried to present a model that would illustrate the point in time when the respective influence seems to be the decisive factor for the type of maturation deficit that is realized. The findings of MÜLLER-KÜPPERS & VOGEL (1965), claiming that an increased incidence of posterior dysrhythmias in a certain family indicates an autosomal-recessive hereditary mode, do not contradict our opinion. Assuming the validity of the mentioned observation, the spectrum of possible causes expands only to the hereditary aspect. JURKO & COLLE (1982) also confirmed the increased incidence in certain families in connection with behavioral peculiarities.

Still under the conventional assumption that a focal EEG-phenomenon, for instance **IRP**, can be interpreted neuroanatomically/neuropsychologically as a residual cortical injury, we questioned its clinical significance in two retrospective, controlled studies (ULRICH & OTTO, 1984a; 1984b; ULRICH & BOHN, 1988). In our hospital, 5% of all inpatients had **IRP**, including those diagnosed as schizophrenics (7%), those with neuroses and personality disorders (2.4%), and those with affective disorders (2%) . Among the patients who were examined computer-tomographically because of the EEG-findings, not one single case indicated a structural lesion that was topographically associated with the EEG-focus. Among the patients with schizophrenic psychoses, the **IRP**-carriers showed, compared to gender-matched control patients:

- a lower age

- an earlier first manifestation of the psychoses

- more frequent anamnestic indications of perinatal complications

- a higher familial incidence of psychiatric disorders

A comparison of the AMDP-documented psychopathology showed a number of statistical differences in distinctiveness at the level of single symptoms that, taken as a whole, indicate an accentuation of hypermotor-expansive tendencies among the **IRP**-carriers. Based on the nosologic unspecificity of **IRP**, we discussed the possible significance of the feature maybe as indicator of a certain pathoplastically effective and prognostically relevant psychobiological matrix at a prephenomenal level. We discussed possible relationships with the *"precursory defect"* (*vorauslaufender Defekt;* JANZARIK, 1959) and *the subtle neuro-integrative defect* (MEEHL, 1962) and tried to prove that carriers of the phenomenon do not necessarily have to develop psychopathological disorders. Further, we examined the question regarding the relationship with the "adult minimal brain damage syndrome" (**MBD**; BELLAK, 1979). The degree of distinctiveness probably plays a role in the evaluation of the individual significance of **IBP/IRP** (**ILP**) as well as all other immaturation indicators,. Typically, the phenomenon will be more pronounced, and in some cases identifiable, when accompanied by a spontaneous or pharmacogenic lowering of the vigilance level.

The most important result of our studies regarding the **IRP**-phenomenon is, in our opinion, the confirmation of our thesis that specific, locally delineable EEG-phenomena do not have a structural correlate and thus do not allow a neuroanatomic/neuropsychological interpretation. However, such common attempts at interpretation are not only inappropriate but, in addition, block the prolific trend-setting perspective of developmental biology. It is important to emphasize this once again, especially with regard to the neuroanatomic research focus in psychiatry reactualized by the modern imaging technologies.

In comparison to the posterior phenomena **IBP/IRP** (**ILP**), the anterior phenomena **IBA/ILA** (Figs. 34, 35), which we have already encountered as state-related manifestations of "pathological functional change", evidently attracted less attention as brain-functional immaturity indicators. HILL (1952) found that anterior-accentuated *runs of rhythmic bilateral 4-7/s activity* (s. a. Table 2) were twice as common in incarcerated violent perpetrators as in control groups. Since this phenomenon can be observed physiologically between the 5th and the 10th year of age (MUNDY-CASTLE, 1951) and often persists into early adulthood, HILL (1952) regarded it as a sign of immaturation, a view shared by LIBERSON (1958).

The research conducted by WILLIAMS (1969) found that the phenomenon was clearly overrepresented in habitually violent persons. This author found the phenomenon either temporo-anterior or frontally accentuated. In two-thirds of the cases, it was bilateral-symmetrical while in the case of asymmetry, it was usually left-accentuated. The frequency, the author indicated, is usually around 4-7/s but can be lower. A simultaneous occurrence of theta- and delta-formations in one and the same EEG represents the rule rather than the exception. This would prove that the frequency is unimportant for the functional significance of the phenomenon.

Especially interesting to us is the comparison of the posterior (**IRP/ILP**) phenomena with the anterior ones (**ILA/IBA**), which were also overrepresented in the examined sample of violent persons, as the anterior phenomena indicated a closer correlation with the personality feature of violence than did the posterior ones. This coincides with ELLIOT'S (1976) findings, claiming that the anterior phenomena are more closely related to the *dyscontrol syndrome*. Although the aforementioned studies make no note of the asymmetrical, usually left-accentuated variant of **IBA**, in particular **ILA**, we still think it is justified to assume an intrinsic relationship between **ILA** and **IBA**. In our view, an important argument for this is that these phenomena and transitional forms often appear simultaneously in one and the same EEG . As far as we know, only BLANC & LAIRY (1961) and BLANC (1962) examined the state-unrelated occurrence of **ILA**. The authors found overrepresentation of **ILA** in persons with character neuroses (*néuroses de caractères*) and assumed a basic *immaturation neuronique* with a predisposition for neurotic decompensation.

With our present, by no means sufficiently supported state of knowledge, we tend to regard flaws in social behavior as the primary deficit associated with **IBP/IRP** (**ILP**) and "impaired impulse control" as the primary deficit associated with **IBA/ILA.**
We also associated an "impulse control impairment" with paroxysmal (epileptiform) potentials (**PP**; Figs. 36, 37). We positioned these in our model, as illustrated in Fig. 26, in the immediate developmental-biological neighbourhood of **ILA/IBA**. In diagnostically

unselected samples of psychiatric inpatients, STRUVE et.al. found a clearly higher rate of suicidal acts in the case history of those with **PP** in the resting EEG than in those without **PP** (STRUVE et al., 1972; 1973; STRUVE, 1983). The suicidal acts of the phenomenon carriers were to a very large extent of the impulsive-reactive nature as opposed to those of the non-carriers. Since suicidal acts based on an impulse probably have a lower success rate compared to the carefully planned ones, it does not surprise us that despite a lowered threshold, the suicide rates among the phenomenon carriers are no higher than among non-carriers.

If an impulse control impairment is the primary defect in the psychological domain of description, the carriers of this EEG-phenomenon should naturally showan increased incidence of the other reflections of this primary defect in addition to the lowered threshold for suicidal acts. Since STRUVE'S et al. research focused on the suicide risk and no other studies exist, we must be content with these assumptions. For obvious reasons, the findings in epileptics are of special interest in this context. Impaired impulse control, which manifests itself in destructive acts, has long been observed in patients with genuine epilepsy (f. i., HILL & POND, 1952; ERVIN et al. 1955; TREFFERT, 1964). GUN (1973) substantiated that such destructive acts can be directed not only outwards but also inwards in a sample of violent prisoners suffering from epilepsy. A significantly higher incidence of suicidal thoughts was observed among the epileptics than among a matched sample of non-epileptics. Furthermore, DAVIS et al. (1975) showed that not the epileptic disease but the exaggerated neuronal synchronization at the functional substrate of the **PP** phenomenon is hereby important in schizophrenics. Compared to schizophrenics without **PP**, those with **PP** manifested a higher incidence of many variations of impaired impulse control, including impulsive suicidal acts. Differences between the groups were considerably more evident in the EEG recorded under the influence of neuroleptics than in the premedication EEG. Whether someone develops **PP** under the influence of neuroleptics depends not only on the kind and dosage of the neuroleptic, but also on individual disposing factors (HELMCHEN & KÜNKEL, 1960; NEIL et al., 1978). In the study by Neil et al. (1978), 50% of the patients with **PP** under neuroleptics treatment did not manifest any **PP** prior to the treatment. This effect is extremely stable intra-individually.

We want to remind the reader of the fact that immaturation indicators, such as **DD**, **IBP/IRP** (**ILP**), and **IBA/ILA,** often become obvious only after a physiological or pharmacogenic lowering of the vigilance level. The findings that schizophrenics with

PP more often present an atypical psychopathological picture (BENTE, 1963; EMDE & METCALF, 1969; VISSER et al., 1964) indicate a pathological significance of **PP** exceeding the phenomenon of impaired impulse control.

Since STRUVE'S findings (1983;1984) are relatively unknown while also remaining unopposed (SMALL et al. 1968; TUCKER et al. 1965; VOLOW et al. 1979), we tried to form our own opinion through a retrospective study involving a sample of psychiatric inpatients with various diagnoses (ULRICH & HEGEWALD, 1990). We excluded only those patients for whom no EEG or EEG disturbed by a distinct artifact was available. Furthermore, we excluded patients treated with clozaril because of the special property of this neuroleptic with regard to the facilitation of **PP**. Of the remaining 1003 patients mostly treated with psychoactive drugs, 51 (5.1%) showed **PP** on an EEG recorded under the customary resting conditions with additional hyperventilation. Only 5 of these 51 patients were epileptics. Thus, the prevalence of **PP** in our sample was approximately twice as high as in the sample studied by BRIDGERS (1987), which also involved 2.6% of psychiatric inpatients. In a sample of healthy young male applicants for pilot training, the prevalence was only 0.5% (GREGORY et al. 1993). This corresponds exactly to the findings by GOODIN & AMINOFF (1984) reported for the general population. Thus, we can conclude that **PP** is overrepresented in a psychiatric population by a factor of at least 5 to 10. After dividing our patients into those with and without **PP** and those with and without prior suicidal acts, we arrived at the following distribution:

		SA	
		−	+
PP	+	25	25
	−	631	281

(n = 962)

Table 4. Bivariate frequency distribution divided into patients with (+) and without (−) paroxysmal (epileptiform) potentials (**PP**) in the resting EEG as well as into those with one or more (+) or no (−) suicide attempts (**SA**) in their case history. For 41 patients, no pertinent data were available.

Statistically significant differences in the distribution indicate that more anamnestic notes about suicide attempts (**SA**) were found for patients with **PP** than for patients without **PP**

(chi^2 = 8.05, $p < 0.01$). These findings basically confirm STRUVE'S et al. (1977) results. Assuming that the psychological defect of impaired impulse control indicated by **PP** should manifest itself not only inwards but also outwards, we examined the relationship between **PP** and selected psychopathological features of the AMDP-system that we use routinely for the documentation of the admission psychopathology of our inpatients. We considered "aggressive," "irritated," "increased drive," "motor restlessness," and "affective labile" as possibly relevant features. No significant relationship was observed in any of these cases.

To evaluate this negative result, we must make the restriction that the AMDP-system as an instrument for the registration of the psychopathological cross-sectional picture and its time course is hardly suitable to provide a reasonably reliable picture of personality traits. A definite answer for the question we stated above requires a prospective study design using special personality inventories.

Of course, theoretically, the higher frequency of suicide attempts in persons with **PP** could also be caused by a basically depressive disposition, a possibility that STRUVE et al. (1977) did not consider. Trying to compensate for this omission under the existing methodical limitations, we considered the AMDP-feature "depressed mood" as an indicator of a depressive state-unrelated basic disposition. It was remarkable that the hypothesis of a relationship between "depressed mood" and the frequency of suicide attempts could be maintained for patients **without PP** ("intraspecific association coefficient" of + 0.76, according to COLE, see LIENERT, 1973: chi^2 = 11.01, $p < 0.01$) but not for the patients **with PP** (association coefficient: - 0.16; n.s.). The highly significant difference between the two association coefficients ($p < 0.001$) indicated that suicide risk cannot be traced to a uniform personality feature but that at least two psychological primary defects are to be distinguished. According to our findings, depressive personalities are overrepresented among suicidal persons **without PP**, and persons with impaired impulse control are overrepresented among suicidal persons **with PP**. Such a differentiation involving the EEG could have some bearing on the question of whether a suicidal person should be treated with psychotherapy or with pharmacoprophylaxis, such as serotonergic substances. To avoid a possible misunderstanding, we finally want to emphasize that **suicidal persons without PP are by far more numerous than are those with PP** - according to Table 4, approximately 10 times as much.

The dynamic rigidity (**DR**) and the dynamic lability (**DL**) were, if regarded at all, by the present studies rather as norm variants than as indicators of brain-electrical immaturity. The possible maturation deficit was considered but not investigated only for the more extreme forms in the one or the other direction (DONGIER et al., 1965; GASTAUT et al. 1960; HILL, 1952; PICARD et al., 1957). This might also be caused by the difficulties associated with categorizations of a continuous distribution of the feature. RÈMOND & LESÈVRE (1957) divided a sample of healthy persons into those with a relatively continuous (group I, 19%) and those with a relatively discontinuous (group III, 32%) alpha background activity and additionally, they formed an intermediary group (group II, 49%). A more pronounced continuity of the background activity was regularly accompanied by a relatively slower and monomorphic frequency of approximately 8-9 Hz as well as by an anterior spreading tendency. The relatively discontinuous EEGs of group III were dominated by low-voltage and desynchronized activity phases with variable beta-amount, sometimes with interspersed theta-waves. The intermediary group II was characterized by a continuously posterior weighted spindle-form modulated 9-11/s-activity. We repeat that we classified the *formative tendencies* associated with group I under the term dynamic rigidity (**DR**) and those associated with group III under the term dynamic lability (**DL**). The vigilance dynamics of the intermediary group II can be termed physiomorphic (**PM**). It now became evident that the persons with physiomorphic vigilance dynamics had comparatively best results in various psychological tests. Persons with **DR** (group I) differed from the two other groups by showing a slower psychological speed, lower reactivity, and higher passivity. The persons with **DL** (group III) were comparatively more reactive, emotionally less stable, more impulsive, and more neurotic in general. These classifications confirm the observations of earlier authors. It was STRAUSS (1945), for instance, who found a lower continuity, amplitude, and regularity of the EEG related to personality-bound anxiety, adaptation difficulties, and increased mental fatigue. SAUL et al. (1949) reported similar findings and additionally emphasized that the EEG-features corresponding to the neurosis cannot be influenced by psychoanalytical treatment. As an extreme form of **DL**, we consider those by no means rare low-voltage-desynchronized EEGs that are often falsely blamed on "psychic tension," where an alpha-rhythm can be found only temporarily in short groups of 1-2 s duration, most frequently upon the closing of the eyelids (Fig. 39)

As we tried to prove in another context, the low-voltage desynchronized activity must be associated with a subvigil intermediary stage B1 rather than with an arousal reaction.

Although this phenomenon did not go unnoticed, for instance, its special relationship with a neurotic symptomatology has been recognized (DONGIER et al. 1965; PICARD et al. 1960; PINE & PINE, 1951), we acknowledge a further need for research. The contrast between the personality features of persons with relatively rigid EEGs and those with relatively labile EEGs could create the impression that only persons with unstable EEG have a disposition for neurotic disorders, as pointed out by RÉMOND & LESÉVRE (1957). The reason for this is probably that traditionally extrovert-active peculiarities of behavior are much more likely to be called neurotic compared to introvert-passive ones. However, according to personality-psychological categorizations, adaptive deficits in the sense of passive-phlegmatic slow movement behavior with adjustment difficulties and possibly depressive disposition can also be found in persons with **DR**.

The quoted findings underline our biperspectivistic perspective of morphodynamics being associated with the current system's state as well as with personality characteristics. As already mentioned, psychiatric EEG-research has thus far largely ignored the question of disposing factors. Besides the hypothesis of depression-predisposing morphodynamics confirmed by numerous findings (see above), we recognize an enormous need for research with regard to schizophrenic psychoses. To this very day, no study systematically investigated the "choppy activity" (Fig.40) that was considered typical for schizophrenia by DAVIS (1941;1942) and that, based on the given characterization, could casually be subsumed under **DL**. Although a reference to "*choppy activity*" can be found in nearly all of the earlier articles on schizophrenia and EEG, the important question of whether the feature is or is not state-related, i. e., constitutional, has not yet been answered. Because of our own observations, though not yet systematized, we cannot share DAVIS' (1942) assumption that the "*choppy activity*" might be a manifestation of an ongoing cortical excitation. Based on routine evaluation, it is our impression that "*choppy activity*," or **DL**, is a relatively stable feature in schizophrenics, which can also be found during psychosis-free intervals and remains unchanged over years. The same is true for the EEG with a continuous, monomorphic, slightly anteriorized and rather slow background activity that point towards **DR,** as noted among schizophrenics. Without being able to prove it with numbers, we consider a certain rough relationship between the EEG-dynamics and the type of the psychosis as a given. For instance, we frequently see a relatively slow EEG pointing towards **DR** in rather weak hebephrenic psychoses. In catatonic pictures, **IBA** or **PP** is overrepresented. A **DL** (or "choppy activity") is found primarily in the remaining majority of the cases, i. e., in the paranoid-hallucinatory forms. The treatment with neuroleptics, of course, makes the systematic study of these relationships considerably more difficult, if not impossible. Therefore, a medication-free recorded EEG is an indispensible requirement in electroencephalographic schizophrenia research. Although there was wide agreement about this in the sixties (BENTE, 1963; FEIGENBERG, 1964; HELMCHEN & KÜNKEL, 1964; ITIL et al., 1966; 1975; IGERT & LAIRY, 1962), no follow-up occurred. Instead, important findings that emerged from these studies were forgotten. Thus, it still is considered true that the relatively slow, monomorph EEG pointing towards **DR** as we find in hebephrenic and chronic forms suggests a relatively poor neuroleptics effect. Moreover, the effect of neuroleptics in patients with **DD** or **IBP/IRL** (**ILP**) is dubious. On the other hand, neuroleptics have a rather positive effect on patients with discontinuous background activity marked by a prevalence of low-voltage subvigil B1-stages corresponding to **DL** and on patients with **IBA** and **PP**. As explained previously, we were able to confirm and specify the existence of a relationship between vigilance dynamics and the therapeutic reactivity to neuroleptics with quantitative methods in a study involving acute schizophrenic patients (ULRICH et al., 1988). While we considered only success or non-success in this correlation study, we found another approach intriguing. This approach is in accordance with the procedure applied by RÉMOND & LESÈVRE (1957) and is based on a classification into three categories depending on the pre-medication EEG-dynamics. Analogous to the findings obtained by these authors, a hypothesis can be formulated and tested, claiming that schizophrenics with physiomorph dynamics (**PM**) who also supposedly possess a comparatively better psychological ability for adaptation have a better therapeutic reactivity and prognosis compared to the patients with dynamic lability (**DL**) and by even better therapeutic reactivity and prognosis compared to those with dynamic rigidity (**DR**). Possibly even a grading of **PM** - **DL** – and **DR** can be established here. After all, our study on the phase-prophylactic effect of lithium in patients with affective psychoses confirmed our view of "physiomorphic vigilance dynamics" as an indicator of a favorable pharmacon effect, among other things (ULRICH et al., 1993).

3. 4. 7 EEG AND PSYCHOPHYSIOLOGY

Psychophysiology consists of correlating objective (physiological) and subjective (psychological) data. The former we owe to the third-person-perspective, the latter to the first-person-perspective. Hence, the two streams of data originate in phenomenal domains being widely different in logical as well as epistemological respect. This has to be considered when trying to interrelate irreconcilable domains of this kind. The two antithetical perspectives can only be conciliated from a metaperspective point of view. It was HEAD'S great and outlasting achievement to become aware of this. In order to exclude any misunderstanding, he chose the factitious term of *vigilance,* which then was not occupied otherwise! He furthermore stressed explicitly that *vigilance* had to be understood as a "theoretical term." "Theoretical terms" cannot be defined by themselves. They needed to define other terms (BATESON, 1982).

From another point of view, it can be stated that Psychophysiology presumes that all psychological processes have a physiological correlate. This basic concept does not require confirmation from empirical findings. It represents, so to speak, the signature of a world view coined by natural science and marks the boundary of convictions of spiritual-magic-mystical provenance.

The situation is completely different, however, if we discuss the **nature** of the relationships between psychological and physiological matters. Many might feel uncomfortable at the mere question of this relationship, since, quite obviously, the "body-mind problem" shines through. This difficult problem is regarded both as unsolvable and irrelevant for research. As evidenced by literature, psychiatric research limits itself to the presentation of statistical correlations between so-called biological and psychopathological data. However, if only a statistically significant correlation is available, such a finding is of questionable value as long as its meaning remains unsettled. All too often, more or less plausible post hoc hypotheses are offered. The problem of the psycho-physiological relationship can be concretized by asking whether and to what degree the subjectively felt alertness/drowsiness is reflected in the EEG. If we consult the literature, we encounter a strange contradiction, which has been in place for many decades between popular opinion and empirically supported knowledge. Still dominant is the concept of a functional isomorphism between the subjective degree of drowsiness and certain objective EEG patterns. GRÜTTNER & BONKALO (1940) already pointed out more than half a century ago that the 14/s spindle-like activity usually associated with the light sleep (stage C, see above) is absolutely compatible with cognitive activities, such as mathematical calculations. FISCHGOLD et al. (1959) thought it remarkable that some subjects were able to keep contact with the experimenter despite unequivocal sleeping patterns in the EEG. KUHLO & LEHMANN (1964) emphasized that low-voltage desynchronized activity corresponding to a stage B1 is not a reliable indicator of subjectively experienced drowsiness. Other authors voiced similar opinions (e.g., LIBERSON & LIBERSON, 1965; MAULSBY et al., 1968; SANTMARIA & CHIAPPA, 1987). In summary, LIBERSON & LIBERSON (1965) stated:

".. a subjective impression of whether one is asleep or not may not be consistent with the apparent EEG pattern."

According to RECHTSCHAFFEN & KALES (1968), the classification of sleep stages cannot be based on the EEG alone. For a valid delineation, additional polygraphically acquired information about motor behavior of eye, pupils and limbs, EKG, blood pressure, and the like, are necessary. Based on the available evidence, the assumption of a one-on-one relationship between feelings of drowsiness or alertness and the EEG cannot be maintained. While there seems to be no doubt about the futility of finding EEG correlates of subjective experiences, such as guilt, feelings, illusions, etc. an electroencephalographic objectivation of the perceived quality of drowsiness or alertness is, for some strange reason, not only considered possible but even taken for granted. This is evidenced through the fact that distinctions, such as "typical alert," "slight drowsiness", and "pronounced drowsiness," are based solely on the EEG (KUGLER, 1981; MATOUSEK & PETERSEN, 1979).

If we question the reasons for this epistemological lapse, it is initially tempting to blame an uncritical interpretation of statistical correlations. Further, it might play a role that drowsiness in contrast to the other mentioned experienced qualities can be arranged on a bipolar continuum with one of the extreme poles unequivocally marked by electroencephalographical correlates of sleep in its different stages. Based on the experienced continuity of the subjectively given quality drowsiness, the inadmissable analogical conclusion about a corresponding objectifiable continuity in the EEG can be made (MATOUSEK et al., 1984). The use of quantitative methods is required assuming that this kind of inner experience can be objectified by means of physical measuring:

„It may be concluded that the EEG method can be employed to measure the vigilance level, and that it has certain advantages over conventional self-rating," and further: *"The EEG method is not handicapped by subjective bias."* (MATOUSEK et al.1984, p. 55-59).

Such a demand ignores the enormous variation characteristic of all introspectively obtained statements. Instead of considering this undeniable fact MATOUSEK et al. (1984) considered it a methodical flaw. Consequently, they also viewed the dubious correspondence between the experience of drowsiness and the EEG patterning as a problem that is solely the result of an inadequate method. Trying to eliminate introspection as a legitimate scientific tool because of its supposed faking of reality, they must inevitably consider mind or psychology in the proper sense and, thus, also psychophysiology as replaceable by physiology.

The common epistemological position, which together with empirism unfailingly leads to contradictions and is rarely explicitly formulated or reflected in the field of psychiatry and psychophysiology, has also been named eliminative reductionism (WERNER, 1988).

A world view as well as an image of humanity that makes no distinction between living and non-living, man-made systems is reflected here (MATURANA, 1982). Only living systems possess subjectivity and, therefore, the capability of experiencing. In addition, they can be objectively described, just as non-living systems. Thus, they can only be understood from a biperspective manner. Both perspectives have their own language, named "mind language" and "brain language" by LASZLO (1972). To avoid epistemological pitfalls, it is of utmost importance to keep the terms belonging to "mind language" and to "brain language" clearly separated. Observing both domains of description simultaneously would give the impression that the physiology of the organism generates its behavior. Thus, a hierarchical multi-layer model is suggested. However, one has to point out that we are dealing here only with an observer-created imagination of an operational causative connection that by no means allows for a phenomenologic reduction. Such a reduction would in fact justify an eliminative reductionism according to which the psychological can be completely replaced by the physiological. A monoperspectival objective analysis is only in accord with non-living systems. A translation of subjective into objective data and vice versa is impossible as a matter of principle because such data originate from logically incommensurable domains (RUSSEL & WHITEHEAD, 1913). Another way to express this idea is that the point of view from which an observing subject makes statements about psychological matters, which can always only concern their own mind, is different from the point of view from which statements about physiological matters are made. The latter embraces all objects, including the own body. Saying that drowsiness is nothing but the lack of a transmitter x at a spot a in the brain or a certain EEG patterning is logically out of question and thus nonsense.

Experiences, such as a certain intensity of subjectively felt drowsiness, are always determined by a multitude of only partially recognizable and in many ways interacting factors. The brain electrical patterns to be designated as *EEG-vigilance* represent thereby only one, although essential, component. Another important factor is the current emotional state or its corresponding multifarious and complex physiological mechanisms.

From the above, we conclude that the assumption of a positive psychological effect of feedback-induced alpha-activity is doubtful, at least. As a matter of fact, the ineffectiveness of such techniques has been proved experimentally quite some time ago (Sacks et al., 1972; TRAVIS et al., 1975; PLOTKIN & COHEN, 1976).

According to EDELMAN (1989), no connection between the frequency power-spectrum of the EEG and mental states exists. In particular, contrary to earlier assumptions, Edelman found no connection among the theta component, specific behaviours, and experiential states. Even if it were possible to cover all objective determinants, their interactive process dynamics could not be considered. Biological systems can be described as *deterministic-chaotic* (SCHUSTER, 1984), i.e., although they are strictly determined in the sense of classical exact natural science, their behavior cannot be predicted.

On the whole, it can be formulated as a basic principle of psychophysiology that a psychological (behavioral-experiential) phenomenon may correspond to various brain (dys)functions, just as seemingly identical brain (dys)functions may correspond to various psychological phenomena. Only if we are constantly aware of this principle, psychophysiological correlation research may prove to be a useful scientific tool, especially for psychiatry.

We are fully aware that the methodological consciousness in psychiatry - probably due to the pragmatic concerns of everyday clinical life - has traditionally never been very pronounced (JASPERS, 1913). Evidence for this may be that it is customary to criticize ambitious or sophisticated research work as "too heavy on theory" while never hearing that it is "too heavy on empirical experience." The development of the Psychiatric EEG entails more than an electrodiagnostic service. In order to develop it as a research tool, it is inevitable that the clinical psychiatry be openminded regarding such a development process. The cooperation of partners with research responsibilities shared by the hospital and the psychophysiological EEG is desirable. To a large extent, the methodological conditions necessary for this scenario must still be created.

The equivalence of empirical experience and theory, generally proclaimed as desirable, indeed does not exist. The prevalent critical attitude towards theory-guided research draws some, albeit very isolated, criticism:

THE THEORETICAL INTERPRETATION OF ELECTROENCEPHALOGRAPHY (EEG)

"It therefore seems more significant today to be raising questions than gathering data" (ANDREOLI, 1992).

For pure empiricists, a researcher discredits himself through the use of terms such as "epistemology" or "theoretical construct." When v. UEXKÜLL & WESIACK (1988) rightly stated that medicine in the 20th century has remained a natural science of the 19th century, this is especially true for psychiatry. About 150 years ago, when psychiatry became a natural science, medicine adopted its methods. However, medicine failed to follow when natural sciences radically changed their understanding of science. The machine model, which is based on classical mechanics, is still dominant as official doctrine. Albert Einstein, according to whom it is our theories that determine what we see and describe- and not the other way round, is a important witness to the primacy of theory over empirical experience in modern natural science. From a certain point, new data no longer clarified a situation but only confused it. FREEMAN (1992) recently summarized the problem in an editorial, which ties into the annual meeting of the "Society of Biological Psychiatry" and the 458 presentations and posters presented there:

"The data were expensive to obtain and are now not worth replicating or even retrieving, because there was little or no theory to specify what to measure, in what ancillary conditions, and with what expected outcomes. This is not the kind of chaos of which we can be proud." (FREEMAN, 1992, p. 1079-1081)

One should, please, start by presenting findings. After that, one might be able to talk about theory. If we follow this recommendation, we must expect incomprehension and rejection for the simple reason that the theoretical explanations that justify leaving the beaten paths necessarily had to be cut short. Further complicating matters is that electroencephalography and psychiatry, after the brief common intial phase for which we have to thank BERGER (1929; 1933) have moved continuously and irreversibly away from each other. Instead of being viewed as a genuine psychiatric research tool, clinical psychiatry considered the EEG today as a dispensable auxiliary tool that belongs in neurology. On the other hand, the administrators of the EEG, who as neuroscientific electro-diagnosticians feel responsible for myo- and neurography too, generally lack any relation to the psychiatry. Thus, we must ask the question who should be in charge of the development of the psychiatric EEG. In our opinion, there can only be one answer: **The psychiatric EEG can only be developed** within psychiatry by psychiatrists with clinical qualifications. Clinical psychiatry must rediscover the EEG as its very own research tool!

3.4.8 ABOUT THE IMPOSSIBLITY OF AN EXTERNAL VALIDATION OF PSYCHOPATHOLOGICALLY DEFINED PSYCHIATRIC DIAGNOSES

Over the years, a substantial number of publications dealt with EEG-correlates of different psychological constructs, such as fear, concentration, absentmindedness, excitement, insecurity, or awakeness or wakefulness, to mention just a few (Low, 1987). However, it was hardly ever possible to clarify whether the observed EEG-effects were related to the specific psychological alterations or to an associated unspecific global functional states. If we assume that the EEG is the result of a partial synchronisation of extended cortical substrates, then it is very unlikely that this method can assess specific psychological phenomena, not to mention specific contents. It seems much more plausible that the EEG allows the distinction of a limited amount of global functional states that show a predilective but not invariant connection with certain psychological constructs, such as those mentioned above. For psychiatry, we can thus conclude that specific EEG-correlates cannot be expected for defined psychopathological phenomena. Nevertheless, the real question that preoccupies many researchers is whether the EEG can differentiate diagnostic entities within clinical psychiatry. Posing this question takes for granted that psychiatric syndromes can be regarded as naturally occuring diseases that we have to acknowledge. Kraepelin's (1920) life-span research showed, unexpectedly, that no such natural disease entities, as for instance measles or diabetes mellitus, exist in psychiatry. Nevertheless, most present authors seem to assume the contrary, i.e., that a psychiatric diagnosis equals a natural disease entity. However, the numbers of those who point to the decades-long inability to validate psychopathologically clearly distinct syndromes on a neurophysiological or neurochemical basis and demand a re-evaluation or a change of the research strategies are growing (f. i., Bentall, 1990; Bhrolchain, 1979; Boyle, 1990; Carpenter et al., 1979; Jackson, 1990; Maas & Kaz, 1992; van Praag, 1990; Wexler, 1992). Such desperately needed new approaches are countered or sabotaged by the already criticized promises of an objective classification of disorders through the EEG. Without any proof or argument, it is stated apodictically:

"*..abnormality profiles are distinct for different disorders*" (John, 1990, p. 251 - 266).

The *abnormality profile* is the result of a statistical comparison between an individual EEG-characteristic and the EEG-characteristic of a "large normative data base."

Consequently, John, who as a mathematician and experimental neurophysiologist of merit was, however, never occupied with clinical psychiatry, named his automatic classification system "neurometrics". This software, which may be incontestable from a formal point of view, is nevertheless methodologically inappropriate.

"We have tried the 'specific disease, specific biology' approach for 40 years without much success. Let us consider a change. It is time to say 'The emperor has no clothes!'." (Maas & Katz, 1992).

In Fig. 41, we tried to show the psychiatric reality with the example of schizophrenic psychoses, which differs from his view. The model claims to be valid also for all other psychiatric disorders. As shown in Fig. 41, the EEG-parameters to be determined for the 3 patients are always within the interindividual variation range of a healthy control population, even if there is a state-specific shift in the characteristic values.

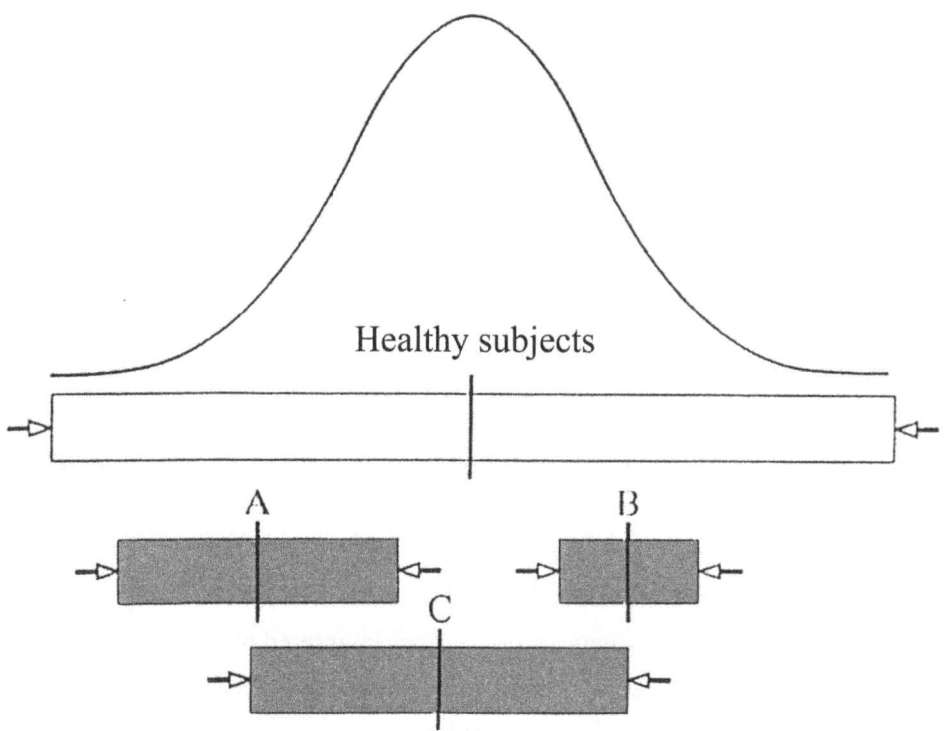

Figure 41. The intraindividual electroencephalographic variation range of the 3 schizophrenic model patients A, B, and C in relationship to the interindividual electroencephalographic variation range of a control population of healthy subjects ("normative data base").

This seems to preclude the diagnostic classification of an individual patient in relationship to a healthy control population. Since the interindividual variation of a population of schizophrenic patients - not shown in Fig. 41 - should be clearly greater than that of a population of healthy people (Garmezy, 1970), it seems quite possible to arrive at a statistical discrimination between the schizophrenics and the healthy people as groups. This fact is unimportant for the classification of individuals of interest from a clinical point of view. The new approach must begin with the definition of disease in the psychiatric sense. Contrary to symptoms, diseases are not phenomena, which can be perceived with our senses and therefore, they are theoretical constructs. The latter, however, are derived or developed from the former. As mentioned earlier, the validity of a theoretical construct depends to what extent it is really derived from an observable pattern and allows for new observations. Diseases show a great variability with regard to their construct validity. As a general rule, the construct validity is lower the more variable the disease appears in all its aspects. Therefore, diseases can be classified according to their construct validity. The schizophrenias as well the other psychiatric pictures have a rather low construct validity. The name assigned to a disease can hide such differences. The self-deception involved is also called *nominalism* or *reification* (see also Ulrich & Hegerl, 1989). Naming "diseases", such as "schizophrenia", gives them a life of their own with real-ontological status, just like the demons that one once thought possessed sick people. Disease is conceived as something that joins the healthy person and changes him or her. This is exactly the picture that characterizes our problem. It is not very surprising at all that clinical practitioners have not developed an awareness of the problem since this has no consequences for the therapeutic practice, which is their primary occupation. However, for the researcher whose task it is not to fight symptoms but to arrive at an external validation of the theoretical construct "disease", it has disastrous consequences if he falls into the trap of nominalism.

In medicine, a certain set of symptoms is recognized as "disease" only when it appears in connection with an objectively and reliably measurable phenomenon. One of the reasons for the overwhelming interest in the external validation of psychopathological diagnoses might be that psychiatry has had to fight from its early beginnings until today to be recognized as a medical discipline. It becomes increasingly clear that the construct validity of our diagnoses is simply too small to make the search for associated pathophysiological mechnisms seem potentially successful. The intensive efforts to define homogeneous subgroups - like the positive/negative or acute/chronic dichotomies - have also yielded hardly any results. However, whether neurophysiologically or neurochemically defined subgroups can be distinguished with respect to the clinical phenomena is doubtful. Despite discouraging failures, today's research strategy still consists of comparing one inevitably heterogeneous group of "normal persons" to a psychopathologically homogeneous but in other aspects also inevitably heterogeneous group of psychiatric patients. was Accordingly, Wexler (1992) coined the witticism of the *pathobiological heterogeneity of psychopathologically homogeneous samples.*

A more recent editorial by Maas and Katz (1992) stated that although RDC and DSM III have improved the diagnostic reliability, they have not contributed to the clarification of pathophysiology: *"Perhaps we have been looking in the wrong places or in the wrong way."* We also will have to consider that differently diagnosed syndromes do not necessarily correspond to an equally different pathophysiology but that the differences in the clinical picture are caused by individually different compensation strategies. Thus, the question is why endogenous psychoses should be any different from exogenous or model psychoses where the relationship between the respective symptoms or syndromes and the premorbid personality has been recognized long since (Birnbaum, 1928; Bonhoeffer, 1912; Leuner, 1962; Schröder, 1912; Walther-Büel, 1968).

In their introduction to the German version of the Diagnostic and Statistical Manual (DSM III) of the American Psychiatric Society, Köhler and Sass (1984) expressed their confidence that the diagnostic precision guaranteed through DSM would become very important for therapy planning. We cannot share their optimism. In a natural science oriented psychiatry, the search for somatic correlates of psychopathological syndromes must be central. Finding such correlates is the condition for a therapeutic intervention guided by rational principles. Since the revisions of psychiatric classification systems done at the conference table are based mainly on opinions and not on results of research - which continually increases the general confusion (Van Praag, 1989) - it is difficult to discover any positive aspects. Van Praag (1992) characterized the DSM as a *premature codification of diagnostic concepts and terms that causes more bad than good.* Zimmermann et al. (1989) criticized the DSM-system, suggesting that experts first allege a certain classification and only then are researchers allowed to examine its validity.

DSM III confronts us with a renaissance of early, long obsolete, Kraepelinian conceptions. Excluding the basic problem of construct validity of psychiatric "diseases," the creators of DSM III postulate implicitly that a finer operationalism will suffice to arrive at valid disease categories. In the face of the hurried obedience at the introduction of the respective latest versions of psychiatric classification systems noticable everywhere,

Heimann (1986) sounds like the preacher in the desert when he warns that *"the fixation of psychiatrists with nosologic specificity complicates a deeper understanding of the relationships between the psychopathological level and the pathophysiological foundations"* (transl. from German).

    The main problem psychiatry is grappling with lies in the difficulty of relating data at the behavior/perception level with neurophysiological/neurochemical data in a **meaningful** way. The all too often heard talk about the breathtaking progress in modern psychiatry seems to be incompatible with a statement of such resignation. However, if we took a closer look, we would realize that all this lauded progress has nothing to do with Heimann's basic problem. Although today we have an impressive multitude of data and knowledge in all kinds of partial areas, we cannot fool ourselves into thinking that we have learned much about the core problem, that is, the pathophysiological validation of psychopathological syndromes. Even the concentration of the research efforts on the central-nervous biochemistry and especially on transmitter mechanisms did not make any change, as the transmitter-oriented researcher psychopathology is nothing but disturbed psychochemistry. Since certain symptoms or symptom complexes can be influenced by interfering with certain transmitter mechanisms, they can be reduced to quantitative deviations of the respective transmitter mechanisms, so goes the argument. Therefore, the pathophysiological validation of psychopathological syndromes can only occur through detailed research of the psychochemistry. Contrary to the current trend, this logic appears rather erroneous rather than compelling. As far as we can see, not a single one of the different transmitter hypotheses could do any justice to the complexity of the mind. Like wooden paths that start out wide and open, these approaches so far always ended in an impenetrable thicket. The reason for the continued attractiveness of the transmitter-psychiatry probably lies in the fact that, contented with partial hypotheses and persevering in bustling modesty, it never raises its eyes to the complex entirety that might cause feelings of insecurity. In addition to this, costly lab technology that investigates the molecular field is still truly scientific.

    From an historical perspective, transmitter-psychiatry is a modern variation of the old humoralpathology. For the humoralpathologists, medical thinking was equal to thinking in fluids. Disease was, as a matter of principle, considered a disturbance in the composition of fluids, a *dyscrasia*. All symptoms would be, as mere ephemeral occurrances, attributed to dyscrasia. Proof of a secret renaissance of this doctrine seems to us to be the almost compulsive reflex noticed in scientific discussions when switching from the clinical but also neurophysiological level to the neurochemical level. Contrary to the predominant paradigm, we consider the transmitters not as determinants but only as compounds to render mind possible at all..

"..the amines, which are themselves servants, so to speak of other ongoing processes" (Freedman, 1992).

To us, psychopathology is the manifestation of certain natural laws following disorganization of a highly integrated functional whole. This, of course, is something entirely different from, for instance, a changed synaptic sensitivity to serotonine or even a whole complex of such partial disturbances that influence each other. It is self-evident that in psychiatric syndromes a multitude of such partial disturbences can be determined. Their proof depends solely on the availability of appropriate procedures and, therefore, on the general state of the technological-scientific development. However, its mere feasibility is far from being an indication for a progress in psychiatric knowledge! Today's still dominant one-sided micro-determinististic "bottom-up" strategy needs as a complementary "top-down" strategy to become heuristically fecund. Such a "top-down" strategy must be grounded in an organismic biological theory in its real and deeper sense. This kind of theory is the condition sine qua non for a meaningful relating of psychopathological and somatic data.

Paradoxically, the "biological" psychiatry still believes that it is able to do without such a theory. In this situation, a reference to the French psychiatrist Ey, thus far unacknowledged by "biological psychiatry", seems as much illuminating as contemporary. Ey's doctrine, which he also called *psychiatrie organo-dynamic* (Ey, 1952) and to which we ourselves owe fundamental inspiration, is rooted in the truly biological way of thinking of the great John Hughlings Jackson (see Taylor, 1958). According to Ey (1952), the usual classification of mental diseases obscured individual physiognomies instead of accentuating them. According to him, the distinction of "organic" vs. "endogenous" cannot be justified. Ey criticized that psychiatry has become stuck in pure note-taking about diseases, with a more detailed analysis of symptoms as the only progress that can be expected. If one wanted to arrange mental illnesses in a natural order, one would have to consider them for what they are, i.e., pathological phenomena corresponding to a certain "dissolution level" (*niveau de dissolution*) or a certain level of "insufficient evolution" (*évolution insuffisante* or *arrêt de développement*). The disorganization mechanism is always one and the same, independent of the etiology that can be toxic or infectuous as well as exogenous or endogenous in nature. Mental diseases differ in the depth, duration, and the rhythm of this disorganization process. Accordingly, one arrives at groupings that do not conform to any of the conventional diagnoses. The clinical differentiation between organic and endogenous mental diseases is unfounded, according to Ey. As psychiatric history teaches, Ey was not the first to question the distinction of organic vs. endogenous. Hoche (1912) already called Kraepelin's endeavours towards disease categories fruitless. Around the same time as Ey, Conrad (1959) stated that nosologic classifications in psychiatry are only pictures viewed with expert's eyes. Entirely in the spirit of Ey, Griesinger (1867) has long before viewed the different clinical forms of mental disease as stages of one specific process. He based this opinion on observations of a regular progression from melancholia, mania, madness, and confusion to idiocy. In this context, the phenomenological regularity in the development of a schizophrenic bout, described by Conrad in great detail, must also be mentioned. Numerous other authors provided convincing empirical proof that the separation of endogenous and exogenous cannot be justified (e.g., Albert, 1950; Barahona-Fernandez, 1956; Büssow, 1939, 1944; Llopis, 1960; Schneider, 1929; Zeh, 1962).

From Jackson's central idea that *"illness does not create,"* Ey concluded that somatic correlates could not be "disease-specific." They could only be modifications of normal-physiologic functions. The focal point of interest for Ey was the transition from wakefulness to sleep, making it possible to observe all dissolution levels in psychiatry in more or less fleeting states, like in statu nascendi. Ey (1967) postulated furthermore a common time structure of *"destruction of the field of consciousness"* on the one hand and the subvigilant intermediary stages that can be delimited in the EEG on the other. We consider this postulate the methodological premise for a psychiatric electroencephalography, which satisfies scientific standards. However, apart from a few exceptions, the path pointed out by Ey has been ignored. The reservations of clinical psychiatry mentioned earlier with respect to the EEG certainly are at least partially responsible for this. However, also in this case, exceptions confirm the rule. In Bente's understanding of psychiatry, which was greatly influenced by Ey's neo-Jacksonianism, the EEG was far more than an auxiliary diagnostic tool. He considered it heuristically fecund as a vehicle for his psychiatric thinking and as an instrument indispensible for scientifically conducted psychiatry, as he once expressed it. The conceptual closeness to Ey is particularly evident in a study about sleep deprivation (Bente, 1969b). This study conducted with healthy volunteers wanalyzed the regularities of the psychophysiological dissolution of functions in the course of time, as it can be observed during a period of complete sleep deprivation of about 100 hours.

Based on the results, Bente concluded, that sleep deprivation is an excellent *physiogenic model* for the study of psychopathological dissolution levels, confirming Ey's theory. The order of dissolution corresponded basically to the one found in an earlier study on central anticholinergica (Bente et al., 1964a). Heinemann (1966) who, like BENTE, viewed long-term sleep deprivation as a *"fitting method for causing psychiatric disturbances in an experimentally controlled way"*, reported similar results with regard to the dissolution order. His subjects showed a sequence of symptoms that ranged from apathetic irritation, lack of initiative, subdued affections, uncooperative irritability and euphoria typified by unfocused ideas accompanied annoyance, sinister mood, paranoid ideas, states of depersonalization to disturbed bodily sensations.

Concerning EEG-correlates of sleep deprivation, Bente's study revealed an initial dynamic labilization in the form of a discontinuous breakdown of the background activity with an increase in frequency and duration of low-voltage subvigil activity states, corresponding to a stage B1. With increasing duration of sleep deprivation, more and more sequences of high-voltage slow waves were observed, corresponding to a subvigil stages B2- B3. Different from the resting EEG of a well-rested subject, where such sequences appear only with increasing recording time preceded by a disintegration of the alpha-rhythm, they were observed here already at the beginning of the EEG. Such findings seem to verify the validity of Ey's conception explicitly. Therefore, further systematic studies of a theory-based correlation of psychopathological dissolution levels and the EEG would have been equally justified and desirable. We are thinking here in particular about longitudinal examinations in psychiatric patients. That such studies directed at the dynamics of the underlying process - except for a few singular attempts (e.g., Helmchen, 1968) - are still missing is certainly a shortcoming.

A primary reason for the lack of effec of Ey's ideas might be that the psychiatrist feels more comfortable with disease classifications that are oriented toward the medical model than with an approach that is rather far removed from the pragmatic way of thinking of the physician. Furthermore, Ey published nearly exclusively in French, and getting a complete grasp of the contents sometimes requires a particularly great effort. Ey would have probably met with greater resonance if he would have countered the *"mere medical note-taking"* with a systematic representation of dissolution levels criticized by him. Fig. 42 is such a systematic presentation. It is based on observations of typical reversible exogenous psychoses. In contrast to the modular models that have regained popularity especially over the past few years (Fodor, 1984), this is a dynamic-integrative model. This means that we can, for instance, talk about a decrease in drive only as long as the dissolution process is limited to superficial functional levels. Once deeper functional levels are affected, the decrease in drive will no longer be recognizable as such, although one can imagine it to be part of a deliriant symptom. Despite its hierarchical order, it would be a mistake to view this sequence as strictly successive.

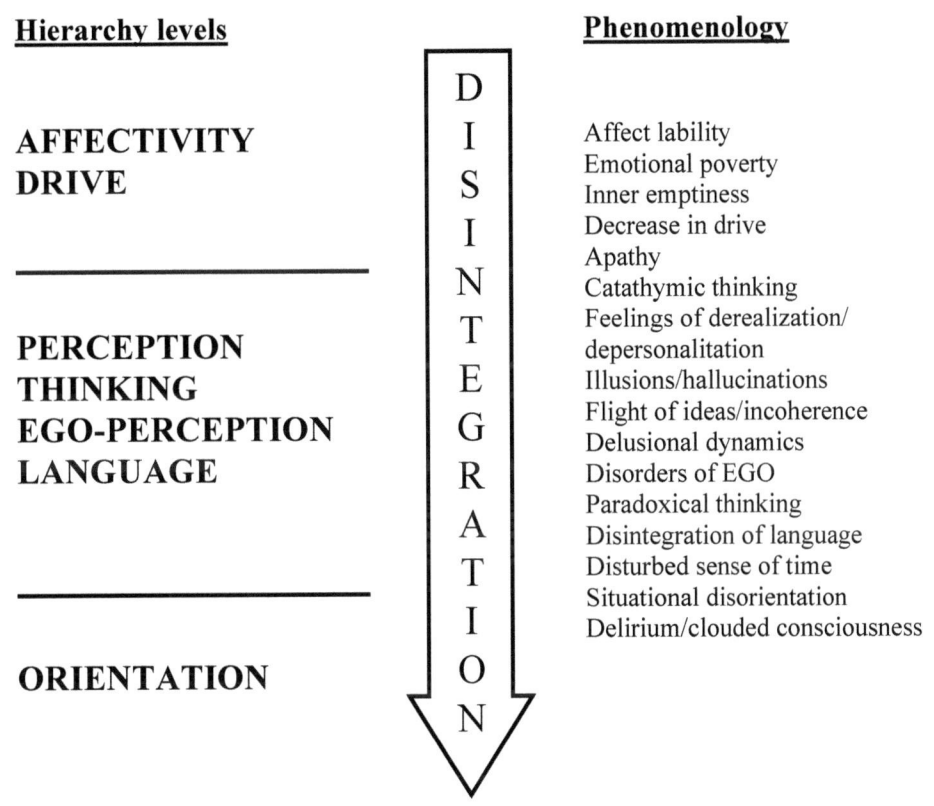

Figure 42. Psychopathology as disintegration of the mind

Since psychopathological syndromes are complex dynamic structures, we must assume that symptoms associated with different dissolution levels can also appear simultaneously. Nevertheless, because of the proportionally different distinctiveness of the symptoms, a characterization and consequently an assignment to a specific dissolution level is usually possible. However, this does not say anything about the possibility of distinguishing between endogenous and exogenous. With respect to this, Bonhoeffer's frequently confirmed dictum "that a clear and complete symptomatologic distinction of the exogenous symptom pictures from the psychological one, otherwise known as endogenous, is not fully feasible" (transl. from German) is still valid.

The quintessential conclusion of the above, which determines our research strategy, is that it is not very promising to use clinical diagnoses to look for EEG correlates, a procedure propagated for instance by Small (1987) in close relationship with DSM III. The argument that different studies conducted on the same topic are comparable only if unified psychopathological classification conventions are observed is not compelling to us. A comparability of clinical pictures by no means indicates the comparability of the associated pathophysiological processes. The argument of comparability, however, presumes a one-on-one classification of clinical picture and process. Since this condition has been proved to be wrong, the research strategy based upon it cannot be correct either. In total agreement with the denosologization of biological psychiatry that Van Praag (1988) demanded, we must consider the full range of variations of psychiatric disturbances and conscientiously keep the diagnostic criteria or categories for inclusion open and flexible. In the following step, an attempt must be made to arrive at pathobiological groupings, possibly through the EEG. Through those patients who at a certain point in time show a specific clinical-electroencephalographic constellation of characteristics, one must attempt to arrive at statements of general importance. These will also offer a more rational approach to therapy, since rigid medication patterns cannot do justice to the dynamic variability of the underlying pathophysiological process (Ulrich & Gaebel, 1987). The fact that research that would comply with the methodological requirements established here is so rare may have its basis in the popular practice of publishing the research findings only if they conform to the presently popular classification conventions (see above).

The correlation of clinical dynamic course with electroencephalographic features is complicated by the fact that as a matter of principle, all state-related varying EEG-features (*state*-indicators) also can be state-invariant, i. e., constitution-related (*trait*-indicators). State-invariant features, which are different from the physiomorphological picture in adults, can be viewed as indicators of a brain-functional maturation deficit if they correspond to a certain infantile or juvenile stage of development. We also have to remember constantly that the distinction between state and trait characteristics is only a model-schematic one. , even *trait* characteristics vary more or less clearly within certain limits as well as from case to case, depending on the actual functional state. Thus certain "trait"characteristics, which are kept in latency by means of compensatory mechanisms, only become apparent after passing a certain threshold of functional deterioration. Finally, we have to consider the possibility that certain trait-characteristics that indicate a maturational deficit disappear belatedly.

In summary, we can state that the development of the psychiatric EEG involves much more than the specific adjustment of a long-known tool to clinical-psychatric necessities. To the extend that psychiatry must be adjusted to the EEG, we are confronted at the same time with a genuine psychiatric undertaking. The fact that it has not been possible to introduce the possibility of a psychiatric EEG into general awareness probably accounts for the fact that clinical psychiatry still considers the EEG as an insignificant auxiliary tool borrowed from neurology for the exclusion of neurological disturbances rather than as the essential psychiatric tool for research for which it was originally introduced in psychiatry.

CHAPTER 4

Qualitative Features of the Psychophysiological EEG : General Principles of Pathological Dissolution of the Organization of Brain Electrical Activity **(Pathologischer Funktionswandel)**

The diagnostic importance of the EEG in organic and especially involutional psychosyndromes is considered rather modest today. A commonly accepted rule of thumb is that more "peculiarities" increase the progressiveness of the underlying process and without progressiveness or chronic state, the EEG would be more or less "normal" (Greenblatt, 1945; Busse & Wang, 1965). Thus, patients with severe mental dissolution can have "normal" EEGs and while undisturbed-looking patients could have "abnormal" EEGs (Bagchi et al., 1956).

Such an assessment may be correct if it is based on neurological criteria about normalcy. However, as we will point out in more detail, good reasons exist for the assumption that the EEG is in reality a very delicate indicator of the pathological functional change that can only be uncovered through refined analysis. Another fact to consider is that with regard to the various EEG-correlates of the brain-organic dissolution and their functional significance, many more open than unequivocally answered questions still remain. Literature proves that although all relevant features have been observed, they have been described and interpreted in very different ways. These features have usually been evaluated as isolated phenomena independent from their morphodynamic context. Isolating operationally defined features certainly meets optimally the legitimate need for statistical processing. On the other hand, following such a largely theory-free approach, we must anticipate the possibility of ambiguous electro-clinical correlations and therefore the risk of drawing the wrong conclusions.

4.1 From the Physiomorphic (PM) to the Diffuse Dysrhythmic EEG (DD)

Considering the example of the EEG in cases of incipient dementia, Bente (1981) distinguished two paths of dissolution (fig. 43, I and II).

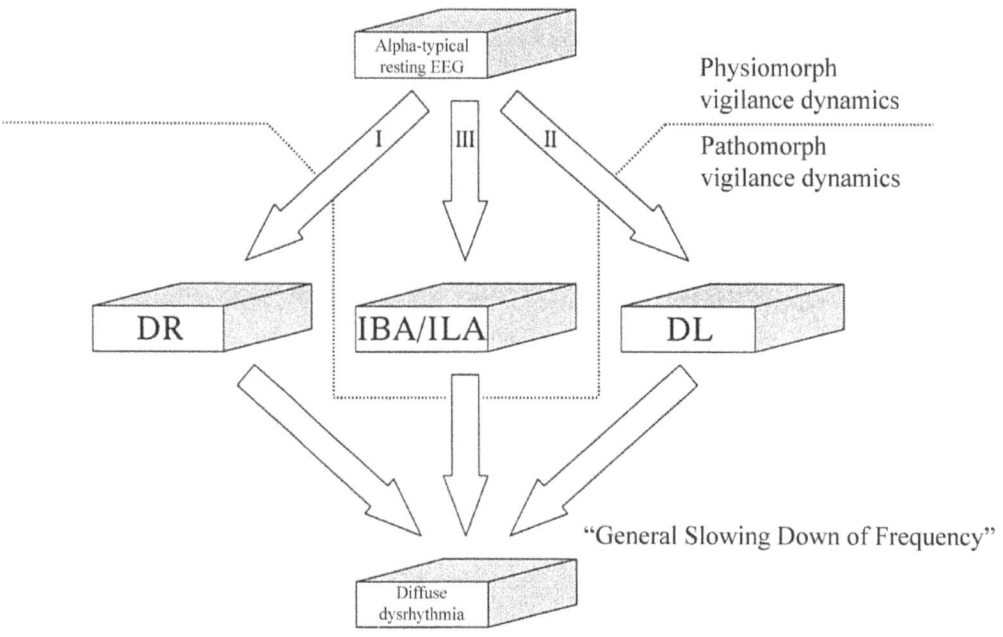

Figure 43. The pathological gestalt change of the EEG

In the first path - named **dissolution via stage A** - the picture of a mid-stage A dominates the resting EEG (stage A1 to A2) (Fig. 43, left arrow I). The second path - the **dissolution via stage B** - is dominated by the picture of a stage B1 (Fig. 43, right arrow II). The patterns themselves have physiomorphic appearance but lack the physiomorphic transition dynamics. They dominate the picture almost stationarily. In both cases, we are dealing with the manifestation of **disturbed vigilance dynamics**.

Bente considered these two modi of functional dissolution (Figs. 44 b and c; 46, 47 being the *morphogenetische Matrix* (morphogenetic matrix) from which, with the progression of the underlying pathological process, the transition to a pathomorph organization develops. This pathomorphic organization results from the disproportion of the diverse *formative tendencies* involved in the evolution of the physiomorphic pattern. Because of the unphysiological persistence of the anteriorly extended background activity that continues past the 5th recording minute, the **dissolution via stage A** is denoted as **Dynamic Rigidity (DR)** (Figs. 44 b, 46). During dissolution, the *formative tendency of the slowing of the frequency* increasingly gains importance. Via a stage of more or less rhythmic theta-activity, the picture of a **Diffuse Dysrhythmia (DD)** is eventually reached (Figs. 52, 68).

During the **dissolution via stage B**, on the other hand, an increase in the discontinuity of the background activity with an increase in frequency and duration of low-voltage activity segments occurs, corresponding to a stage B1. In this case, we talk about Dynamic Lability (**DL**, Figs. 44 c, 47). With continuing dissolution, the *formative tendency of desynchronization* gains importance.

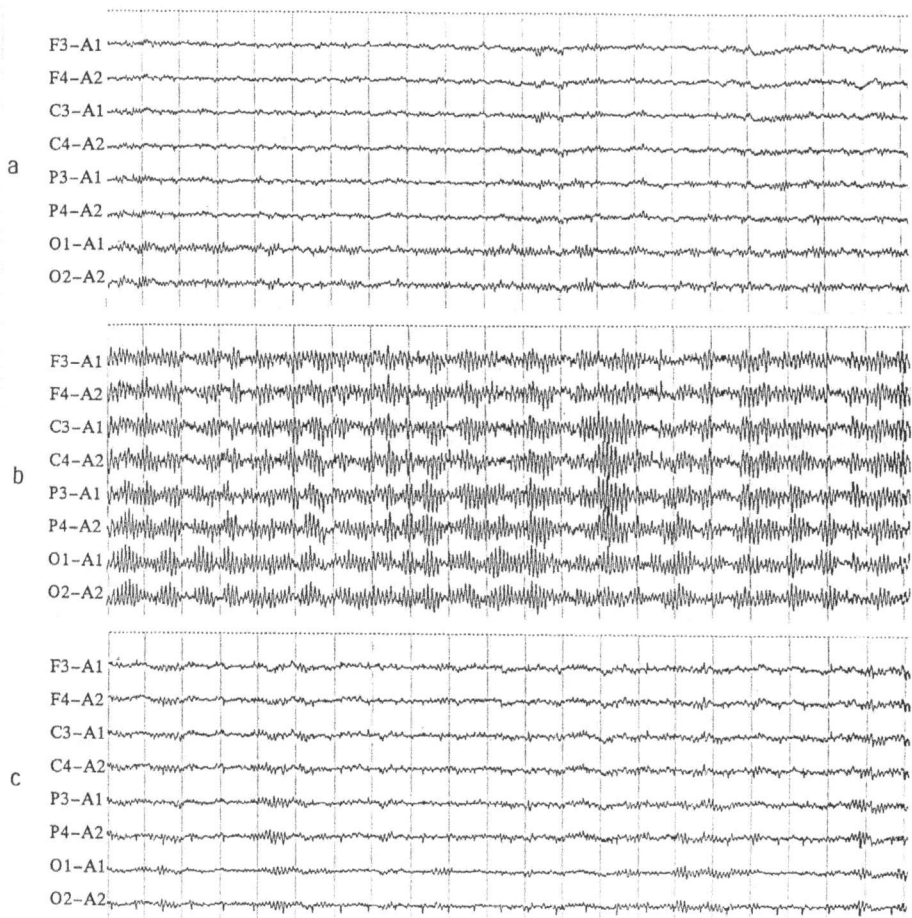

Figure 44. Representative recording examples taken from the first minute (reference to the ipsilateral ear).
a) Physiomorphic dynamics (**PM**): Mostly continuous 9/s alpha-activity with posterior maximum, largely corresponding to a stage A1.
b) Dynamic rigidity (**DR**): Continuously anteriorized, relatively monomorphic and slightly slower 8.5/s activity corresponding to a stage A2. This picture does not show any change during the 15 minute recording at rest.
c) Dynamic lability (**DL**): Discontinuous 9.5/s alpha-activity of varying degrees of anteriorization. Abrupt transitions to more or less lasting low-voltage desynchronized phases corresponding to a stage B1. This picture does not show any significant change during recording either.

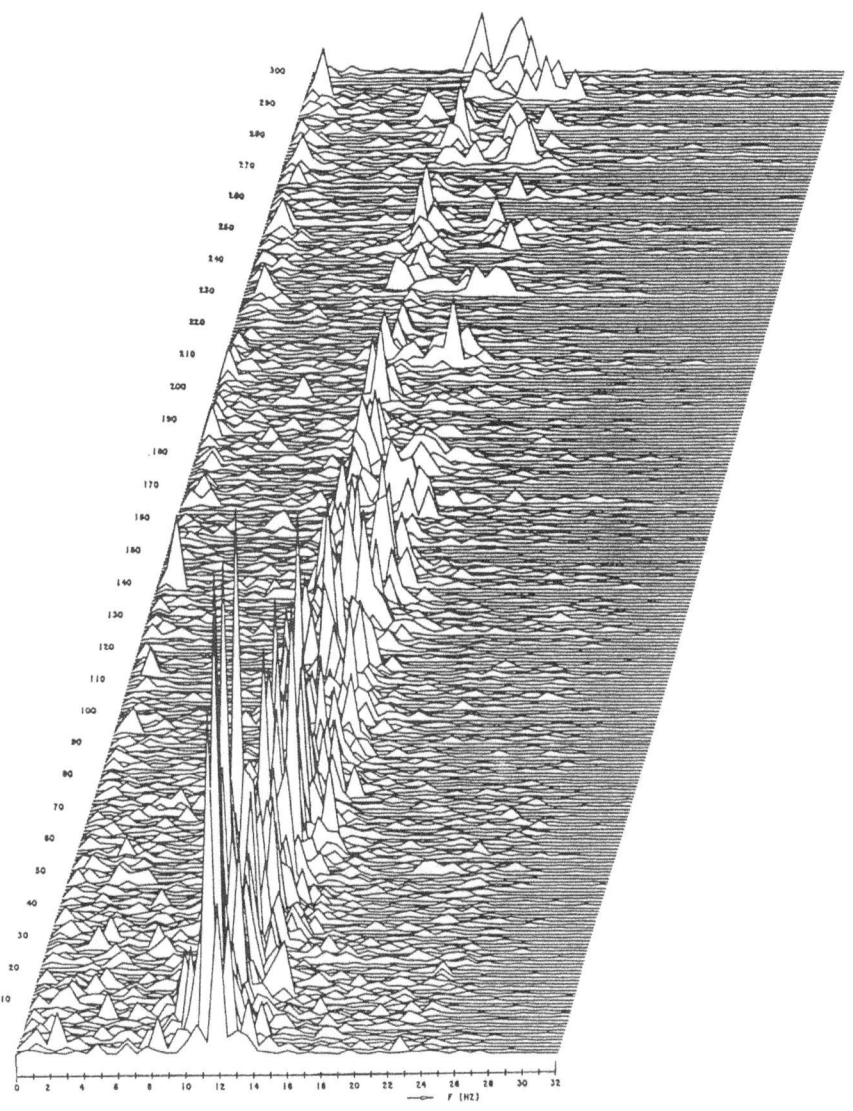

Figure 45. Chronospectrogram of physiomorphic vigilance dynamics (**PM**, see Fig. 44 a). In staggered formation, 300 power spectra (derivation O2-A2, FFT-analyzed, frequency range 0-32 Hz) are shown for consecutive 2-s epochs of a 10-minute resting record. The spectral alpha-component of 11.5 Hz is most pronounced at the beginning of the recording (stage A1) and remains at a high level until approximately epoch 150 (i.e., until the 5th minute). After that, we see a progressive Alpha dissolution corresponding to an increase of subvigil B-stages.

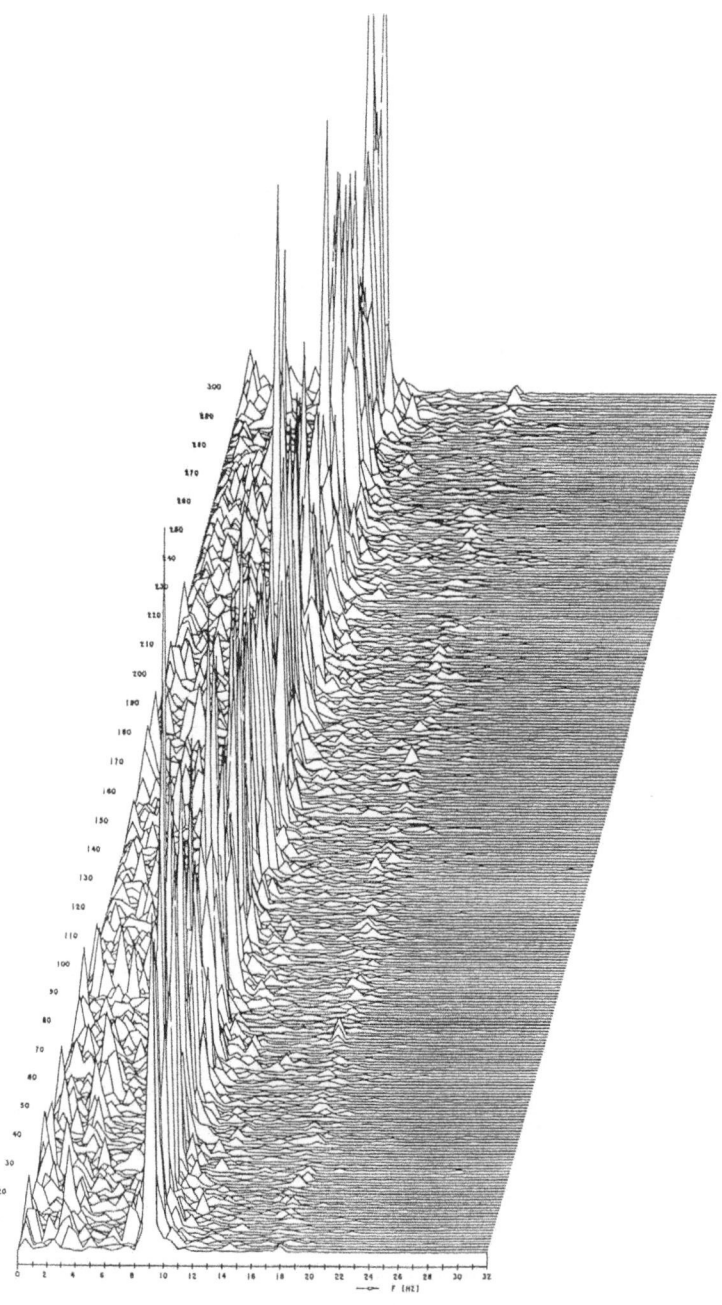

Figure 46. Chronospectrogram of a Dynamic Rigidity (**DR,** see Fig. 44b). The very distinct alpha-activity of stable frequency (derivation 02-A2) remains unchanged during the 300 epochs of the 10-minutes resting record. No increase of subvigil B-stages along with recording time is expected physiologically.

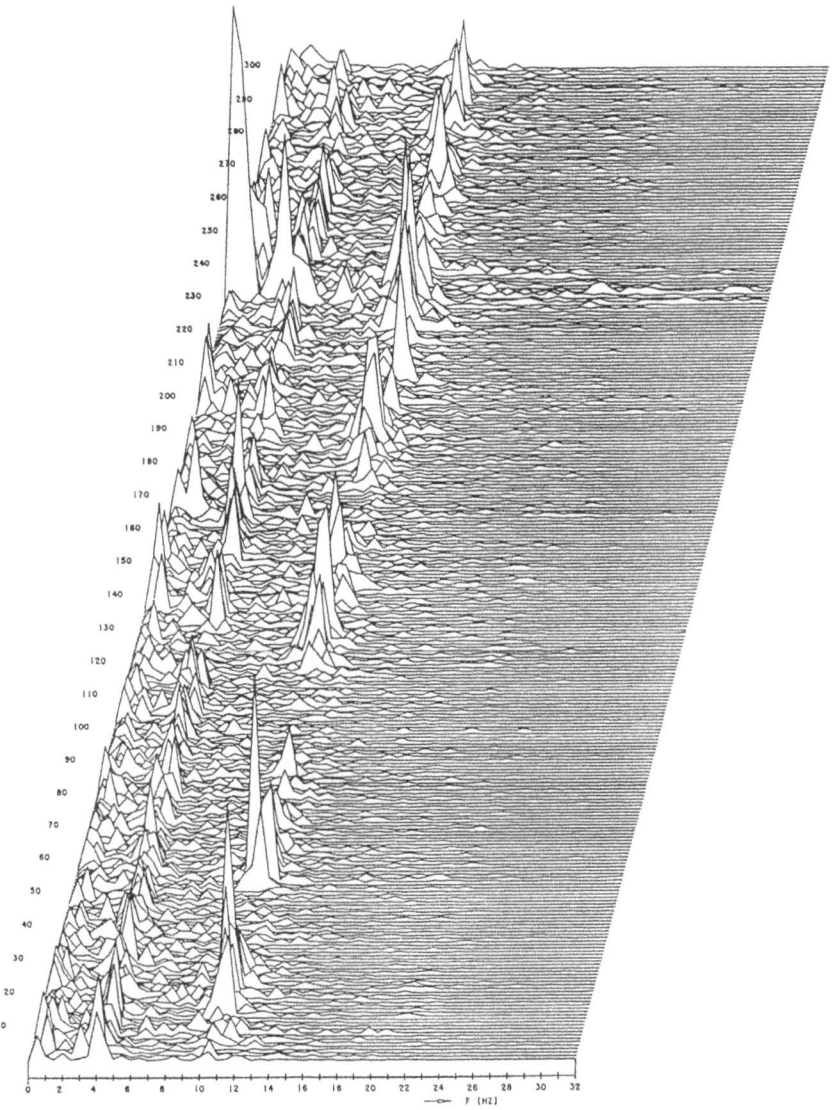

Figure 47. Chronospectrogram of a Dynamic Lability (**DL**, see Fig. 44c). A discontinuity of the 10-12/s background alpha-activity (derivation O2-A2) prevails from the beginning of the recording until the end without any trend towards change.

Thus, the picture of a *polyrhythmic frequency dissolution* results comprises, in most cases, a beta-component. Through the progressively increased proportion of slow activity, the picture of a Diffuse Dysrhythmia (**DD**) is eventually reached. **DD**, which is conventionally viewed as the typical correlate of organic brain syndromes, also represents the common final stretch of those two dissolution paths (**DR** and **DL**) that start with the disturbance of the vigilance dynamics.

However, we believe that in addition to the two paths stressed by Bente, another one with initially largely untouched vigilance dynamics exists. This third dissolution path (Fig. 43, arrow III) manifests itself in the intermittent occurrence of pronounced sub-alpha-, theta-, as well as delta-groups under mostly physiomorphic vigilance dynamics. Attempts to find the most fitting terminology for this pattern, which occurs in many variations, have led to the already discussed terminological confusion (3.3.4). We treat these patterns (IBA/ILA) as pathomorphic variations of an A-stage.

The long accepted belief, dating back to older authors such as Duensing (1949) and Faure et al. (1951), which views IBA and ILA as an expression of processes close to the diencephalon, the upper brain stem, and the fossa posterior is regarded as obsolete today. These patterns, subsummarized by us as **IBA** (**I**ntermittent **B**ilateral **A**nterior) or as **ILA** (**I**ntermittend **L**eft **A**nterior), are the result of an increase in the voltage, deceleration, synchronization, and anteriorization (mostly temporalization!) that are characteristic of the mid- and late A-stages. At the same time, a tendency for a discontinuous pattern dissolution corresponding to stage A3 can be observed. Bente (1964b) considered the „focal" left anterior sub-alpha groups encountered especially in older patients to be a pathomorphic variation of the late A-stage (stage A4). Based on our observations and even more on certain experimental findings (see below), we deem it justifiable to also consider all those phenomena as pathomorph variations of a late A-stage that have a similar morphological basic pattern but a different frequency.

Kornmüller (1941) was able to show inhalation of a nitrogen-oxygen mixture equal to that at an altitude of 7500 meters, a characteristic sequence of stages, in the EEG of healthy volunteers under experimentally induced hypoxia. After only a few minutes, a more distict increase in alpha-amplitude and alpha-continuity was observed in anterior-temporal ratger than posterior. This was followed by a stage characterized by groups and sequences of rhythmic anterior sub-alpha and later theta-waves with higher amplitudes. Signs of altitude sickness, that is, of an impairment of consciousness affecting the adaptive behavior eventually occurred in connection with initially still rhythmic 3-4/s-waves that grew increasingly irregular with augmented topographical generalization so that in the final stage, the picture of a diffuse dysrhythmia resulted. With the reintroduction of fresh air, the EEG changes disappeared in reverse sequence and often very rapidly. As a result of an extended hypoxia, often an additional stage of low-voltage desynchronized activity preceding the reappearance of the posterior alpha-activity could be observed. Kornmüller's findings were later largely confirmed by Goetze (1950) as well as by Jung (1953). We consider this an excellent experimental model of a *pathologischer Funktionswandel* (pathological functional change). Fast motion-like EEG demonstrates the sequence of all phases that we associate with psychiatric disorders (see below).

The observations that classifiable conspicuities are often the only EEG modification in diffuse encephalopathies under **IBA** support the view that this indeed constitutes a dissolution path of its own (Schaul et al., 1981 a; b). Because of a frequently observed simultaneous incidence of intermittent bilateral anterior (**IBA**) and focal intermittent left anterior groups (**ILA**) in the same EEG, especially in patients with involutional syndromes or under long-term lithium prophylaxis, we wondered about a possible intrinsic relationship. Our observations and interpretations coincide with those of Rice et al. (1990):

"Patients with mild-to-moderate dementia primarily exhibited a focal abnormal left temporal slow activity pattern , whereas patients with severe dementia exhibited a more diffuse slow activity pattern ..." and further, *"These data suggest that focal, left anterior temporal EEG slow activity might be a sensitive indicator of the milder stages of SDAT".*

During earlier systematic examinations, we came across certain regularities (Ulrich et al., 1983). EEGs with **ILA** usually show an asymmetrical voltage generation with a left-sided amplitude accentuation of the posterior alpha-activity at the beginning of the recording. The anterior spreading of the background activity, corresponding to the stages A1 and A2, also shows a left side accentuation (Figs. 12, 34). The formative tendency of frequency deceleration associated with the A-stage that is already physiologically more pronounced in the anterior than posterior regions, as well as the formative tendencies for voltage increase, lend the left anterior alpha-groups a semblance of circumscribed left anterior foci of lesional origin. These "foci," just as their bilateral variation (**IBA**), can have a rather diverse morphology, depending on how the formative tendencies involved in their genesis are proportioned. The spectrum reaches from groups of focal left anterior rhythmic alpha- and sub-alpha-waves, high-amplitude rhythmic 6-7/s-waves, and irregular

4-6/s-theta-waves to irregular delta-waves. If one disregards the morphogenetic context, then a misinterpretation indicating circumscribed brain damage is suggested.

Numerous studies have emphasized an increased occurrence of intermittent left anterior and also, to a large degree, temporo-anterior and frontally localized groups of slow waves of varying frequencies observed in samples of elderly patients (Arenas et al., 1986; Barnes et al., 1956; Busse, 1973; Busse et al., 1954; Busse & Obrist,1963; Gschwend & Karbowski, 1970; Harvald, 1958; Hughes, 1960; Helmchen et al., 1967; Koufen & Gast, 1981; Mundy-Castle, 1962; Obrist, 1975; 1976; Obrist & Henry, 1958; Rice et al., 1990; Silverman et al., 1955). In general, it was unclear why the focal changes occurred almost exclusively on the left side:

"... *around 70 years, the absence of any unilateral right-sided discharges and the emphasis on the left side is curious ...*" (Hughes, 1960).

Despite intensive research efforts, a structural correlate could not be found. The opinion that is still dominant nowadays is expressed in a quote by Obrist (1976):
"Little is known about the exact origin of focal temporal abnormalities in elderly people."

It is practically proved that **ILA** has no relationship with left- or right-handedness nor to hemispheric dominances, that neither aphasia nor left-hemispheral diminished blood flow exists, or that fatigue as well as hyperventilation facilitate the manifestation of the phenomenon, which disappears with the transition to light sleep, i.e., stage C. Several authors thought it peculiar that the positive correlation between age and frequency of occurrence is limited to 40 to 60 years olds. Beyond the age of 70, there was no longer any evidence of a frequency increase (Busse, 1973; Obrist & Busse, 1965; Silverman et al., 1955). An explanation for this, as well as for the seemingly paradoxical finding, is still missing, although an independent research confirmed that **ILA** is found less frequently in samples of gerontopsychiatric patients with obvious mental impairments than in control groups of healthy or inconspicuous elderly people (Silverman et al., 1955; Torres et al., 1983). According to Obrist (1976), to whom we owe the majority of the findings concerning the **ILA**-phenomenon, no connection exists between the morphological distinctiveness of **ILA** and the degree of a possible mental performance deficit. In his view, such deficits exist only if **ILA** appears in the context of a diffusely increased irregular slow activity, *"when it involves adjacent areas or becomes part of a diffuse disturbance, chronic brain syndrome is more probable."*

This observation conforms to the dissolution order conceived by us in which **ILA** proceeds into a diffuse dysrhythmia (**DD**) via bilateralization (**IBA**). This dissolution order also explains why the positive correlation between **ILA**-incidence and age is no longer existent beyond the age of 70 years. If the severity of involutional syndromes is determined by age, from the statistical point of view, we would have to expect, after a certain age, an increase of bilateralizations (**IBA**) as well as generalizations (**DD**) of the **ILA**-phenomenon limited previously to the left brain. Throught the expansion of "focus" - in our opinion unwarranted - an increase in bilateral foci is also mentioned: "*the incidence of bitemporal foci increases with age*"(Hughes & Olson, 1981). The unilateral and therefore in the proper sense focal **ILA** phenomenon becomes increasingly infrequent in very old people on account of bilateralization and generalization.

We also must take into account that a temporal focus of a certain extension can remain undiscovered for technical reasons during recording. For bipolar array montages with relatively narrow distances between the electrodes, this can be understood easily. The same problem, however, can also occur with ear-reference recording, where the potential under the reference electrode is probably very similar to that of the temporal region. This can be deduced from the usually small amplitude of the leads T3-A1 or T4-A2 (s. a., Zschoke et al., 1990).

The typical **ILA**-phenomenon that gains its morphological distinctiveness against the background of an otherwise more or less physiomorph EEG marks a relatively early dissolution stage in the process we sketched (Fig. 43). This explains why studies (e.g., Breslau et al., 1989; Drachman & Hughes, 1971; Oken et al., 1992; Visser et al., 1987; Wang et al., 1970;) showed no evidence or only minor evidence of functional deficits in the subjects showing **ILA**. Possibly, performance deficits actually to be expected remain inapparent on account of a sufficient degree of compensation, an explanation that we also considered for the involutional beta-activity in connection with a **DL**.

The external validation through performance tests is usually viewed as a proof of the pathognostic relevance of a specific EEG-feature. This implies that these performance tests are more sensitive indicators of a pathological functional/performance change than are EEG-features. The opposite possibility, though equally plausible, is strangely never considered. In this case, one of course could not assume the clinical insignificance of the EEG-feature from the failure of the external, i. e., behavioral validation. We find it necessary to emphasize this, especially considering the above-mentioned contradictory opinions of the clinical significance of **ILA**.

If the ongoing dissolution process resulted in the bilateralization of ILA postulated by us and thus in the occurrence of bilaterally symmetrical, anterior-accentuated groups and sequences of high-amplitude rhythmic waves (**IBA**, Figs. 35, 36), we would usually also observe an obvious deterioration in performance. Thus, **IBA** has been long considered as almost pathognomonic for the advanced stages of Alzheimer's disease (e.g., Gordon & Sim, 1967; Krankenhagen & Köhler, 1973; Letemendia & Pampiglione, 1958). Authors who paid attention to lateral asymmetries referred exclusively to a left-sided focus. Krankenhagen and Köhler (1973) found seven times as many left foci as right foci in their Alzheimer-patients and claimed that a structural lesion could not be established for any of the patients with such "focal" signs. The popular practice that regards these "foci" after rejecting a structural lesion as "functional" in origin does not make much sense. Aside from the fact that such an interpretation does not provide any new insights, one must remember that the **functional diagram** EEG, as a matter of principle, represents only functional lesion. To avoid misunderstandings, we prefer to interpret these patterns in our clinical reports as local **manifestations of a global functional disturbance.** It should be mentioned that although rare, the mirror-image right-sided eqivalent to the **ILA** can also be observed..

The predilection of particularly the left brain half to the alpha-anteriorization and the associated focal accentuation of slow waves is less of a mystery if we remember that the EEG, even from the physiological perspective, is in no way organized symmetrically and that this fact in all likelihood can be explained with the generally accepted neurodynamic inequality of both brain halves. We can, for instance, assume that the readiness for synchronization of the cortical neurons differs between the left and the right hemisphere. It has been known for some time that left-sided discharge foci are much more frequent than right-sided ones in genuine epilepsy (Takahashi et al., 1963). In 90% of the cases, Metrazol in epileptics with bilateral foci leads to a left-sided prevalence of the paroxysmal activity (Ajmone-Marsan & Ralston, 1957).

Our interpretation is supported by observations that **ILA**, with the advancement of the pathological process, shows a tendency for generalization, starting with a bilateralization (e.g., Rice et al., 1990). Thus **ILA** and **IBA** seem to be different degrees or stages of a uniform dissolution process. That the hypoxia experiments did not show any EEG-asymmetry might have its reason in the fact that during the experimental, fast motion –like *pathological change of function*, intermediary stages remain inapparent. **ILA** can be possibly associated with lesser dynamics or intensity of the underlying pathophysiological process compared to **IBA.** It is possible that compensatory mechanisms also play a role.

Our model of morphologically distinct dissolution paths signifies a fundamental departure from the usual procedure that utilizes a single characteristic, such as a dominant frequency or a sum score formed by several single features, as a quantitative indicator of a global functional disturbance. In this case, one assumes, without any evidence, the existence of a linear relationship between the degree of the functional dissolution and the change of the index variable. However, since the pathological gestalt modification of the EEG at best occurs linearly **within** the individual dissolution stages, attempts for an electroencephalographic validation of involutional decline of the mental performance level have to be viewed very skeptically. Indeed, very few scientifically supported findings exist in this area. An important question for which we do not yet have a definite answer is why different dissolution path are chosen in different cases. The preexisting conditions, just as psychotropic drugs, may have a significant effect on the kind of EEG-modifications that have to be expected. Another question yet to be tackled is whether the distinct dissolution paths can also be associated with different psychopathological pictures. Assuming that the respective dissolution path is determined by the premorbid organization of the EEG and that this premorbid organization corresponds to specific behavior dispositions, such different psychopathological pictures can certainly be expected.

THE THEORETICAL INTERPRETATION OF ELECTROENCEPHALOGRAPHY (EEG)

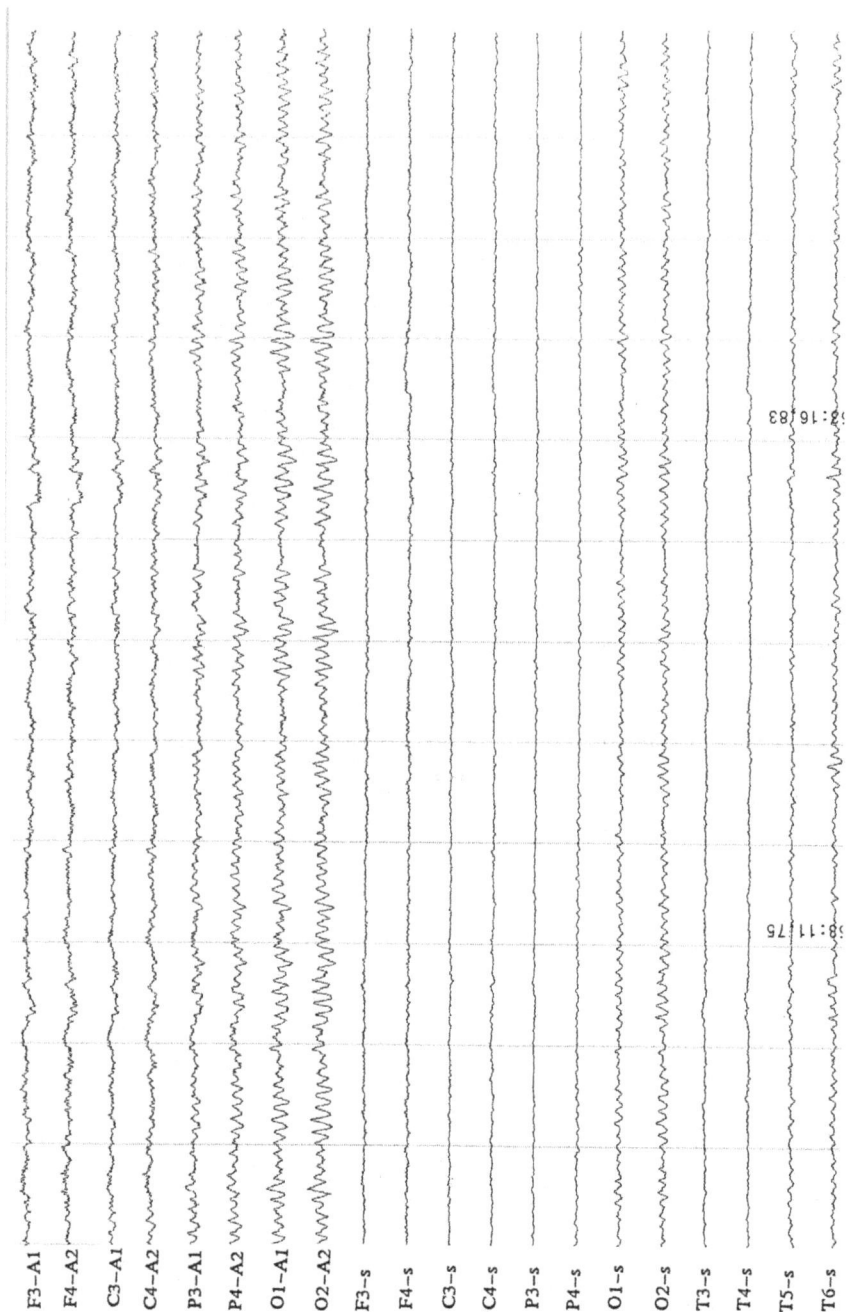

Figure 48. Ideal-type (Physiomorphic, **PM**) of organized EEG (5th minute) with a continuous, slightly spindle-form modulated and entirely posterior-accentuated 8.5/s alpha-activity (Figs. 48-62 identical derivation schema).

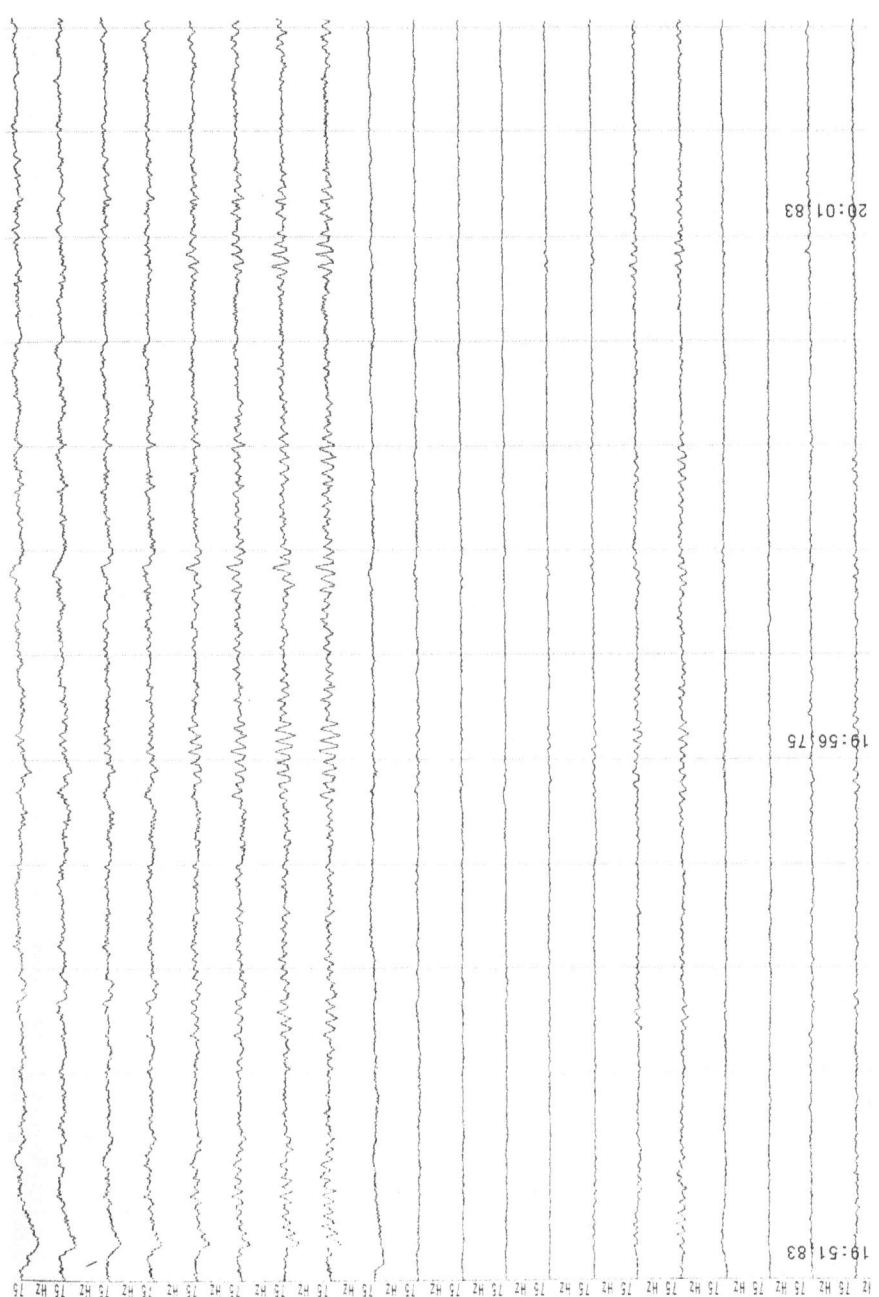

Figure 49. Ideal-type (Physiomorphic, **PM**) of organized EEG later on in the recording time (12th minute). Compared to the beginning of the recording, increased discontinuity of the still posterior-accentuated alpha-activity, due to frequent transitions into low-voltage desynchronized activity, corresponds to a stage B1.

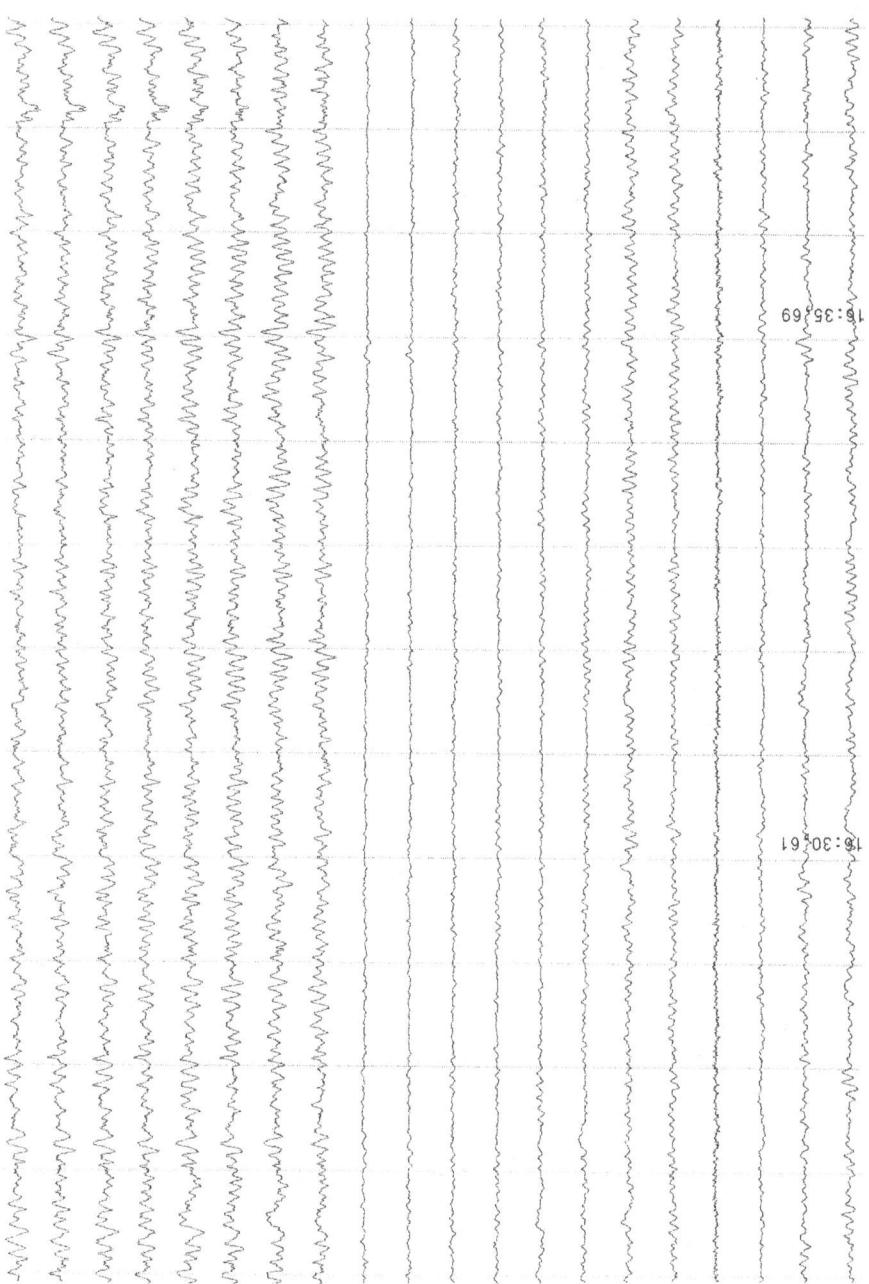

Figure 50. Slight Dynamic Rigidity (**DR**): Alpha-activity with frequency variations around 9.5/s with a medium-level intermittently occuring anteriorization corresponding to a stage A1-A2.

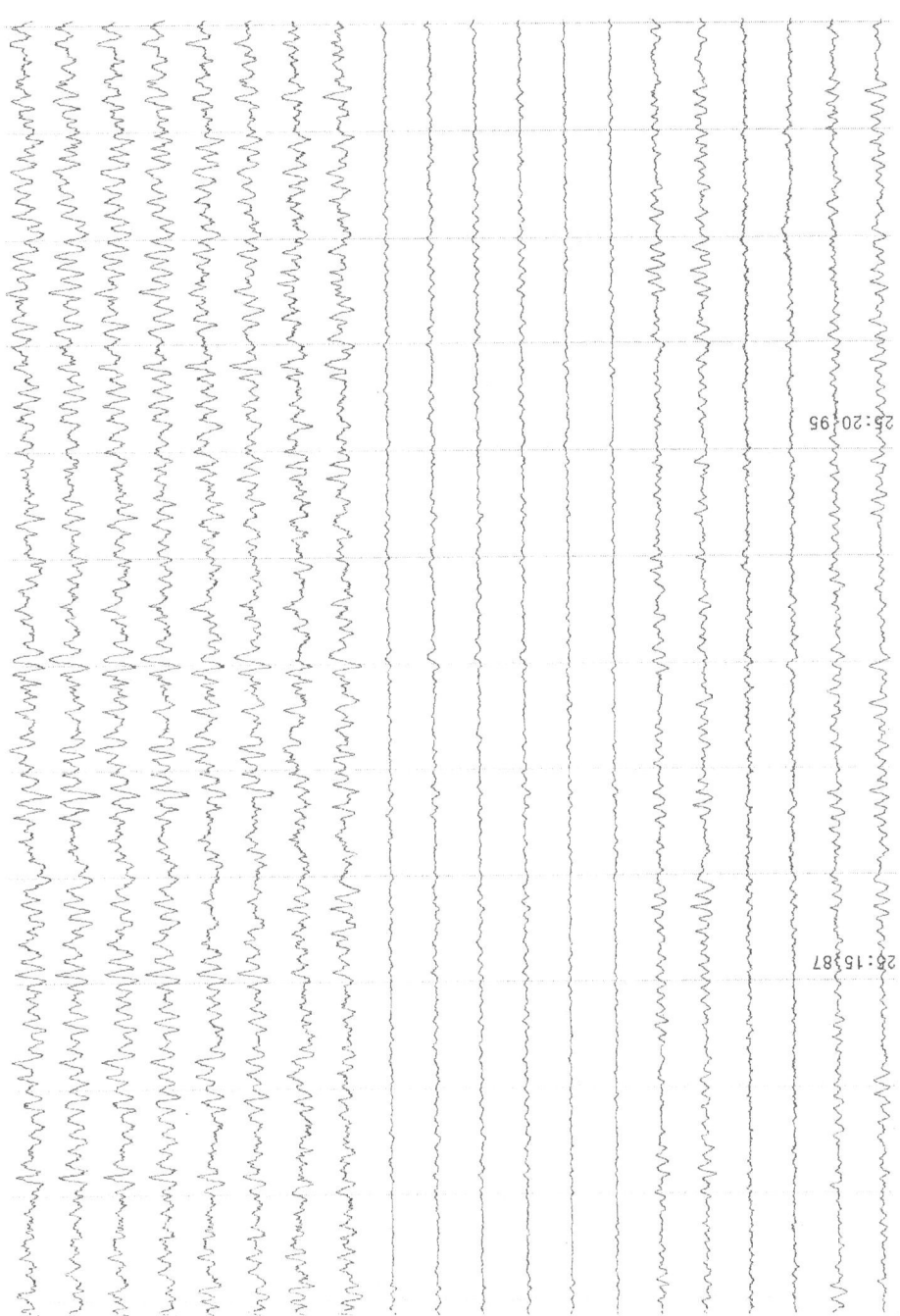

Figure 51. More pronounced Dynamic Rigidity (**DR**): Alpha-activity with frequency variations around 8/s with accentuation of the slower frequency components with anteriorization corresponding to a stage A3.

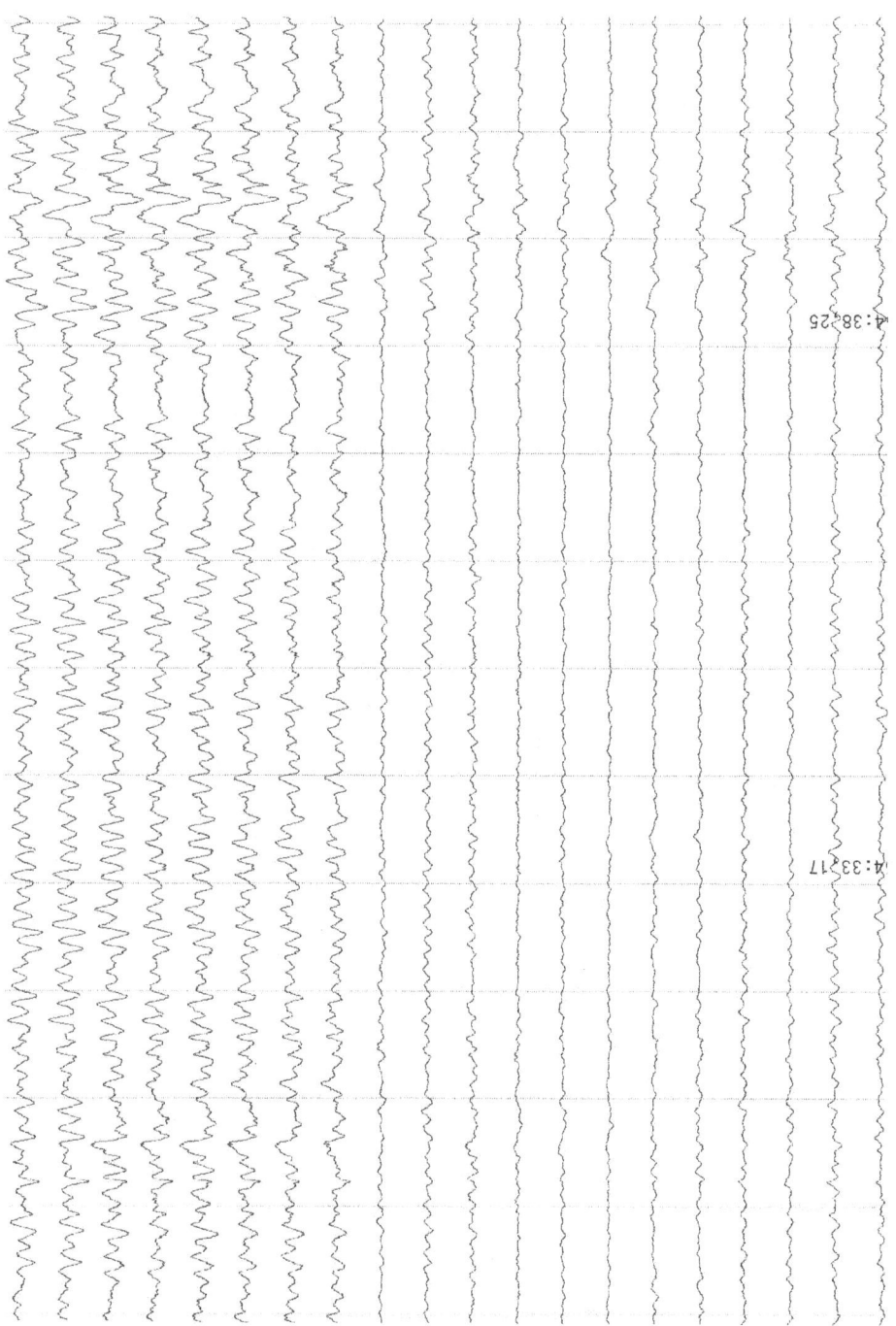

Figure 52. Dynamic Rigidity (**DR**) in transition to diffuse dysrhythmia (DD). Groups and sequences of a rhythmic 6.5/s-activity of anterior accentuation (corresponding to a stage A4) alternate with irregular theta-/delta-activity.

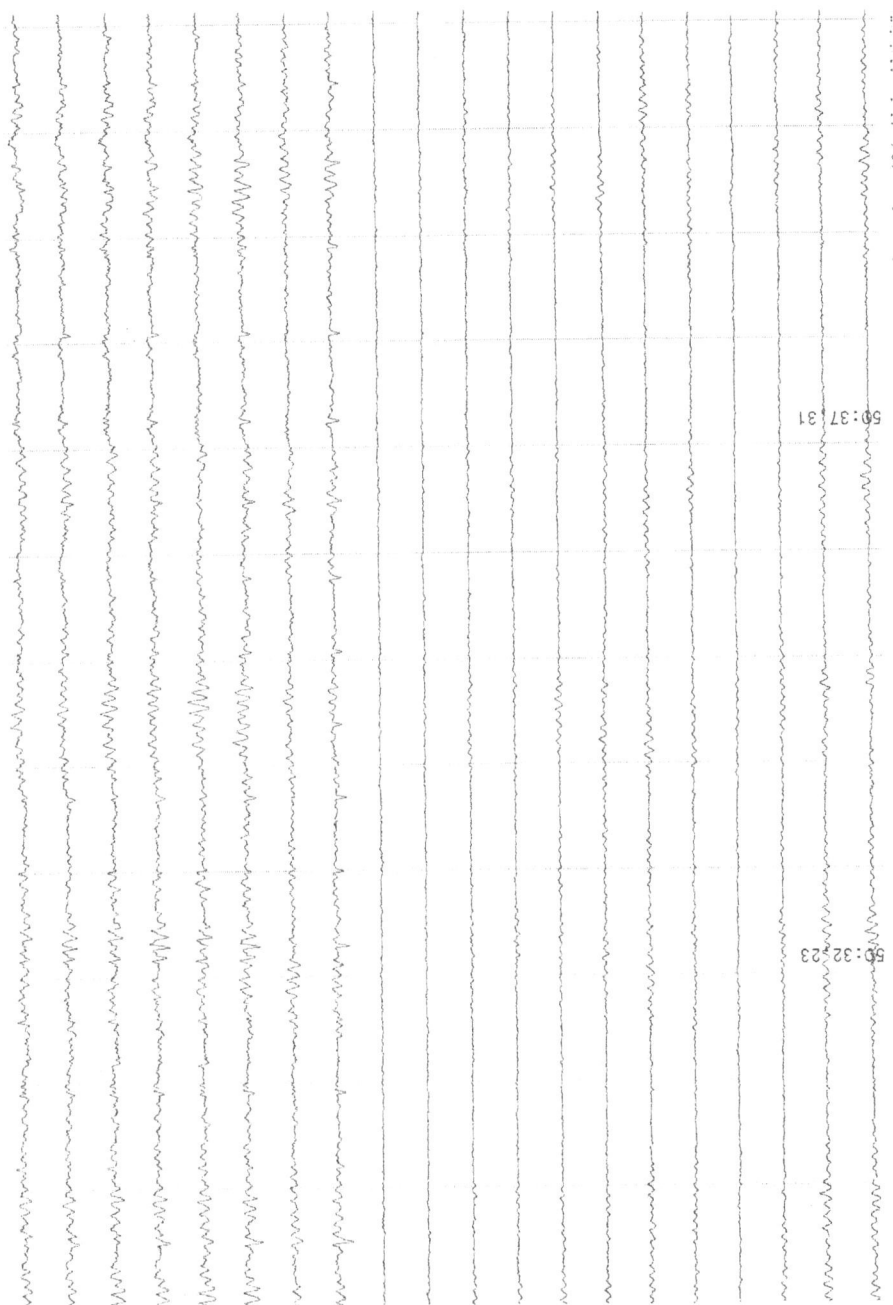

Figure 53. Medium-degree Dynamic Lability (**DL**). Already at the beginning of the recording (2nd minute), only discontinuous, 10/s alpha-activity differing in degree of anteriorization were delineated in groups and sequences dominated by low-voltage desynchronized B1-stages.

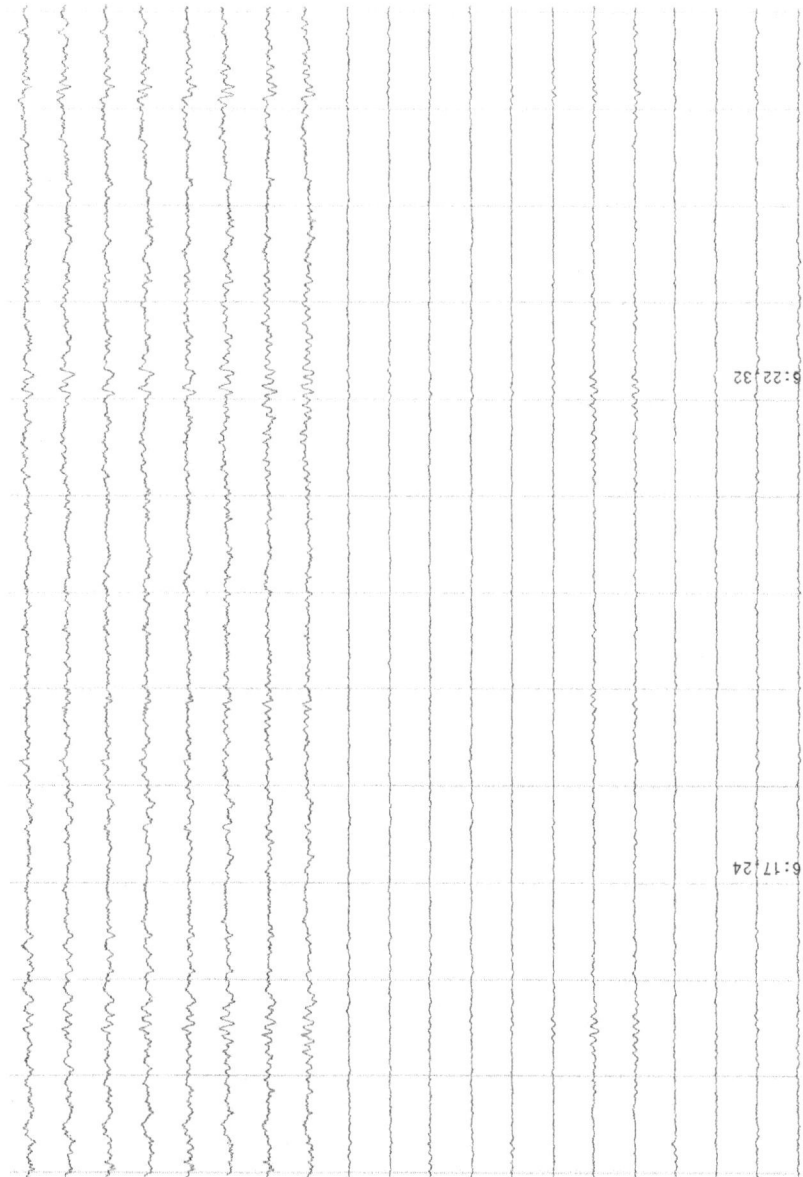

Figure 54. More pronounced Dynamic Lability (**DL**). Already at the beginning of the recording (2nd minute), lower-voltage desynchronized activity prevails, sometimes in connection with irregular theta activity, corresponding to stages B1-B2.

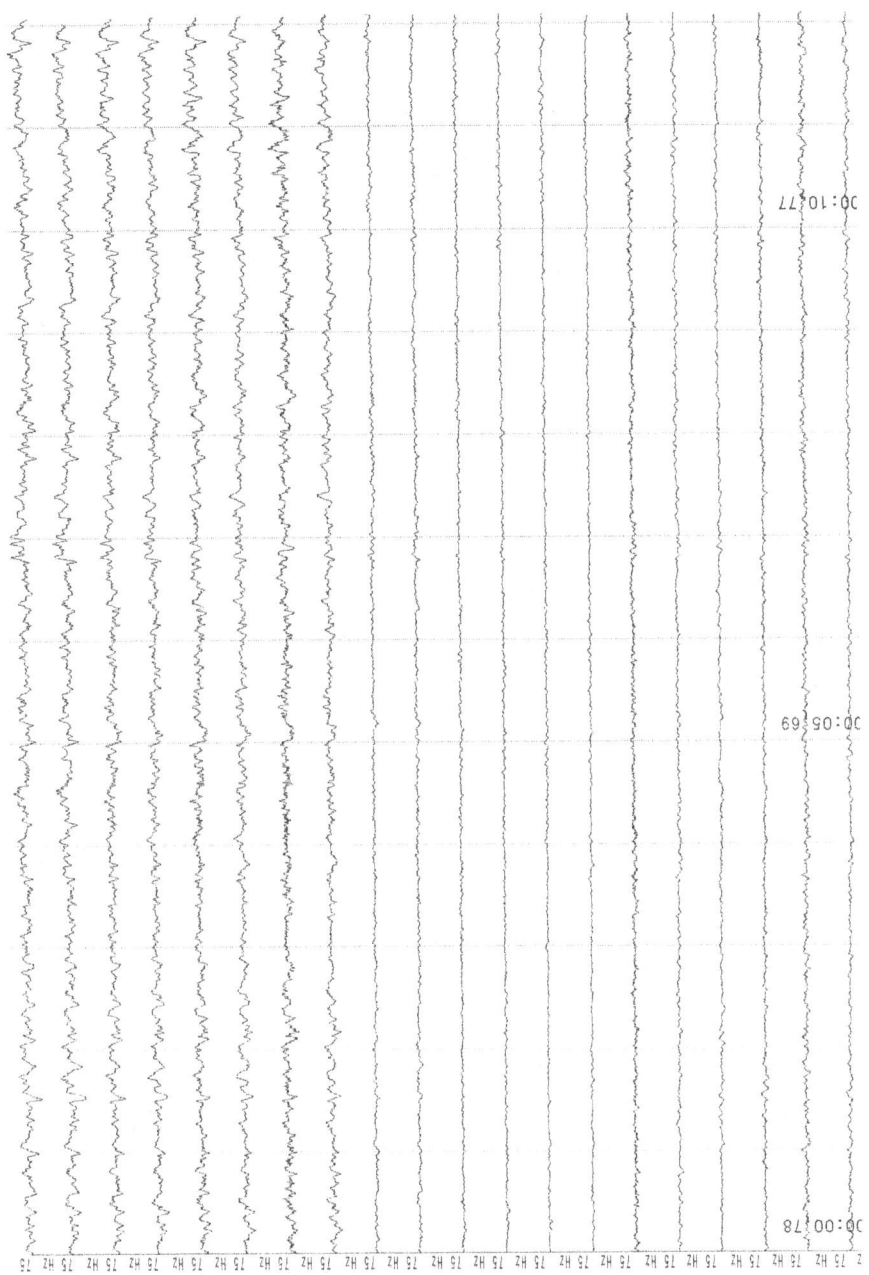

Figure 55. Dynamic Lability (**DL**) in transition to Diffuse Dysrhythmia (**DD**). A relatively low-voltage activity is temporarily subseded by an irregular mixed theta-/delta-activity. It is almost impossible at this point to clearly delineate subvigil intermediary stages.

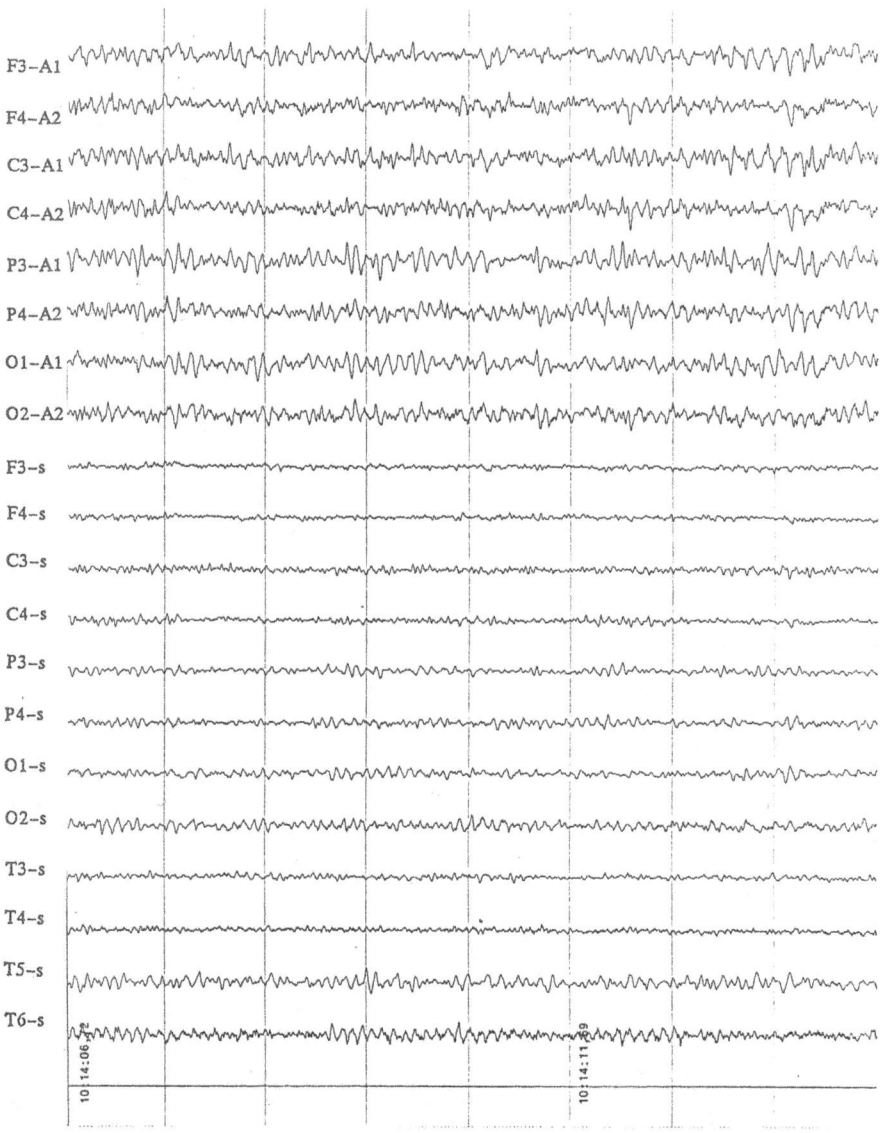

Figure 56. Pathomorphic variants of the A-stage (**ILA/IBA**). Frequency-variable alpha-activity around 8.5/s with a left-sided amplitude dominance - clearly recognizable during the first 4 seconds - develops into a short group of focal 6/s-waves (**ILA**) with left-anterior dominance.

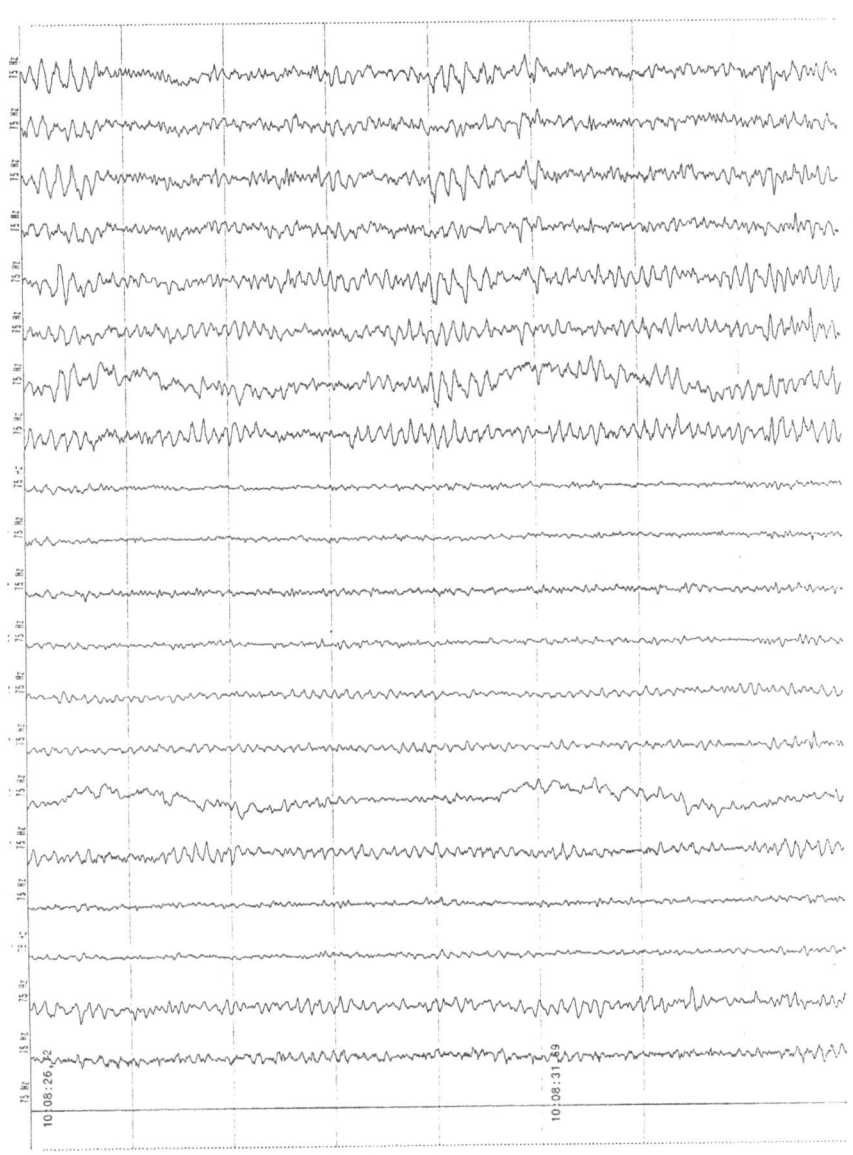

Figure 57. Pathomorphic variants of the A-stage (**ILA/IBA**). A group of rhythmic focal 7/s-waves with left-anterior dominance is followed in the 5th second by a group that also extends to the posterior regions.

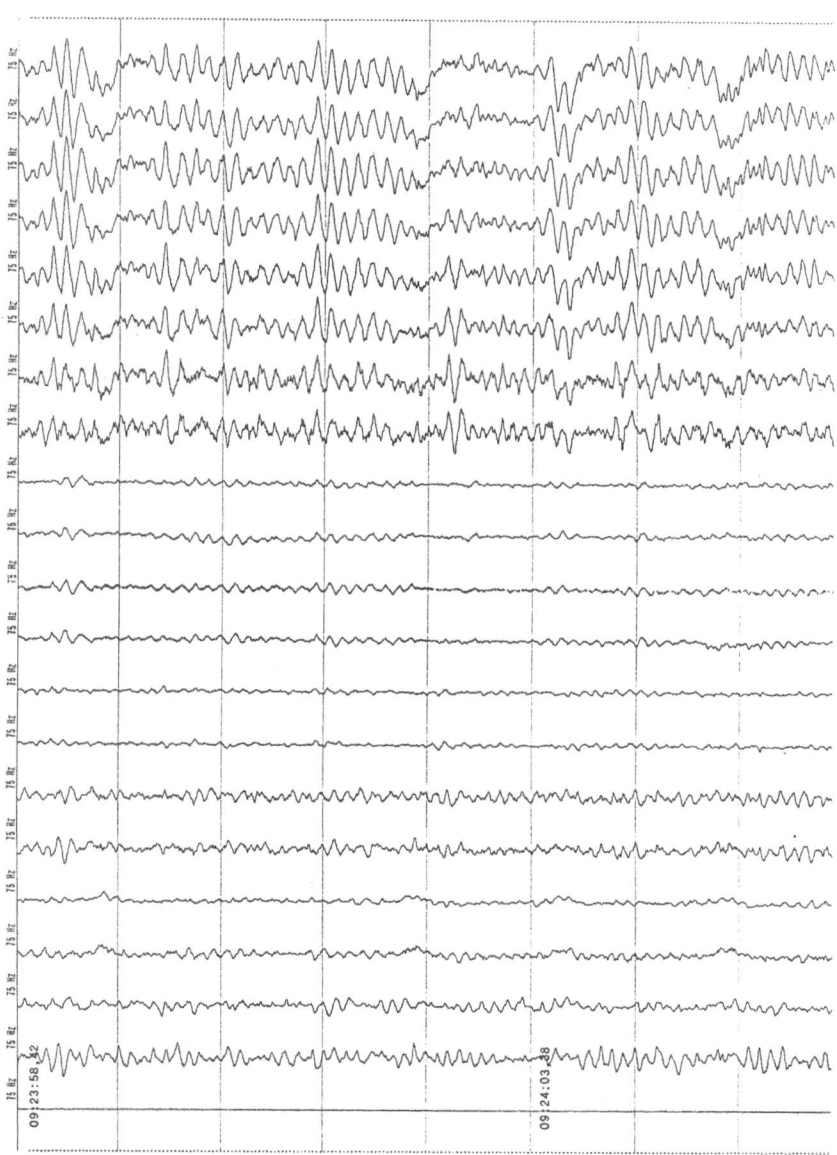

Figure 58. Pathomorphic variants of the A-stage (**ILA/IBA**). Groups and sequences of rhythmic, bilaterally symmetrical 7/s-waves (**IBA**). A 9-10/s alpha-activity largely hidden in the reference derivations can be detected in the source derivations above the posterior regions. The same patient is shown in Fig. 73, two weeks after reanimation; Alpha/theta-Coma (H.H. 56 y. EEG-nr. 877/92).

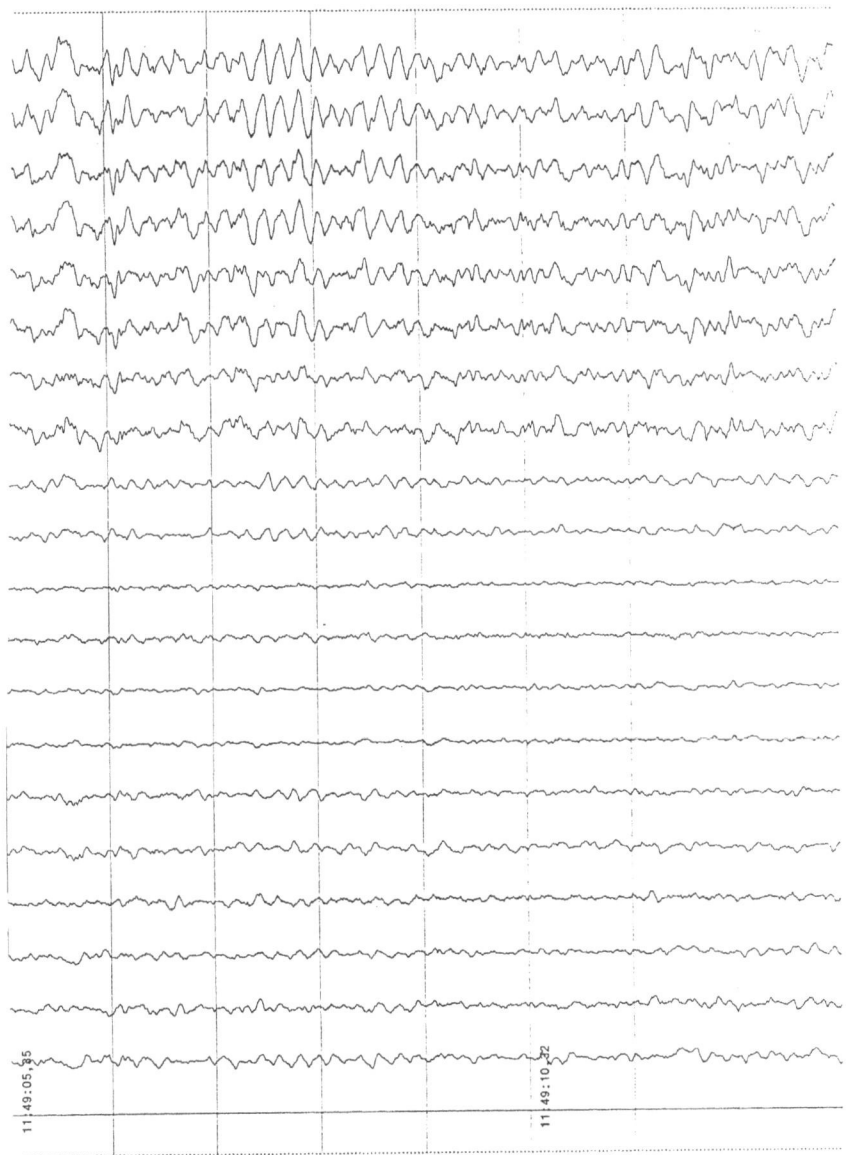

Figure 59. Pathomorph variants of the A-stage (**ILA/IBA**). Intermittent groups and sequences of a moderately rhythmic bilaterally symmetrical 5/s activity (**IBA**) with transitions into diffuse-dysrhythmic activity. Alpha-activity cannot even be distinguished in outlines.

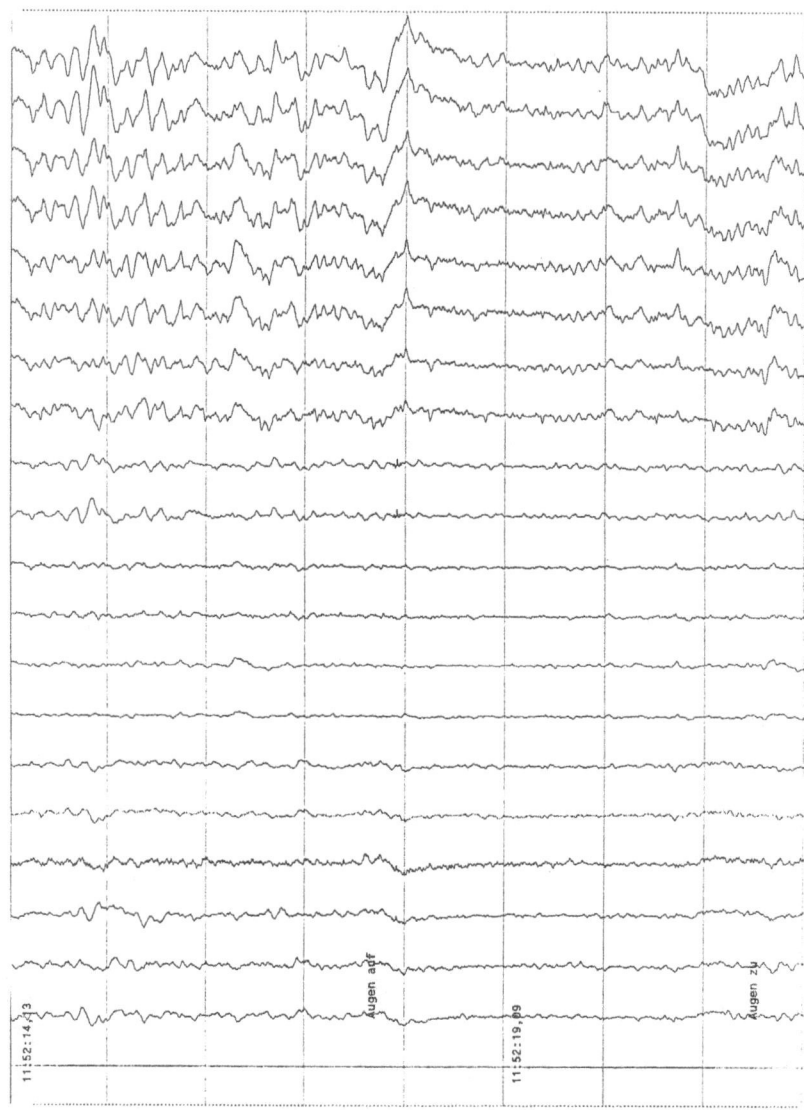

Figure 60. Pathomorphic variants of the A-stage (**ILA/IBA**). During the first 4 seconds, a transition from a moderately rhythmic higher amplitude anterior and bilaterally symmetrical 5/s activity (**IBA**) to a generalized diffuse-dysrhythmic activity that is blocked by the opening of the eyes is evidenced. Two seconds after the opening of the eyes, a passing 0.5 second posterior 9/s alpha-rhtyhm is shown.

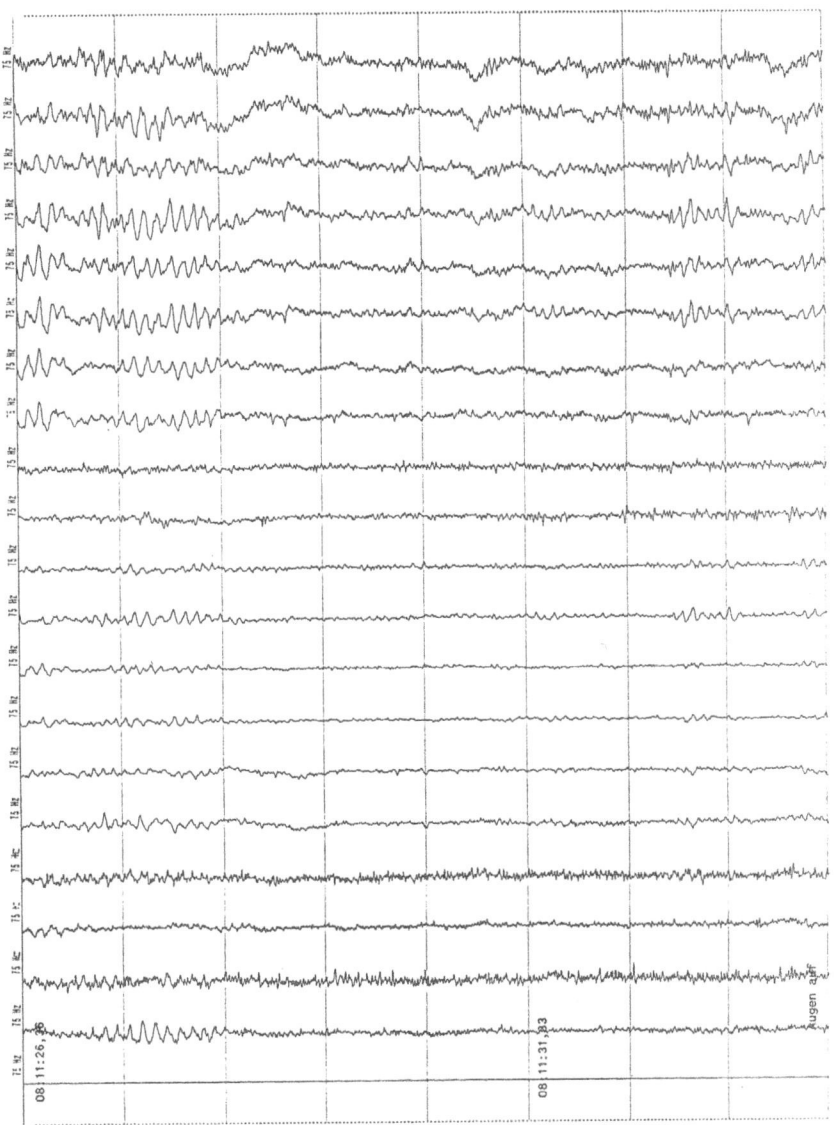

Figure 61. Pathomorphic variants of the A-stage (**IRA/IBA**). Frequency-variable rhythmic activity around 7.5/s with right-accentuated anteriorization during the first 2 seconds. Shown here is the relatively rare mirror-image equivalent to the **ILA**-phenomenon pictured in Figs. 34, 56, 57.

THE THEORETICAL INTERPRETATION OF ELECTROENCEPHALOGRAPHY (EEG)

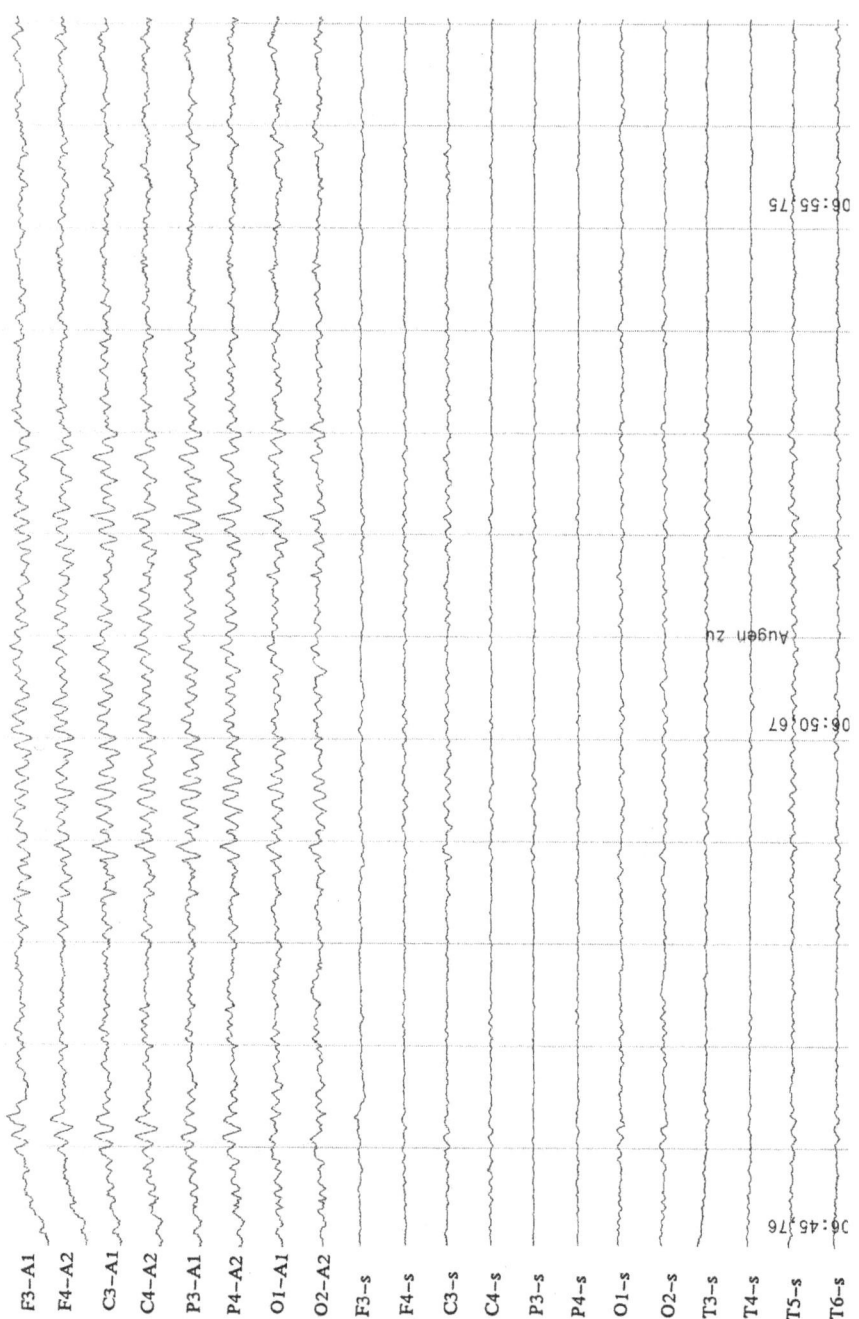

Figure 62. Mixed form of a pathomorphic gestalt change. A low-voltage desynchronized activity corresponding to a stage B1 develops into a passing phase of rhythmic anterior-accentuated bilaterally symmetrical 7/s-waves. This example contains elements of all three dissolution paths.

Finally, it must be mentioned that sometimes the definite association of an EEG with one of the three dissolution paths is difficult, since the elements of the different paths can combine among themselves. We guess that such infrequent cases do not question the foundations of the ordering function of our model (see Fig. 43).

Apart from the possible practical-diagnostic value, our model also has implications for pharmaco-electroencephalography. In the efficacy test of a supposed nootropicum, a positive effect will manifest itself in patients with baseline **DR** in a directional change towards **DL** and in patients with baseline **DL** in a directional change towards **DR**. Since we must assume that a random sample of patients will always include some with dissolution via the A-stage (**DR**) and some with dissolution via the B-stage (**DL**), the consideration of the baseline condition is of great importance. However, one must expect false-negative group results if one relies primary and exclusively on mean values from spectral analysis, as is common practice. Since a change in the direction of **DL** is usually accompanied by a decrease of the mean spectral alpha-power as well as an increase of the beta and sometimes theta-power while a change in the direction of **DR** is evidenced by inverse shifts, one would inevitably fail to recognize an existent favorable effect in the group statistics. Since with primary quantification, the retrograde correlation of the calculated power values with the morphodynamics of the raw signal is totally out of question, one would not even question such a false-negative result. Therefore, it seems advisable to revise all thus far conducted EEG-studies regarding nootropical effects, which ignore the baseline condition. In two of our studies with the calcium-antagonist Nimodipine (Ulrich, 1987; Ulrich & Stieglitz, 1987), we demonstrated that the nootropical effect of this substance would not have been recognized if the baseline condition had been ignored.

In our attempt to first get the undivided interest of the reader in our model of morphologically distinct dissolution paths, we have deliberately not mentioned an important fact thus far. The fact is that all EEG-characteristics, **DR, DL,** and **IBA/ILA** - described as dissolution correlates - can also be observed in completely healthy persons as constitutional variants in the sense of a "trait" characteristic; therefore, the observation of those characteristics can be associated with a pathological functional change only if supported by either additional clinic information or course observations. This means that there will always be cases where the electroencephalographic evaluation of a pathological functional change must remain uncertain because of constitution-related peculiarities.

4.3 From the Diffuse-Dysrhythmic EEG (DD) to Brain-Electrical Inactivity

A disorganized diffuse-dysrhythmic EEG (**DD**) is pathognostically ambiguous. Disease-specific or only pathognomonic wave forms do not exist.

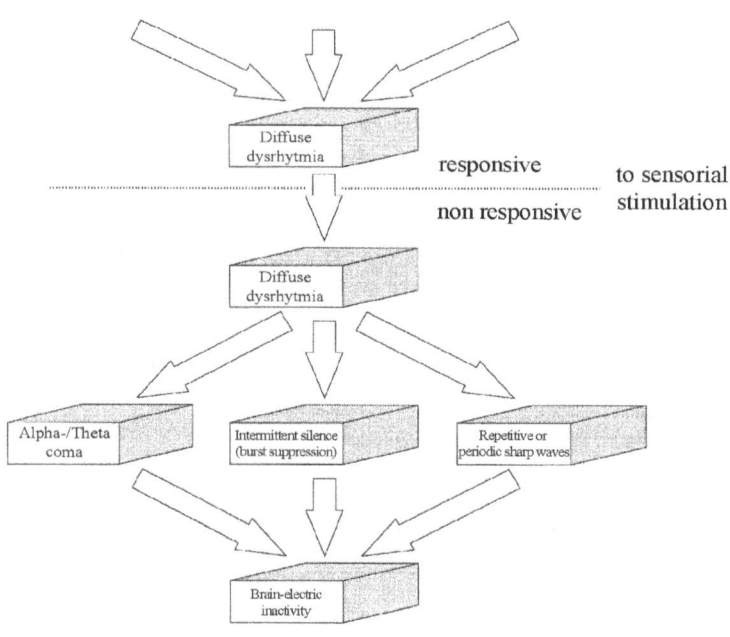

Figure 63. *The pathological gestalt change of the EEG.*

Our dissolution model discussed in the previous chapter (Fig. 43) can be extended beyond the diffuse dysrhythmia (**DD**), as shown in Fig. 63.

Contrary to older assumptions, one cannot conclude hepatic encephalopathy (Small, 1986; Glaze, 1990) from "triphasic" waves (Fig. 64) nor Creutzfeld-Jacob disease (Smith & Kocen, 1988; Schlenska & Walter, 1989) from periodic or repetitive sharp waves (Figs. 65, 66). However, distinctions are possible according to the disintegration level. This is reflected primarily in a pathological change of the physiological dynamics. With progressive dissolution of functions, the delineation of subvigilant intermediary stages becomes increasingly difficult. With an increase of diffusely interspersed irregular theta-activity (Fig. 67), the complete picture of **DD** (Fig. 68), characterized by polymorphous delta-activity, finally develops. However, the evaluation of the functional dignity of a **DD** cannot be based solely on the **SR-EEG**. In any case, reactivity tests by means of visual, acoustical, or somalgetic stimuli are indispensible. These tests usually allow the distinction between a **DD** either as a result of **severe encephalopathy** or as a result of **psychotropic medication**. Medication-induced (e.g., typically by carbamazepine or clozaril) **DD** that can reach considerable degrees with usually no recognizable deficit in the domain of behavior/experience can be significantly reduced by sensorial stimuli (Fig. 69). In the case of encephalopathic **DD** however the sensorial reactivity is usually rather limited, inconsistent, or missing (Figs. 70, 76). The extent of the reduced reactivity allows conclusions about the extent of the functional dissolution. Here, the high variability of the responses to stimulation in repeated tests must be considered. Therefore, a reliable decision cannot be based on a single test. For unconscious patients, the most effective sensorial stimulus has proved to be loud handclapping close to the ears. Startling reflexes caused by this manoeuvre that are evidenced in the EEG by high-amplitude with often sharp potentials should not be confused with brain-electric phenomena.

With preexisting high-amplitude delta-activity, sensorial stimuli typically cause a decrease in amplitude possibly accompanied by a frequency increase. However, in the case of a flat curve, an activation of single or grouped high-amplitude slow waves can also occur (Fig. 75) while no consistent relationship exists between EEG-reactivity and behavioral reactivity. The possible causes of **DD** that are of interest to the psychiatrist are listed in Table 5.

Table 5. Causes for a diffuse-dysrhythmic EEG (DD)

- Psychotropic medication (see Chapter 4.5)
- Other chemicals or drugs
- Electro-convulsive treatment (ECT)
- Metabolic poisoning (uremic, hepatic, acetonemic, etc.)
- Hypoglycemia
- Post-ictal state with kown or unknown epilepsia
- Hypoxia/anoxia (state after reanimation)

- Brain injury

- Degenerative brain disesases

- Acute encephalitis

In the case of a non-reactive diffuse-dysrhythmic EEG, the patient usually suffers from clouded consciousness or is completely unconscious. However, no consistent relationship between the depth of unconsciousness and the severity of the **DD** has been found. Therefore, the extent of a **DD** cannot be used to draw conclusions about the degree of global brain dysfunction. In an extensive observations of patients with brain trauma, Lorenzoni et al. (1975) found only a slight *Allgemeinveränderung* in as much as 10% of the deeply comatose. On the other hand, they found a severe *Allgemeinveränderung* in as many as 14% of the subcomatose patients. The authors also referred to the possibility of discordant courses where a clinical improvement of the patient is accompanied by an increase in the degree of dysrhythmia.

As a brain-electrical correlate of an apallic syndrome, the **DD** usually shows a periodic change from faster higher-amplitude (5-6/s) to slower lower-amplitude (2-3/s) activity. The first is regarded as a sleep activity and the latter as a waking activity (Silverman, 1963; Butenuth & Kubicki, 1975). This is generally explained by the observation that waking stimuli, applied during the phases of higher-amplitude 5-6/s activities, induce a lower-amplitude irregular 3-4/s activity. If, in an apallic patient such a basic distinction between waking and sleeping activity is impossible, the prognosis is considered to be particularly bad. An even lower dissolution level than **DD** is represented by the three EEG pictures (Figs. 73, 74, 75) and the non-reactive diffuse dysrhythmia (Fig. 72).

In the Alpha-coma-EEG, we are faced with what seems to be an inconspicuous alpha-organization at first glance (Fig.72), or in rarer cases, a more or less rhythmic 5-7/s theta-activity (Fig. 73). According to the definition, the physiomorphic posterior voltage dominance is missing, just as is the sensorial reactivity. Even though this definition generally fits, there are also cases with posterior voltage dominance or sensorial reactivity (Fig. 74). As a clinical correlate of the electroencephalographic alpha-coma, we find either a non-reactive coma or an apallic syndrome. Pathogenetically, this is most often a case of irreversible brain stem damage caused by pinching of the brain stem in the tentorium notch.

As a variation, which is typically only fleetingly encountered, we would like to mention the so-called **spindle-coma** (Jasper & Van Buren, 1953; Okada & Inoue, 1992). Here, an 11-14/s spindle activity of frontal accentuation, which corresponds to light sleep stage C, dominates the picture. This EEG pattern can be observed in comatose as well as in slightly somnolent patients.

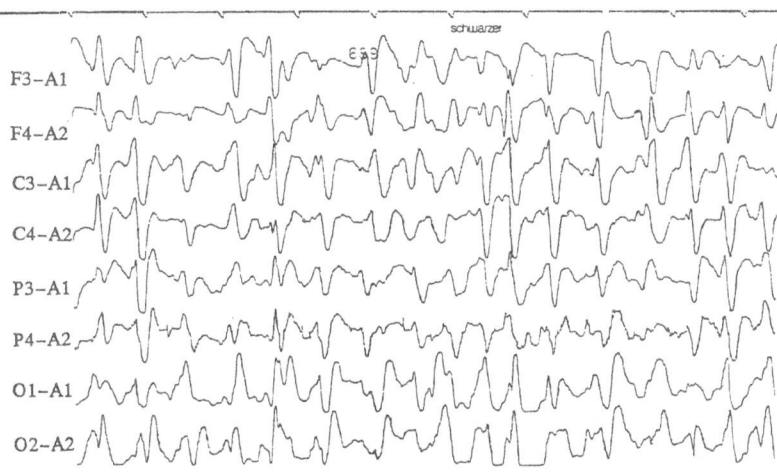

Figure 64. Diffuse-dysrhythmic EEG with „tri-phasic" waves. State after reanimation in case of heart infarction, severe clouding of consciousness (D.A. 64 J., m., EEG-nr. 891/93). Figs. 64-81 identical derivation schema.

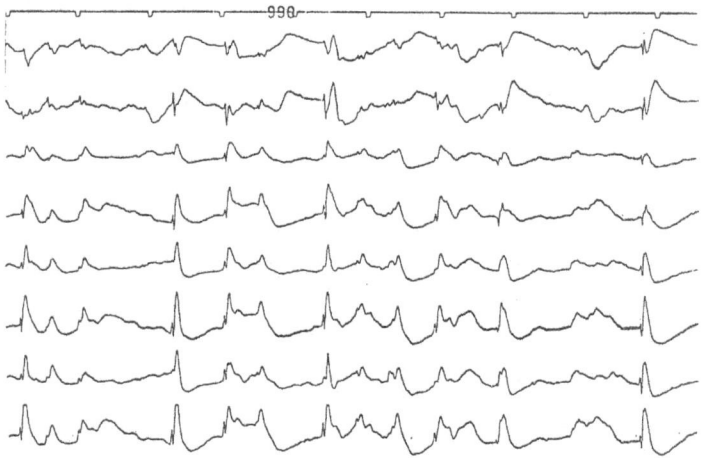

Figure 65. Periodic complexes of steep waves combined with irregular slow waves. State after reanimation in case of heart infarction, non-reactive coma (K. P., 78 J., m., EEG-nr. 682/93).

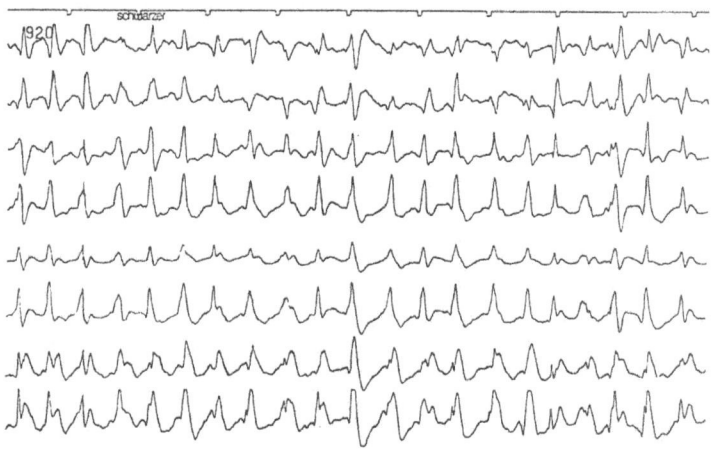

Figure 66. Repetitive sharp waves with a discharge frequency of 1-2/s. Encephalitis of unknown origin, severe clouding of consciousness (I. P., 58 J., f., EEG-nr. 752/93.

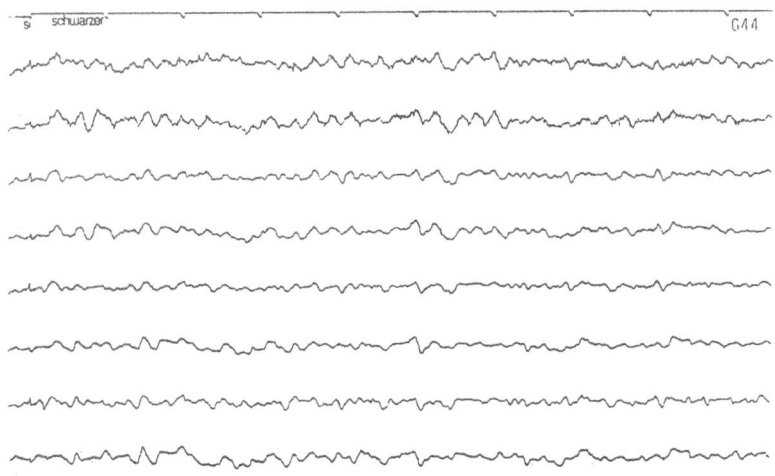

Figure 67. Light to medium diffuse dysrhythmia dominated by an irregular 4-5/s theta-activity of alternating topographical accentuation and sporadically superimposed alpha-waves around 9/s. Senile dementia, no clouding of consciousness (A. B., 83 J., f., EEG-nr. 506/91).

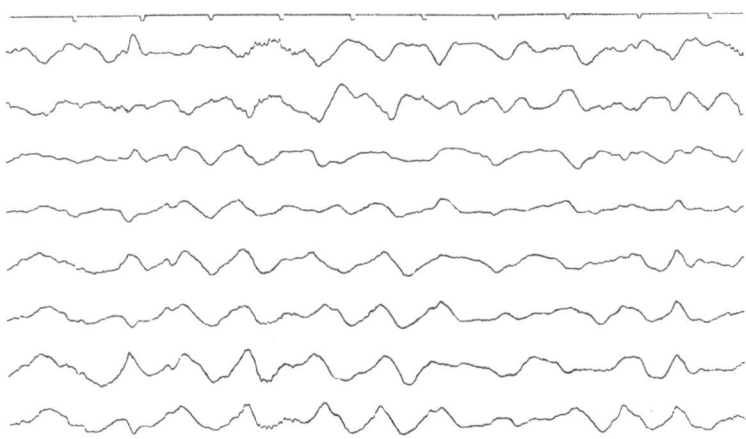

Figure 68. Full picture of a diffuse dysrhythmia characterized by polymorphous 1-2/s delta-waves. Senile dementia, medium clouding of consciousness (B. P., f., 82 y., EEG-nr. 102/90).

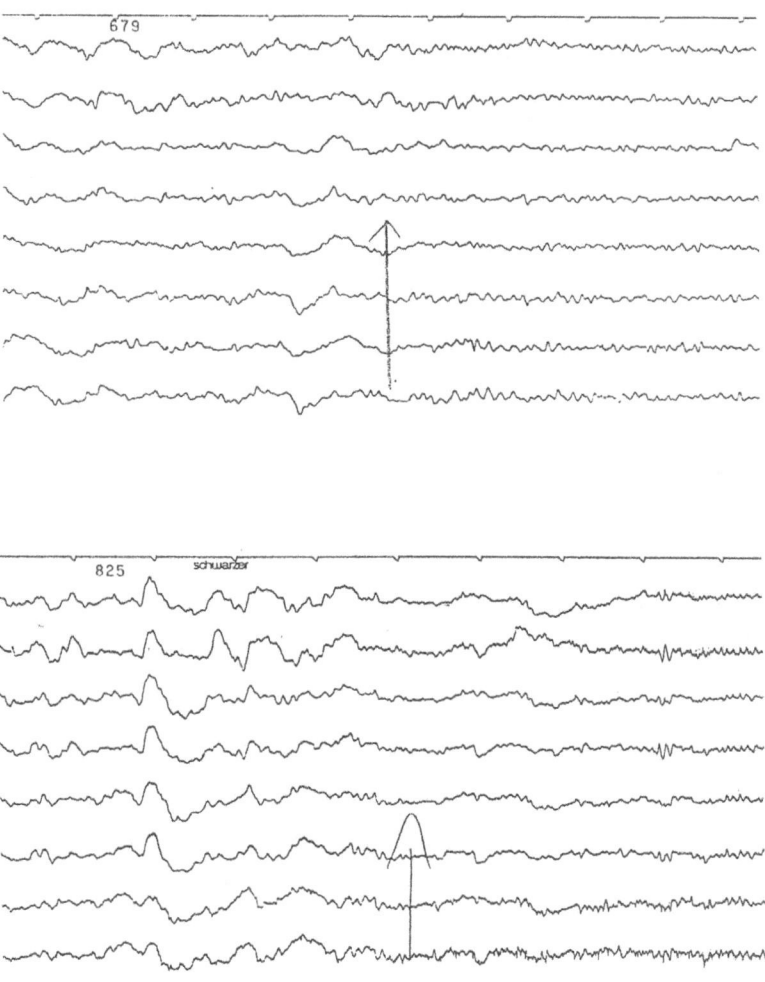

Figure 69. Above: Diffuse dysrhythmia (**DD**) with senile dementia, distinct reactivity to sensorial stimulation (hand clapping (E.D. 85 y, f. EEG 205/91. Below: Diffuse dysrhythmia (**DD**) caused by carbamazepine with drug-specific reactivity to sensorial stimulation (hand clapping) (K.R. 63 y. f. EEG-1003/92).

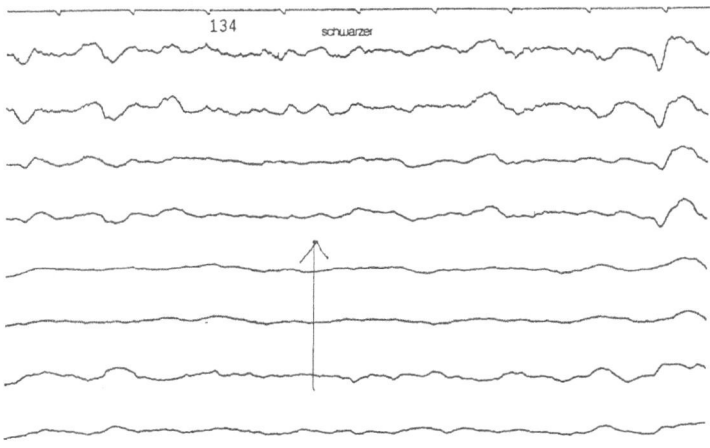

Figure 70. Pronounced dysrhythmia in non-reactive coma without sensorial reactivity (hand clapping). State after reanimation from asystolia in status asthmaticus (E. P., 47 y., f., EEG-nr. 105/93).

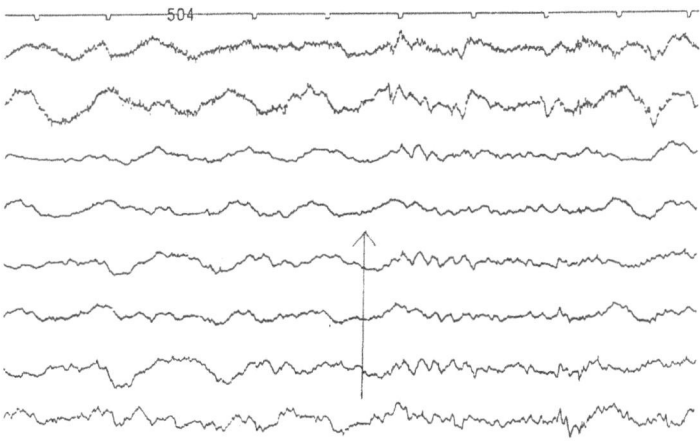

Figure 71. Pronounced Diffuse Dysrhythmia (**DD**) in apallic syndrome after brain-trauma with paradoxical sensorial reactivity: Upon hand-clapping, a rhythmic 4-5/s theta-activity temporarily appears with preexisting close-to-baseline delta- and sub-delta waves (K. A., 33 y., m., EEG-nr. 623/92).

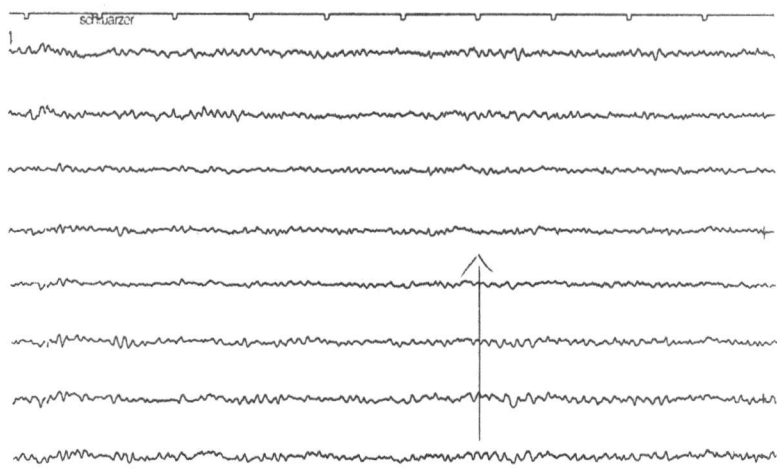

Figure 72. Typical alpha-coma with apallic syndrome after reanimation: 9-10/s-rhythm without topical accentuation and without any reaction to sensorial stimulation (hand clapping and painful stimuli) (W.V., 44 y., m., EEG-nr. 657/93).

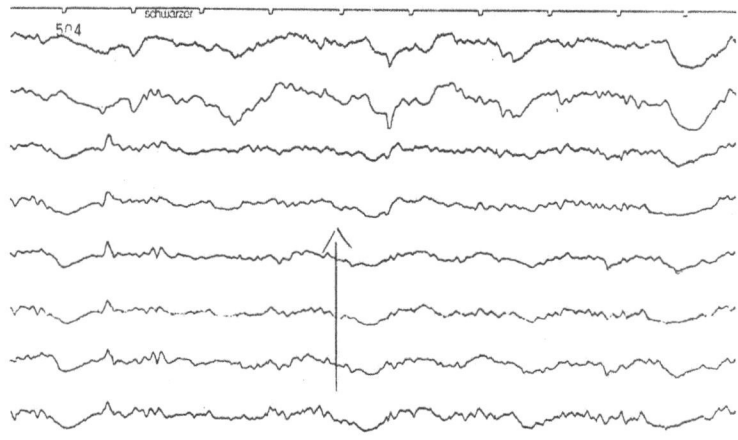

Figure 73. Alpha/theta-coma with apallic syndrome after reanimation; irregular theta- and delta-waves (H.H 56 y.m.EEG-nr. 772/92).

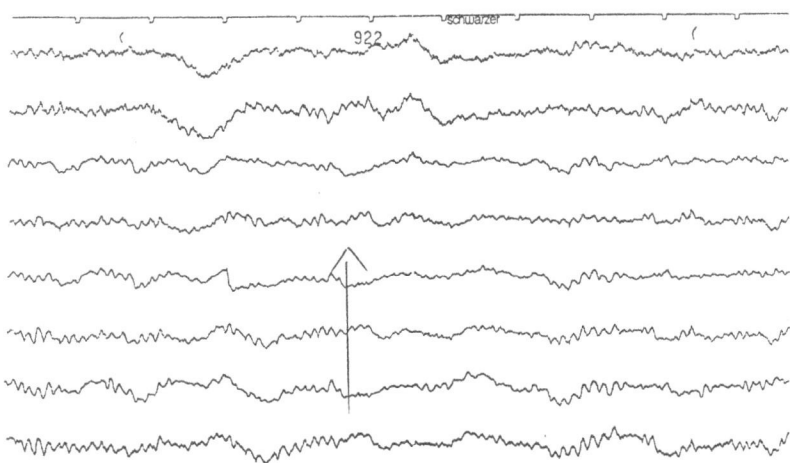

Figure 74. Atypical alpha-coma with apallic syndrome after reanimation: Slightly discontinuous 9/s alpha-activity with posterior accentuation, corresponding to a stage A1, attenuated temporarily and only partially by sensorial stimulation (hand clapping) (E. D., 67 y., m., EEG-nr. 1003/92).

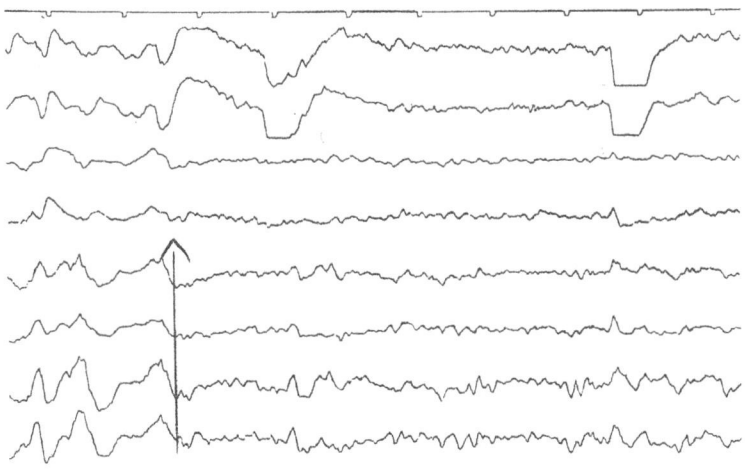

Figure 75. Diffuse Dysrhythmia (**DD**) with largely maintained sensorial reactivity. Medium severity clouding of consciousness, partially-complex seizures beginning approximately 36 h before recording ((H. P. 58y, f. EEG-nr. 802/92)..)

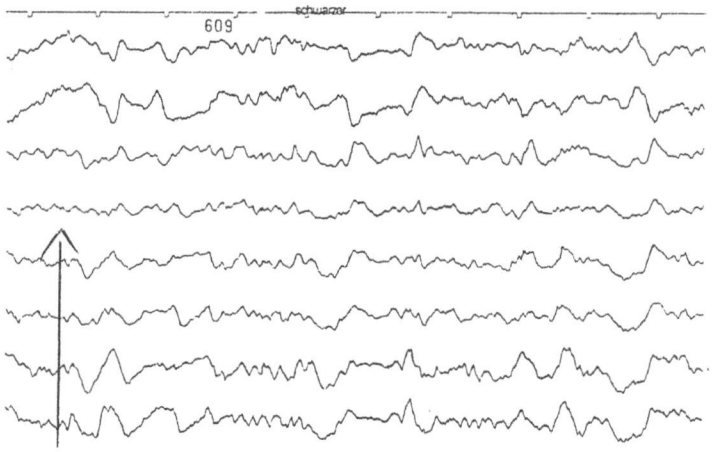

Figure 76. Diffuse Dysrhythmia (**DD**) without sensorial reactivity. Anticonvulsive benzodiazepine-medication increased clouding of consciousness (EEG-nr. 837/93).

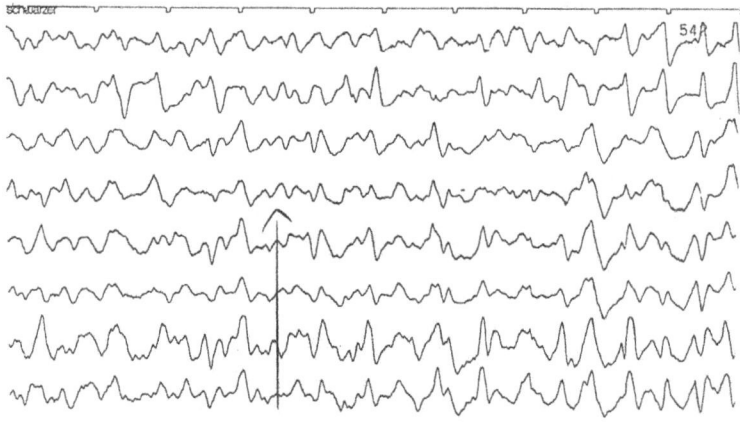

Figure 77. Diffuse Dysrhythmia (**DD**) with sharp and partially tri-phasic waves without sensorial reactivity (EEG-nr. 870/93).

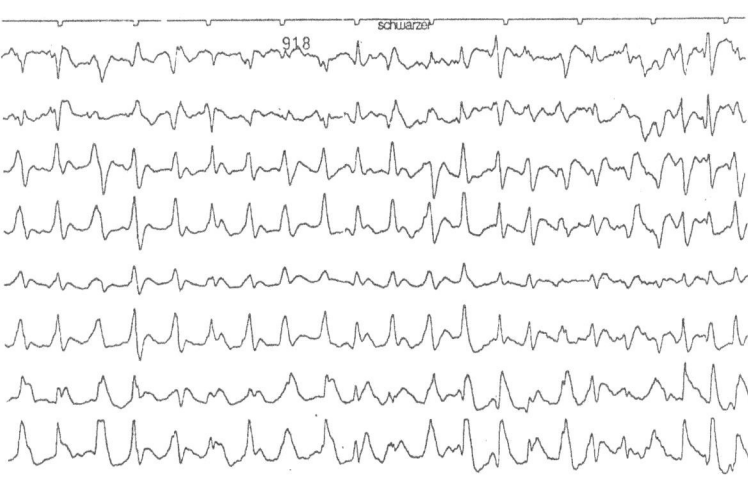

Figure 78. Rhythmic activity in the form of repetitive sharp waves with a discharge frequency of 1-2 Hz. Clinical deterioration towards coma (EEG-nr. 883/93).

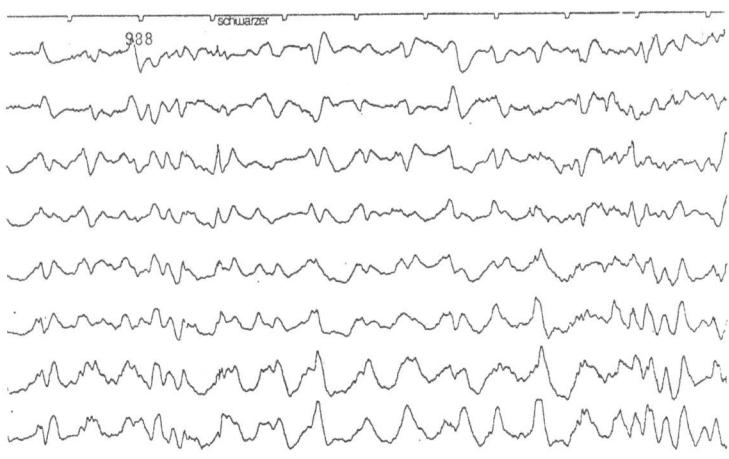

Figure 79. Diffuse Dysrhythmia (DD) with regained partial sensorial reactivity; distinct improvement of the state of consciousness (EEG-nr. 912/93).

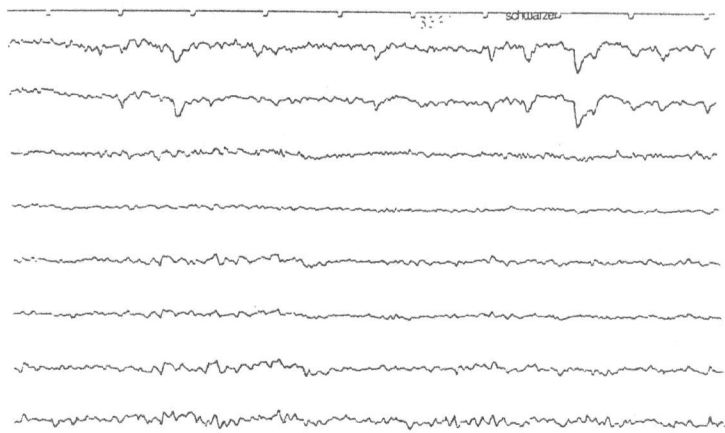

Figure 80. Slight theta-dysrhythmia, dominating is a frequency-variable activity of 8-9/s providing evidence of general recovery transfer to a general nursing unit (EEG-nr. 945/93).

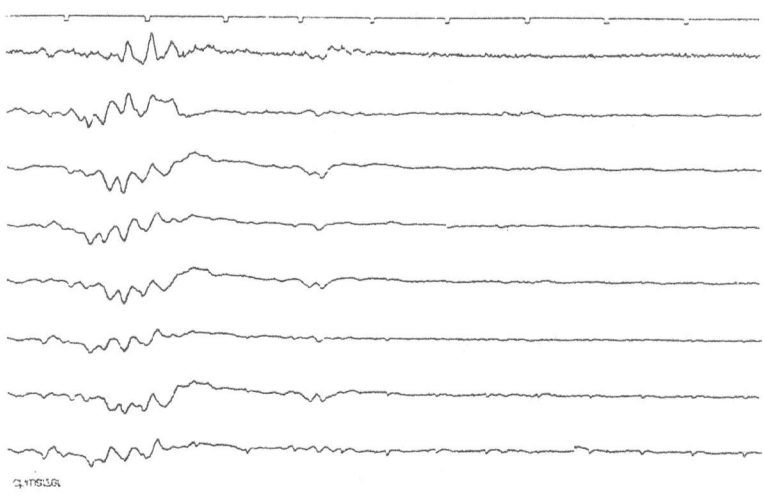

Figure 81. Intermittent activity at brain-electric silence ("burst supression activity"). State after polytrauma, non-reactive coma (K. K., 32 y., m., EEG-nr. 901/93).

The uni- or bilateral repetitive or periodic sharp waves or sharp- and slow-wave-complexes are considered a "signum mali ominis" (Figs. 65,66). Special predilection-types of the *Periodic Lateralized Epileptiform Discharges* (**PLED**) described by Chatrian et al. (1964) and the cerebral bigeminy (Bertolucci & Silva, 1992) can be defined. Such patterns characterize stages of the severe and sudden progressiveness of a pathological process. Thus, with Creutzfeldt-Jacob disease, we find, for instance, subacute sclerozing panencephalitis and hemorrhagic-necrotizing encephalitis, but also the progressive loss of functions after anoxia and periodic paroxysmal potentials or complexes the frequency and periodicity of which increase steadily until death (Au et al., 1980; Brenner et al., 1975; Burger et al., 1972; Butt et al., 1982; Kuroiwa & Celesia, 1980; Pampiglione, 1962; Saunder & Westmoreland, 1984; Smith et al., 1975; Upton & Gumpert, 1970; Westmoreland, 1982). Cases where such patterns regresstowards physiomorphic organization (**PM**) via a **DD** are rare (e.g., Fig. 79). Intermittent brain-electric silence ("burst suppression"-activity, Fig. 81) must be considered a preliminary stage of complete brain-electric inactivity if it is not a reflection of intoxication by hypnotics or narcotics. Only in cases where intoxication has not caused extensive and irreversible anoxia damages can a favorable prognosis be considered following the proof of such patterns. From a developmental-biological perspective, relationships among these dissolution patterns can be established to resemble formally similar phenomena in prematurely born babies termed "tracé alternant" (Monod & Tharp, 1977) and interpreted as a manifestation of a brain-functional maturation deficit (Wilder-Smith & Karbowski, 1992).

4. 4 INVOLUTIONAL PSYCHOSYNDROMES AND HEALTHY AGING

In this chapter, we would first like to recapitulate the findings presented thus far concerning the topic of EEG and degenerative organic psychosyndromes. Then we will try to demonstrate that the features, regarded thus far in isolation, can be understood as stages of an unitary dissolution process that can be subdivided further.

The brain-organic dissolution has forever been equated with a slowing down of the dominant frequency. Berger (1933) first described such a slowing down in patients as senile dementia. He clearly rejected the idea of a merely age-related phenomenon. Because of considerable constitution-related individual variations in the frequency of the background or basic rhythm, a slight to moderate slowing can only be assessed in comparison to a premorbid base-EEG. To this day, a relatively slow alpha-activity discovered in older people is termed as "according to age." Such an evaluation is based on the negative linear correlation between age and basic rhythm frequency, which is found by comparing extensive groups and starts around the 6th decade. This seemed to prove the dependency of the basic rhythm frequency on the physiological process of aging (Matejcek, 1980). However, for several reasons we must assume that this slowing is much more likely associated with various pathological processes, which become more frequent with increasing age than with the normal-physiological process of aging (Duffy et al., 1984; Fazekas et al., 1953; Giaquinto & Nolfe, 1986; Katz & Horowitz, 1982; Oken et al., 1989; Prinz et al., 1982; Sokoloff, 1966; Torres et al., 1983). Giaquinto and Nolfe stated a decrease in frequency related to mere aging as being extremely minute, if it can be documented at all, "... *data do not support the hypothesis of a continuum from aging to dementia, as has been supported by anatomical considerations.*" A convincing argument against such an assumption of continuity is contained in the EEG-findings of very old people. There are centenarians with a seemingly absolutely "normal," even fast dominant alpha-frequency (Green et al., 1986; Hubbard et al., 1976). The situation with regard to the faster frequency components appears confusing. Thus, both the increase and decrease have been described as involutional-typical. Each attempt at interpretation must consider statistically founded group-level findings that from about the 5th decade on, a steady increase of precentral-accentuated beta-activity occurs. This linear trend comes to a standstill and, at higher age, is even reversed (Busse, 1983; Duffy et al. 1984; Greenblatt et al., 1944; Obrist, 1975; Obrist & Busse, 1965). A possible reason for the positive age correlation of the early-senium beta-increase could be the increase of cerebro-vascular processes that cane be expected at this stage of life. A review of the literature reveals that only the findings from Duffy et al. (1984) support such an assumption. Other studies reported contradictory findings, indicating that geriatric patients with mental deterioration manifested a performance level that increased with increasing beta-proportion in the EEG (Barnes et al., 1956; Coben et al., 1983, 1985; Frey & Sjörgen, 1959; Mengoli, 1952; Noll, 1952; Obrist & Henry, 1958; Obrist et al. 1961; Prichep, 1983; Silverman et al., 1955; Thompson & Wilson, 1966; Williamson et al., 1990). This, however, says nothing about the situation in mentally healthy old people. Thus, the conclusion that low-voltage beta-activity is a favorable sign in seniors (Obrist, 1975; Obrist & Busse, 1965) seems appropriate only for functionally impaired patients. In mentally intact seniors, a higher beta-proportion cannot be used as an indicator of undisturbed brain function because until the 5th decade, no beta-activity of any significance can be observed. This suggests that beta-activity in senior patients is more likely to be viewed as a positive sign and that its disappearance indicates a progression of the involutional process. However, the question about the functional significance of the reappearance of rapid activities together with signs of clinical involution is still an unsolved riddle.

Unanswered questions also remain with regard to the typically intermittent left anterior groups (**ILA**, see above) of sub-alpha-, theta-, but also delta-waves (Busse et al., 1954) relatively frequently observed in the age involution. With regard to their age-relatedness, there exist analogies with rapid activity. Here, too, we are dealing with a feature that in the beginning, age involution shows a rather evident rise in frequency and comes to a standstill in the 7th decade (Busse, 1973; Obrist & Busse, 1965; Silverman et al., 1955). Furthermore, the feature was found more frequently in groups of functionally intact seniors rather than in groups of functionally disturbed patients of the same age (Silverman at al., 1955; Torres et al., 1983). Some authors reported feature-correlated performance deficits (Hughes et al., 1971; Visser et al., 1987; Wang et al., 1970).

Another feature that many authors consider to be involution-typical is the low-voltage desynchronization activity more or less superimposed by fast beta-waves (see above). According to the descriptions (Duffy et al., 1984; Gschwend & Karbowski,1970;Mengoli, 1952; Mundy-Castle et al., 1954; Mundy-Castle, 1962; Obrist, 1954;), this feature possibly overlaps at least partially with the aforementioned feature of increased beta-proportion.

The rather frequent feature of the anterior spreading of alpha-activity (see above) in involutional psychosyndromes has been mentioned only by few authors (Gaches, 1960; Justiss, 1969; Oken et al., 1989), which may reflect the negligence of the topographical aspect. We also must not omit to mention that some authors (Bancaud, 1961; Bancaud et al., 1955; Daumezon & Lairy, 1957; Lairy & Fischgold, 1953;) viewed dynamic parameters, for instance, the degree of alpha-continuity in an EEG recorded over 20-30 minutes under the usual resting conditions, as especially informative. There are, thus far, two reasons for which evaluation of the pathognostic dignity of the aforementioned features has been so difficult. First, investigators depended essentially on on a "trial and error" strategy of statistical correlation because of the lack of a theory of electroencephalographic morphodynamics. Second, no sufficiently sensitive, feasible test-psychological indicators of the dysfunctional change of the brain can be used for an external validation of the EEG features. As every clinician knows, the global-intuitive judgement of the physician, especially with the diagnostically problematic organic psychosyndromes of lower intensity, is often far superior to the "scores" derived through test-psychology (Fähndrich et al., 1981; Fischer & Jacobi, 1978; Hartje & Orgass, 1972).

If we focused on the dynamic aspect of the dissolution of brain electric organization, two contrary ways can be distinguished (see Fig. 43), namely the dissolution via the **A-stage** corresonding to **Dynamic Rigidity (DR)** and the dissolution via the **B-stage** corresponding to **Dynamic Lability (DL)**. Gaches (1960) was the first to describe what Bente (1981; 1982) later called the dissolution via the **A-stage**. Gaches compared various neurological patient groups and observed an age-correlated spreading of the alpha-activity to the frontal regions that started after the age of 50. This anterior spreading was most pronounced in a patient group with cerebro-vascular insufficiency. It deserves special mention that Gaches also included the wider morphological context, contrary to the common manner of viewing the EEG. For instance, he recognized the close relationship among anteriorization, continuity increase, and slight slowing of the alpha-activity. For him, this triad was the manifestation of a basal synchronization tendency: "*Il nous parait s'agir d'un phénoméne trés général de synchronisation progressive ...*"

The excellent gift of observation of this author, who otherwise did not become prominent, is also evidenced by his identification of another, entirely different involution-typical phenomenon, such as the increasing rarefication of background alpha-activity in connection with an increase of the fast beta-activity.

According to Obrist and Busse (1965), Gaches' triad is an "*interesting and largely neglected aspect of the senescent EEG.*" Their request for further research, however, did not meet with any resonance. Obviously ignorant of Gaches' work, Justiss (1969) reported a negative correlation beween the performance in the Porteus-labyrinth test and the amount of semi-quantitatively measured anterior 7-13/s alpha-activity. The findings were based on a geriatric sample with a median age of 76 years. In complete agreement with Gaches (1960), but also in obvious ignorance of his publication, Oken et al. (1989) found an age-correlated increase of alpha-anteriorization starting in the 6th decade. Since this finding did not seem plausible, the authors thought that a methodical artifact was the reason for this phenomenon. With the same lack of consideration for earlier literature, Dierks et al. (1991) debated whether or not the Alpha-anteriorization might be usable as an early indicator of demential processes. Reason for this was the discoveryof an anteriorization of the alpha- and beta-activity that accompanied less serious forms of dementia, which was also confirmed by Breslau et al. (1989). That the triad described by Gaches and encountered daily by every EEG-interpreter without being noticed plays such a subordinate role in the medical literature most likely has its reason in the still predominant penchant for the isolating detail analysis. From perceptual psychology, we know that only that is perceived for which we have the respective perceptual schemata. Perceptual schemata, however, are built only for what is considered important. The non-classifiable goes unnoticed! To some degree, a technical aspect of the recording method might be responsible for the relative disregard of alpha-anteriorization as an important part of **DR**. It cannot be a coincidence that in all studies showing alpha-anteriorization, ear reference was used for the derivation. Simultaneous ear reference and source derivation as described by Hjorth (1980) provide simple proof that alpha-anteriorization corresponding to a stage A2 or A3 can only be found in the derivations with ear reference.

Whether the expansion occurs in the direction of the temporal or fronto-central regions appears to be an individual characteristic without pathognostic relevance. It should be emphasized, especially considering the highly popular, equally premature and inappropriate neuro-anatomical interpretations of topographic EEG-records.

As with every typification, we cannot expect only typical examples for the dissolution via the A-stage. The fully developed and complete triad of anteriorization, continuity increase, and slowing of the alpha-activity (Figs. 44b; 46) is rare compared to incompletely developed forms. Often, only an isolated anteriorization or a slight slowing is noticed.

Under certain conditions, findings of a dissolution-correlated frequency slowing in the alpha-range allow one to assume a **DR** with quantitative methods, i.e.,with the Fourier spectral-analysis. Since the physiomorphic transition from stage A1 to stage A2 and, even more so to A3, is already accompanied by a slight decrease of the dominant alpha-frequency, an increase in the proportion of mid and late A-stages must lead to a slowing of the alpha-frequency averaged across the entire EEG.

Finally, our model of the different dissolution paths also allows an explanation of observations of mental deterioration without the associated EEG-slowing (Stoller, 1949). In such cases, the dissolution occurs not via the A-stage (**DR**) but via the B-stage (**DL**) or the pathomorph variants of the A-stage (**ILA/IBA**, s.a. Fig. 43). Conducting a study with outpatients of the geronto-psychiatric department, we attempted to find a psychopathological correlate of the **DR** (Ulrich et al., unpublished manuscript) with an outpatient sample of patients. Since an earlier study involving patients with depressive syndromes had already revealed certain correlations (Ulrich & Brand, 1993), we could now test certain hypotheses. The study included all outpatients of the Gerontopsychiatric department from 1986-1991 of whom a routinely recorded resting EEG and an AGP-documented psychiatric evaluation (CIOMPI et al. 1973) from approximately the same time period existed. Overall, 151 patients, 119 women and 32 men with an average age of 74.7 years ±7.23 met these criteria,. The definitions of the AGP-items allow a comparison of geronto-psychiatric and psychiatric studies. After assuring anonymity, the microfiche-stored EEGs were classified in one of four mutually exclusive categories, after careful reassessment:

- physiomorph dynamics (**PD**)
- dynamic rigidity (**DR**)
- dynamic lability (**DL**)
- diffuse dysrhythmia (**DD**).

The classification was based on markedness thresholds, as exemplified in Figs. 51 (**DR**), 54 (**DL**), and 68 (**DD**).

Because of our findings in depressive patients (Ulrich & Brand, 1993), among senescent patients with **DR,** we expected a relatively higher frequency of the items: inhibited thinking (15%), affective rigidity (8%), retarded thinking (55%), lack of drive (62%), and disordered memorization (76%). The percentages listed in parentheses refer to the persons showing the AGP-item independent of the EEG classification. Because of the low frequency of patients exhibiting the first two AGP-items, a hypothesis test appeared to make sense only for the remaining three items. We replaced the melancholy-typical feature "inhibited thinking" with the involution-typical item "perplexed" found in 62% of all patients. Independent of the respective data-collecting modus, we treated the EEG and psychopathology features as alternative data in the sense of "present" or "not present."

EEG	lack of drive		retarded thinking		disordered memorization		perplexed	
	no	yes	no	yes	no	yes	no	yes
PM (n = 23)	12	11 (48)	13	10 (43)	12	11 (48)	10	13 (56)
DL (n = 39)	16	23 (59)	20	19 (48)	19	20 (51)	21	18 (46)
DR (n = 51)	17	34 (67)	23	28 (55)	15	36 (71)	11	40 (78)
DD (n = 38)	12	26 (68)	10	28 (73)	3	35 (92)	16	22 (58)
	$\chi^2 = 3{,}25$ ns		$\chi^2 = 6{,}65$ $p < 0{,}10$		$\chi^2 = 18{,}94$ $p < 0{,}000\,1$		$\chi^2 = 10{,}51$ $p < 0{,}02$	

Table 6. Bivariate frequency distributions of 151 geriatric patients among the mutually exclusive EEG-categories: physiomorphical dynamics (**PM**), dynamic lability (**DL**), dynamic rigidity (**DR**), and diffuse dysrhythmia (**DD**) on the one hand and the AGP-items "lack of drive," "retarded thinking," "disordered memorization," and "perplexed" observed as present (yes) or not-present (no), on the other hand. The numbers between parenthesis indicate the percentage within the EEG-categories.

As expected, the examined items, with the exception of "perplexed," were observed most frequently in patients with **DD**. Overall, 92% of these patients suffered from "disordered memorizaton". For the patients with **DR**, on the other hand, the feature "perplexed," observed in 78% of the cases, appeared to be typical while it was found in only 58% of patients with **DD**. Since "perplexed" corresponds to a confusion experienced by the patient, it seems plausible that with increasing degrees of disturbance expected with **DD**, the ability for introspection required for the registration of the perceptive quality "perplexed" no longer exists. Therefore, "perplexed" might thus far be neglected sensitive indicator of a light- to medium-degree pathological functional change. Because of the observed correlation with the EEG, **DR** could be considered an objective indicator of such a medium degree of deterioration. This seems to be confirmed by the fact that the percentage of "disordered memorization" in patients with **DR** (71%) lies exactly between the percentage of patients with **DD** (92%) and those with **DL** (51%) or **PM** (48%). Although it deserves to be mentioned that the patient group with **DL** clearly seemed less disturbed than that with **DR**. The disturbance level of the **DL** group could not be distinguished from the disturbance level of the **PM**-group. These findings support the assumption that compared to the dissolution via the A-stage (**DR**), the dissolution via the B-stage (**DL**) is characterized by a higher compensation capacity. Although every EEG-textbook contains examples of curves that impressively document Gaches' triad of the **DR** in various exogenous psychoses, the phenomenon went widely unnoticed. A true treasure trove is Christian's (1975) textbook. Most of the curve examples meet the recording-technical requirement for the depiction of alpha-anteriorization, being ear-references. Furthermore, the recording examples are sufficiently long, ±10 seconds, to allow an evaluation of the degree of continuity, i. e., the dynamics. All of the following descriptions refer to this textbook:

> Fig. 188. Cor pulmonale: 7-8/s activity with continuous anteriorization (corresponding to a stage A2)
>
> Fig. 212. Encephalitis: Course depiction; regression of an initial diffuse dysrhythmia; after two weeks, continuous anteriorization of an 8.5/s activity (corresponding to a stage A2); 7 weeks after the beginning of the disease still medium-degree anteriorization (described as "largely normal")
>
> Fig. 213. Encephalitis: Course depiction; regression of an initial diffuse dysrhythmia; after 4.5 weeks pronounced anteriorization of an 9/s activity (described as "still phases of slight Allgemeinveränderung but mostly rather stable alpha-rhythm")
>
> Fig. 223. Abacterial meningitis: In the third week of disease continuous anteriorization with a pronounced frequency dissociation between the posterior 9-10/s rhythm and the anterior 7-8/s rhythm (described as "slight Allgemeinveränderung")
>
> Fig. 224. Pneumococcic meningitis: Course depiction; regression of an initial diffuse dysrhythmia; 17 weeks after the beginning of the disease pronounced anteriorization of a 9/s activity (described as "slight Allgemeinveränderung").

Consulting the existing literature, we learn that only short and partial aspects of DL attracted attention, but not the most conspicuous feature in our opinion, namely the long term variability of the curve pattern over time which indicates real DL. Furthermore, these partial aspects were considered, without further examination, as age-related or normal for aged persons (e.g., Gschwend & Karbowski, 1970). Thus, we read about an age-correlated increase of low-voltage activity phases or a decrease of the alpha-proportion, as well as an increased discontinuity of the alpha background rhythm - usually in connection with an increase in the beta-proportion (Davis, 1941a; Duffy et al. 1984; Gaches, 1960; Gordon, 1968; Mengoli, 1952; Mundu-Castle et al., 1954; Obrist & Henry, 1958; Obrist & Busse, 1965; Wiliamson et al., 1990; Zimkina et al., 1965). As any interpreter familiar with the EEGs of elderly people should know, such features are common in the involutional age. Plenty of quotes support this fact:

"It might be conservatively estimated that 50 per cent of all elderly people show at least traces of low-voltage Beta rhythm in one or more leads" (OBRIST & BUSSE, 1965).

Or:

"The majority of elderly people show curves of either unstable frequency, with many low-voltage beta-waves or with an over-all slowing of frequencies" (Gschwend & Karbowski, 1970, transl. from German).

We cannot afree with Gschwend & Karbowski's (1970) statement, which assumes that the aforementioned EEG-features found in clinically healthy persons belong to the age norm because no proof exists of a true correlation between age and EEG-parameters. Moreover, the term normalcy is, in all its vagueness, not only useless but counterproductive for a clinical electroencephalography that considers itself a science and whose primary goal can only be to define brain-electric indicators of an **incipient** pathological functional or performance change.

Since the phenomenon of an increased variability of electroencephalographic pattern dynamics (**DL**) is rarely mentioned in literature, we enter unknown terrain with the question about its pathognostic relevance. Certain indirect clues can be derived from the research concerned with partial aspects of **DL**. For instance, beta-activity has been a well researched partial aspect. As we pointed out earlier, the decrease in voltage and the desynchronization that correspond to the subvigil stage B1 are facultatively accompanied by an increase of fast beta-waves, i.e., the "subvigil" beta-activity. Thus, it seems possible to deduce, "cum grano salis", a Dynamic Lability (**DL**) from a described or quantitatively assessed increase of fast beta-activity and vice versa.

We have already discounted the general opinion that an increase in beta is always associated with an "arousal" occurring, for example, during mental efforts or after insufficient psychological relaxation. We must not forget that there are clearly identifiable subvigil B1-stages with but also without significant beta-activity. Thus, we can conclude that the subvigil beta-activity cannot be considered a constitutive part of a lowered electroencephalographic vigilance level. We are more likely to consider Bente's (1964b) hypothesis claiming that the subvigil beta-activity is the manifestation of a *"subliminal counter-regulatory rise of the vigilance level"(transl. from German)*. Thus, a further lowering towards the late B-stages, as characterized by irregular theta- and delta-activity, is countered. Explaining the beta-increase with the dissolution via the B-stage (**DL**) elucidates all those seemingly contradictory findings of increased or decreased beta-activity in elderly people with or without clinical symptoms. Thus, the increase of low-voltage and desynchronized activity observable from approximately the 5th decade seems to be the manifestation of an incipient's pathological functional change (*Pathologischer Funktionswandel*) in the sense of a dissolution via the B-stage (**DL**). This development is often accompanied by an increase in fast beta-activity. This increase is the expression of counter-regulatory mechanisms that prevent a further lowering of the vigilance level. Such observations should explain why numerous researchers found a positive correlation between mental performance level and the amount of beta-activity in samples of slightly disturbed patients (e.g., Wiliamson et al., 1990). In slightly disturbed patients, the beta-proportion functions as an indicator of the activated functional compensation mechanisms. It points to a neuroadaptive syndrome that is clinically unapparent at first sight. With the progression of the underlying pathological process, the exhaustion of the compensation capacities is evidenced by a decrease of the beta-activity and an increase of the theta- and delta-activities. The formerly positive correlation between mental performance level and the amount of beta-activity disappears.

The composition of the sample quite significantly determines the direction of the correlation between mental performance level or performance deficit on the one hand and the amount of beta-activity on the other hand. The negative correlation between mental performance level and beta-activity found by Duffy et al. (1984) in a sample of clinically inconspicuous, at most slightly disturbed persons, corresponds exactly to the expectations that can be derived from our premises. A negative correlation can also be postulated for a mixed sample of older and younger healthy people.

4.5 Dynamic Rigidity (DR) and Dynamic Lability (DL) with Exogenous Psychosyndromes

Fig.82 shows the EEG assessed on the second day after admission of a patient who was initially diagnosed as suffering from a reactive state of excitation due to a hysterical personality. At the time of the recording, mood swings and diffuse neurasthenic symptomatology were prevalent. Because of a pronounced **DR** at a dominant frequency of 9/s (Fig. 82), the exclusion of a neurological disorder was recommended. The ensuing liquor serology delivered proof of Borrelia encephalitis. The test-psychological examination that also occurred only because of the EEG-findings showed slightly slower cognitive performance. After a ten-week stay at the hospital and antibiotic treatment, physiological EEG-dynamics had normalized with an alpha-background activity accelerated to 10/s, now posterior-accentuated as well as slightly spindle-form modulated (Fig. 83). The patient appeared completely inconspicuous from the psychopathological perspective at the time of the second recording. In retrospect, it seems probable that without the EEG, the true diagnosis would have failed, since after all, the symptomatology did not necessarily seem "organic"! However, we must emphasize explicitly that both such morphodynamically different EEGs (Figs. 82, 83) would conventionally have been considered "normal," i.e., viewed as such in most EEG-labs.

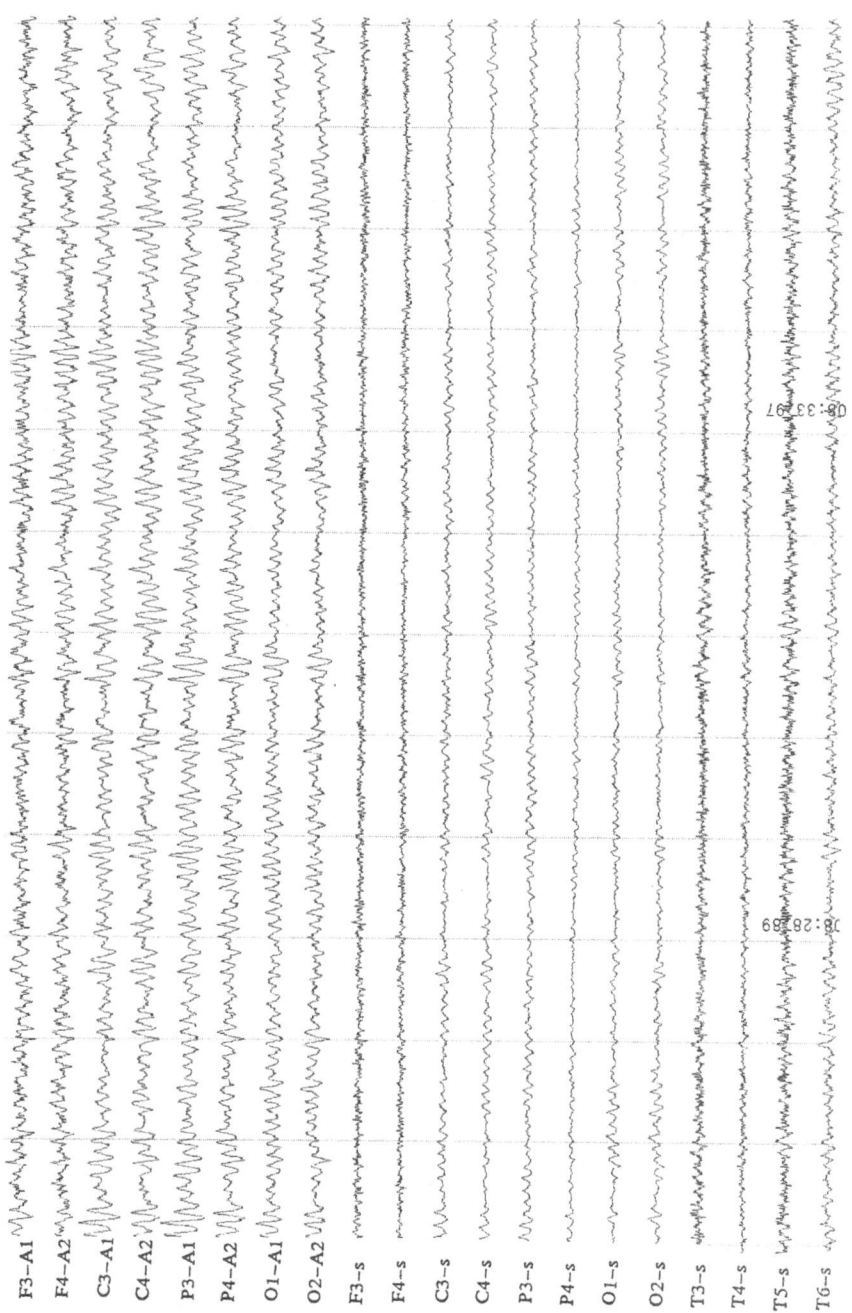

Figure 82. Continuously anteriorized (in the reference and source derivation) 9/s activity - picture of a Dynamic Rigidity (**DR**). Diagnosis at admission as inpatient: Reactive state of excitement in hysterical personality (D.R. 47 y., f., EEG-nr. 952/91) (Figs. 82-84 identical derivation schemata).

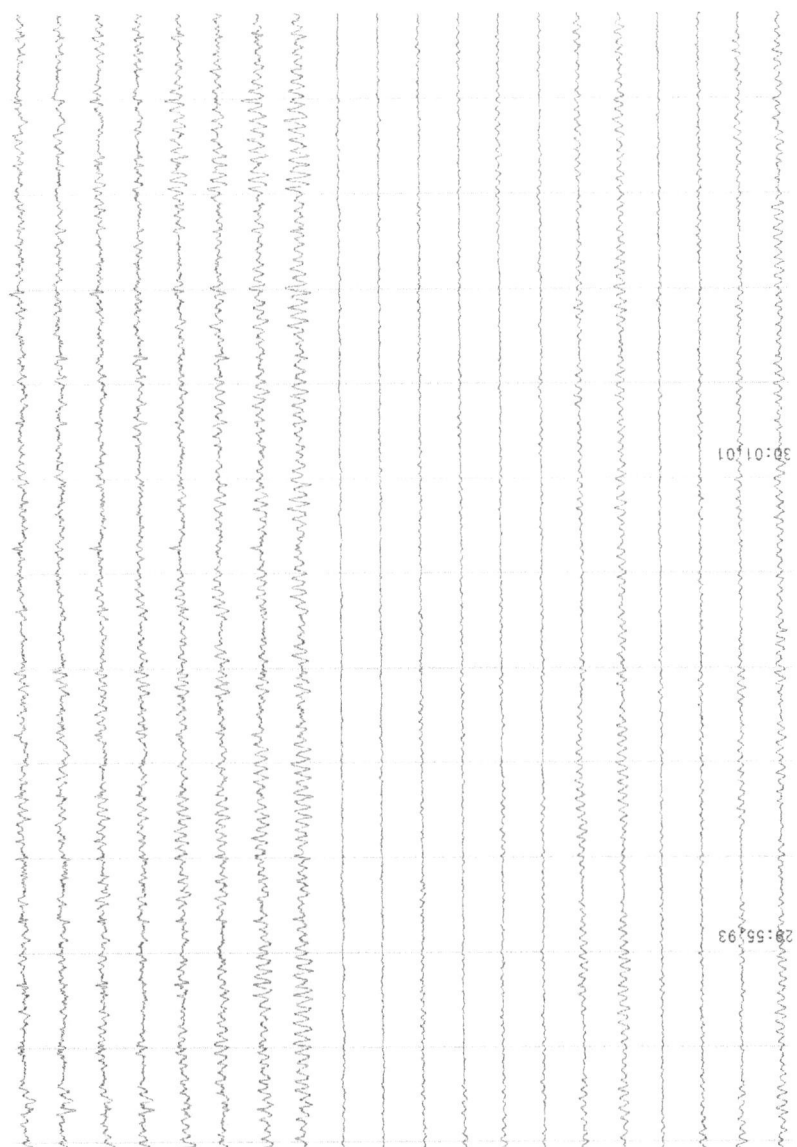

Figure 83. Typically organized EEG with a posterior-accentuated 10/s alpha-activity. The same patient as in Fig.82 after a ten-week antibiotic treatment of Borrelia encephalitis after a tick bite that was diagnosed with liquor serology; at this time psychopathologically insignificant (EEG-nr. 1247/92).

THE THEORETICAL INTERPRETATION OF ELECTROENCEPHALOGRAPHY (EEG)

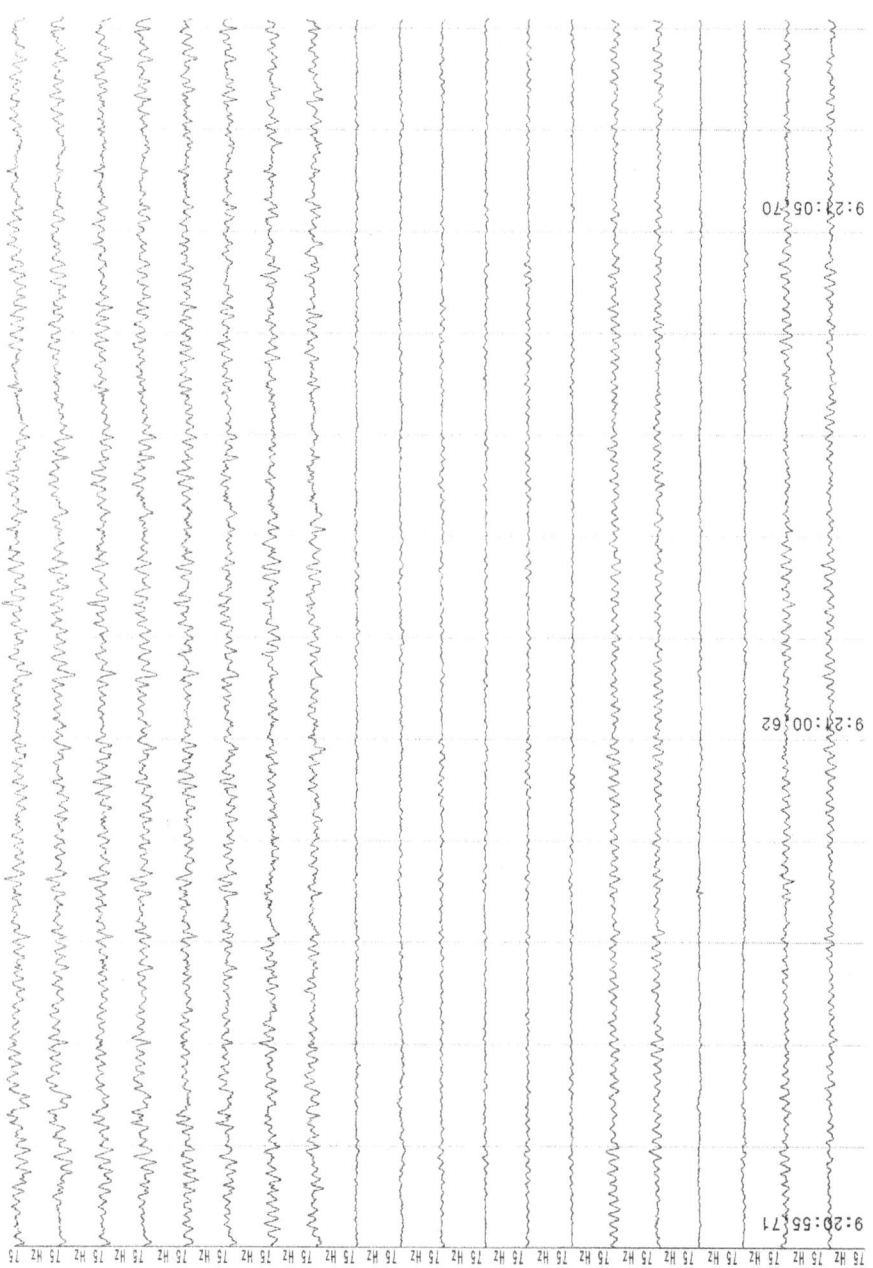

Figure 84. Continously anteriorized 8-9/s alpha-activity typical of Dynamic Rigidity (**DR**); pat. admitted because of suicide ideation with AIDS-related symptom complex; mild cognitive impairment (W. W., 38 y, m., EEG-No. 847/92).

Fig. 84 belongs to an HIV seropositive patient with an "AIDS-related-symptom-complex" who was admitted to the psychiatric ward because of acute suicidal tendencies. We again see the typical picture of **DR** with an apparently slightly reduced and continously anteriorized 8.5/s activity. The **DR** seems to play an important role here based on our experiences rather than solid evidence with HIV seropositive patients with psychiatric symptomatology. We could add any number of equally instructive cases to prove quite convincingly that the growing disdain of the EEG is a regrettable development that must be stopped. They showed that apart from its possible usefulness as a psychiatric research tool, its practical-diagnostic usefulness as a tool for neurological screening has not yet been exhausted.

Bente (1964b) conducted the only systematical research on the potential importance of the dynamic-labile EEG (DL) outside Gerontopsychiatry with a mixed group of neurological and psychiatric patients. Bente defined DL as the discontinuous background rhythm with predominant subvigil activity corresponding to the stages B1-B3. From a total of 1040 patients, those with acute brain trauma, i. e., who suffered the trauma less than 6 months previously, were excluded while 164 (15.7%) showed such a DL. Overall, 50% of patients suffering from postconcussional syndrome as well as non-traumatic brain damages showed the DL, which indicates a clear overrepresentation. These findings confirm, rather nicely, older, somewhat anecdotal observations claiming that prevailing low-voltage segments - an essential partial aspect of DL - reflect a typical residuum of brain trauma (Lairy & Benbanaster, 1954; Lechner, 1957). Oddly enough, the phenomenon of post-traumatic low-voltage, significant for giving expert opinions on questions of financial compensation, is no longer mentioned in the literature conducted in the past two decades. Christian (1975) opined that the findings of Vogel (1970) that low-voltage EEGs have a genetic basis play a role here. However, Vogel's findings also consider that low-voltage EEGs with other than genetic bases also exist. A low-voltage EEG allows neither the conclusion of a postconcussional syndrome (Janzen & Müller, 1955; Jung, 1953; Meyer-Mickeleit, 1953;) nor a genetic variant. On the other hand, the traumatic genesis of an EEG-phenomenon cannot be rejected with the argument that this phenomenon can also be observed in healthy people who never suffered brain trauma. In Bente's study (1964b), patients with DL could be distinguished from patients without DL by their fatigue, lack of drive, listlessness, and sleeping problems, in addition to a wide array of vegative disturbances. Bente related these symptoms to an *exogenous reaction type* or, more exactly, to a *pseudoneurasthenic syndrome* sensu Bonhoeffer (1912). Bente, who considered low-voltage merely a partial aspect of an underlying disturbance of morphodynamics, correlated the post-traumatic **DL** with an alteration of baso-diencephalic functional circuits.

According to our model of various dissolution paths (see Fig. 43), we claim that **DL**, as a predilection type of a pathological functional change that is widely independent from the effect of noxa, can be encountered in situations other than post-traumatic syndroms. Indeed, a number of studies in literature can be used as empirical proof of the justification of this claim. EEGs that fulfill the criteria of a **DL** according to the given visuo-morphological charcterization, i.e., based on curve examples, have repeatedly been described as correlates of endocrinous psychosyndromes. Krankenhagen et al. (1970) considered the "partial beta-type" with the curves showing a pronouncd **DL** as typical of Cushing syndrome. The authors only paid attention to the (subvigil) beta-activity but not to the discontinuity of the alpha-background activity in connection with the prevalence of low-voltage desynchronized B1-stages, which is decisive from our perspective. According to Hess (1954) and Christian (1975), a low-voltage EEG with prevalent fast frequencies - this description, too, indicates a **DL** - must be considered a typical correlate in a primary hyperthyreosis. Especially instructive to us is the case description of the recovery from a psychosis induced through triiodothyronine abuse. The initial acute thyreotoxic psychosis corresponded to a largely diffuse-dysthyhtmic EEG. The curve example of the 4th day shows a pronounced **DL** and that of the 9th day a medium **DL**. After complete clinical remission on the 21st day, physiomorphic vigilance dynamics (**PM**) are displayed.

Idiopathic narcolepsy with its pathognomonic **DL** holds a special position, since it does not represent a *pathological functional change* but rather a primary regulatory disturbance of vigilance dynamics. According to research by Heyck and Hess (1954), Roth (1959), as well as based on our own observations, a **DL** characterized by abrupt stage changes and late B- and even C-stages can be found in most narcoleptics. It goes without saying that such an EEG in itself is pathognostically unspecific and that it gains its clinical importance only in the clinical context, just as all other EEG-features.

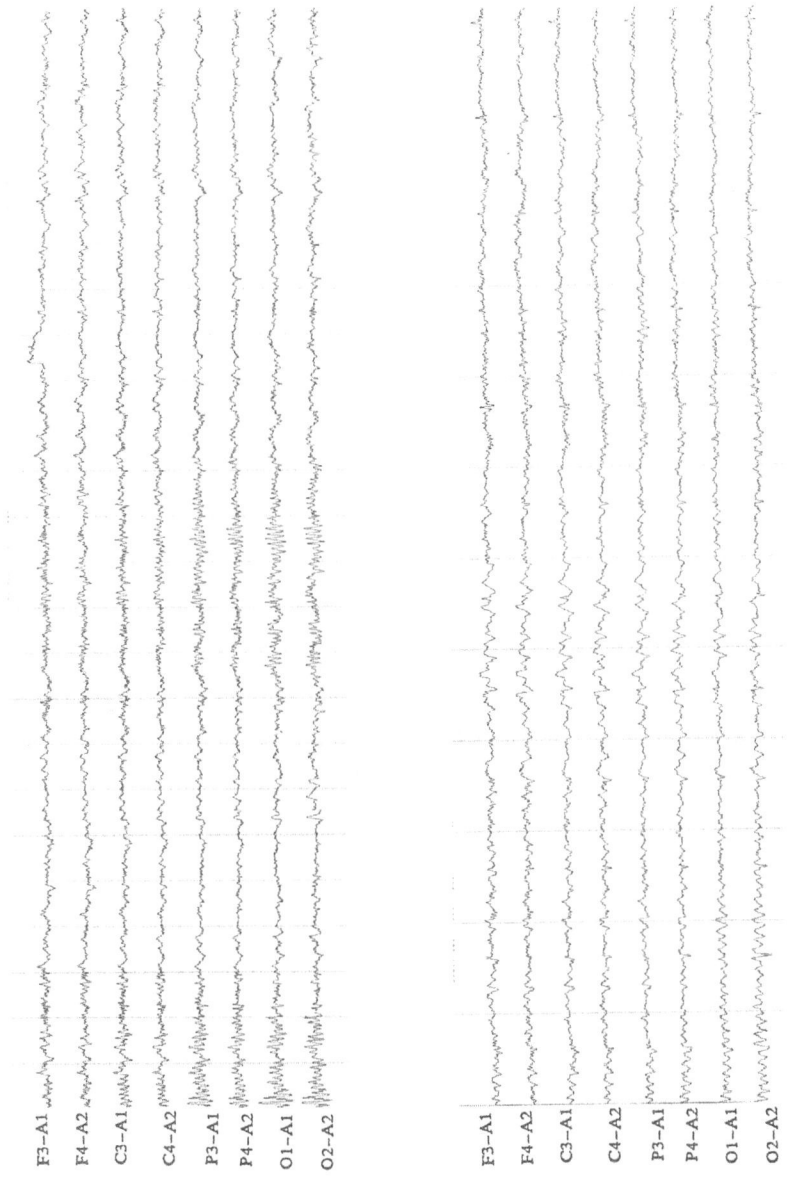

Figure 85. Dynamic Lability (**DL**) in essential narcolepsy.

<u>Above</u>: 24 1-s epochs (24 s segment) of the first recording minute; in the 3rd second, abrupt transition of a posterior 9.5/s alpha-activity (stage A1) to a low-voltage irregular activity of approximately 7/s occurs, corresponding to the stages B1-B2, followed by a spontaneous and again abrupt restitution of the posterior alpha-rhythm and finally another mid to late B-stage.

<u>Below</u>: 24 1-s epochs (24s segment) from the same EEG; in the 4th second, abrupt transition of a posterior alpha-activity to anteriorly accentuated polymorphous delta waves corresponding to a stage B3 occurs, followed by low voltage desynchronized activity corresponding to stages B1-B2 (K.P. m. EEG nr. 501/92 and EEG nr. 599/92); Figs. 85-92 identical montages.

Statements such as those by Walsh et al. (1982) or Daly (1984) that the EEG is irrelevant in the diagnosis of idiopathic narcolepsy are based on their observations that low voltage EEGs with only a small amount of Alpha waves (corresponding to **DL**) may also be observed outside of narcolepsy.

The temporary occurrence of **ILA** in *exogenous reaction types* has been proved numerous times. The clinical spectrum reaches from "exhaustion" of somatic or psychological genesis (Blanc & Lairy, 1961; Blanc, 1962) to after-effects of electro-convulsive treatment, (Schulz et al. 1968; Volavka et al., 1972; Strömgren & Juul-Jensen, 1975), addiction treatment (Van Sweden, 1984), and to AIDS (Gabuzda et al., 1988; Parisi et al., 1989; Riedel et al., 1992; Tinuper et al., 1990). Overall, 6 out of 22 patient presented by van Sweden (1984) with mental impairment as part of a withdrawal syndrome after tranquillizer abuse, temporarily showed an **ILA**-phenomenon:

"When global EEG dysfunction receded localized slow wave activity over the left temporal regions could still be noted for several days or weeks."

On account of this characteristic course, the authors considered **ILA,** without referring to but in agreement with similar assumptions of earlier authors, as indicative of a certain stage within the regression of a disturbed global brain function.

Out of 103 HIV-positive patients examined by Riedel et al. (1992) at various stages of the disease, 18 showed a left focus and 7 a right focal accentuation of slow waves. Assuming a binomial distribution, this is a statistically significant difference. The assumption that the observed left "foci" are to be considered as **ILA** and thus, according to our model, **local manifestations of a global functional disturbance**, is also supported by the fact that these foci were associated with memory loss significantly more than the right foci.

EEG-modifications that are casually subsumed under **IBA** from their description are considered typical correlates of metabolic and toxic encephalopathies (Foley et al., 1950; Jacob et al., 1965; Köhler & Petzold, 1974; Kuroiwa & Celesia, 1980; Penin, 1971; Schaul et al., 1981 a; b; Zurek et al. 1985), diffuse degenerative encephalopathies (Gloor et al. 1968) and cerebral compression (Daly et al., 1953). Of special interest to us is the occurrence of **IBA** under acute hypoxia as well as hypoglycemia (Saunders & Westmoreland, 1984). Here, at least, **IBA** cannot be viewed as immediate reflection of the functional impairment of hypoxia- or hypoglycemia-sensitive substrates. If this were the case, cognitive stress, implying an additional need for oxygen and glucose, would have to lead to even clearer evidence of **IBA**. In reality, however, the opposite is the case. A simple wake-up stimulus, such as opening the eyes, is capable of completely blocking **IBA**. Permanent cognitive load has a similar effect. This leads us to conclude that **IBA** is a reaction schema (Fig. 43) representing a specific disintegration level that is not directly dependent of the triggering noxa. This explanation conforms to the occurrence of **IBA** in acute as well as chronic diseases. Reaching or passing a very specific disintegration level is probably the only determining factor for the manifestation of **IBA**, regardless of the kind of noxa or the intensity and speed of its effect. This places us in opposition to Penin (1971) who considered *parenrhythmias* as an indicator of process acuity.

4. 6   Dementia of the Alzheimer Type (DAT)

Neuropathologists essentially agree that the destructive process underlying **DAT** must have been active for 10-30 years before the appearance of first clinical signs of cognitive impairment (Braak & Braak, 1991; 1995; Hyman, 2004; Mayeux, 2000; Ohm et al., 1995; Smith et al., 2007). To make a diagnosis, one has to distinguish an early preclinical period covering at least a decade and the ensuing clinical phase. Up to now, only the beginning of the clinical phase can be diagnosed through psychological testing. Therefore, early diagnosis of **DAT** is misunderstood as an early diagnosis of its main symptom, i.e., dementia. *"Clinically apparent **AD**, however mild, represents end stage disease"* (Knopman, 1998). From the discrepancy between extensive neuronal loss and the lack of clinical signs, one has to infer functional compensation. It is estimated that 5-10% of the original cortical neurons are sufficient to guarantee inconspicuous cognitive performing, provided a low momentum of the disease process (Braak & Braak, 1991;1995; Beyreuther et al., 1993). The fact that early diagnosis of **DAT** indicates end stage of the disease has hampered Alzheimer research for many years.

A perspectivic change is being heralded by a recently published book titled **"The Living Brain and Alzheimer's Disease"** (Hyman et al., 2004). In contrast to former mainstream publications, the authors postulate a diagnosis of **DAT** within the preclinical stage. Assuming that certain neuropathologic changes shown by people aged 50-60 years indicate the beginning of a pathologic process, it was concluded that this clinically silent process must have lasted between 10 and 30 years (Beyreuther et al., 1993). Subsequent to clinical manifestation, the disease lasts about another 5-15 years until death. If one adds preclinical and clinical period, a pathologic process progresses over 30-50 years.

The fact of clinically inapparent stage in brain diseases with slowly progressive pathology (so-called low *momentum*) has been well known in neurology since about 100 years (v. Monakow, 1914). This is reflected by the manifold of explanatory terms, e. g., *Neuroadaptation, Neuroplasticity, Neuronal Reorganisation, and Functional compensation*, among others. The heuristic potential of slowly developing or remitting pathologies has not been given proper attention for a number of reasons. The main reason has been that mainstream research generally dismisses conceptual frameworks, such as armchair philosophy. Nevertheless, theoretical considerations are indispensable for a meaningful use of the available technology. Instead of the often promised "major breakthrough", we have to accept after years of data driven research and ambiguous (peer-reviewed) unconfirmed research publications, that the then favoured technology was inappropriate. Today, for example, there is a far-reaching agreement that the great expectations in quantitative EEG analysis have been disappointing. Nearly all studies on Alzheimer's pathophysiology are based on the *let's- try- it-and- see* strategy. No arguments were given why these but no other quantitative EEG- parameters were assessed. Literally, not a single studythat would rely upon hypotheses about the functional **meaning** of visually or quantitatively distinguished EEG-features can be found. Thus, it is not amazing that EEG was being discredited over the last two decades. As a rule, the authors restricted themselves to an estimation of frequency power values by means of Fast Fourier Transformation (FFT), dispensing with any kind of information about recording-time dependent changes, be it across time course of one single EEG under resting conditions (**SR-EEG**) or between EEG recordings repeated over weeks or months (for example, Brenner et al., 1987; 1989; Coben et al., 1983; Duffy et al., 1989; Erkinjuntti et al., 1988; Johanneson et.al., 1979; Jordan et al., 1989; Penttilä et al., 1985; Soininen et al., 1989; Stigsby et al., 1981).

A rule-confirming exception is the approach of Soininen et al. who longitudinally evaluated patients with slight to moderate dementia. Only patients who deteriorated within a 12 months observation period showed the expected general slowing down frequencies. The authors inquired about how it can be that patients with distinct dementia may present with normal EEGs and concluded that simple spectral analysis probably does not deliver the kind of information that is needed to obtain differences across repeated measurements. We are entirely in agreement with this opinion, which led us to a more profound exploitation of relevant EEG-information. Since the EEG, by its nature, reflects the self-organized neuronal mass activity of the cortex, no other investigative or diagnostic tool should be more appropriate.

Notwithstanding the wealth of well established visual EEG findings accumulated in various neuropsychiatric disorders over the years (Ulrich, 1994), the significance of EEG with **DAT** is being regarded as rather low.

Moreover, we have to state a general decline of expertise in clinical or psychophysiologically oriented EEG. To give only one example, in spite of an abundance of confirmed research results, the erroneous belief in age-dependence of EEG (in adults), especially of the **dominant background activity,** seems to be revitalized (Ulrich, 1994). This kind of ignorance is fostered by the so-called *Normative Databases,* which are the core of the well known software-packages for quantitative EEG analysis advertised worldwide (Thatcher, 2011). Interestingly, already Berger (1933) disputed an age-dependent slowing of frequencies. Meanwhile the alleged causal age-dependence has been invalidated convincingly by painstaking quantitative studies (4.4). Former studies supporting an age-dependence suffered from the notorious mistake of confounding a group-statistical correlation with causation. Today, this group-statistical correlation does not reflect years of **age** but rather the age-bound increase of **morbidity** (4.4).

On the one hand, it is obvious that the brain changes its structure with the years, just as any other organ does. This is reflected by some minor functional changes in the EEG, which are of such a small order of magnitude that they may be neglected in comparison to morbidity-dependent changes. Even with very old but healthy people, the life-span slowing of the basic rhythm does not amount to more than 0.25 cps (Giaquinto & Nolfe, 1986).

If it is correct that clinical symptoms are not seen before the cortical neurons have been destroyed to a great deal (see above), one may postulate that EEGs recorded repeatedly with certain intervals woul reveal a trend towards disorganization. It is amazing that such studies have not been performed up to now! A slowing of the basic rhythm, either alone or along with an increased dysrhythmia, is by no means the only **age-correlated** (but not **age-caused**) EEG-indicator of functional impairment. A further characteristic correlated with older age, due to age-bound higher morbidity, is a **desynchronized low voltage EEG** with alpha waves occurring only sporadically or in bursts and shortlasting groups (Castle et al., 1954; Davis, 1941; Duffy, 1984; Gaches; 1960; Gordon, 1968; Gschwend & Karbowski; 1970; Mengoli, 1952; Mundy-Obrist & Busse, 1965; Obrist & HENRY, 1958; Williamson et al., 1990; Zimkina et al., 1965). Some authors subsume it under "Beta-type" -or "Flat desynchronized" and consider it as a pathognostically irrelevant constitutional variant to be observed in about 10% of a sample of healthy adults. From a descriptive point of view, we prefer to speak of a **dynamic labile EEG (DL).** Independent of the terminology, it is important to always keep in mind that an EEG with sparse and discontinuous Alpha activity and abrupt transitions into longer lasting low voltage Beta activity dominated episodes is compatible with cognitive health or a very mild impairment at most.

Over the years, repeated recordings of EEG showed am unchanged low voltage EEG of fully alert and cognitively as well as emotionally stable subjects.
Such interpretation, as a variant of "normality", does not fit when such an EEG clearly shows up as a *state*-dependent in people suffering from neuropsychiatric disturbances (Ulrich, 1994). Thus, we have to distinguish between a low voltage EEG representing a *state*-dependent pathological feature and a low voltage EEG as an outlasting *trait* without any direct clinical relevance (3.4.6).

Visuo-morphologically *trait* **dependent** low voltage **DL** resembles, to a high degree, *state* **dependent** low voltage **DL**. Some contextual peculiarities may support this distinction.

- The spatio-temporal EEG picture (the dynamic *Verlaufsgestalt*) of *trait*- dependent low voltage EEG is more uniform across time.
- In contrast, *state*-dependent low voltage EEGs become increasingly distinct along with recording time. Furthermore, the transitions between the sparse Alpha activity and longer lasting episodes of desynchronized low amplitude activity occur more abruptly with the former.
- The mean proportion of alpha activity is far smaller with *trait*-low voltage EEG compared to *state*-low voltage EEG.
- A low voltage episode lasting longer than a few seconds indicates *state*-dependence, i.e., lowered EEG-vigilance stage B1, as defined by Roth (1961). The B-stages are generally associated with relaxation or diminished alertness. A more or less pronounced preponderance of 20-30/s Beta activity has been interpreted as a reflection of an excitatory counterregulatory mechanism protecting the subject from falling into sleep unwillingly (Bente, 1981; Sterman, 1984; van den Bergh, 1997). Moreover, Bente (1981) speculated that this mechanism might be important with regard to the compensation of cognitive performance deficits in preclinical **DAT**. A number of independent observations of decreasing Beta-activity along with cognitive deterioration in **DAT** patients

supported this speculation. According to Bente, a **DL**-EEG in elderly but otherwise cognitively intact people heralded a so-called **Dissolution via Stage B** (*Abbau über das B-Stadium*). This interpretation is inconsistent with Lindsley's neurophysiological "arousal" interpretation, which still has its adherents in psychophysiology. Accordingly, a low voltage desynchronized EEG corresponded to a feeling of tension or anxiety. however, much evidence shows that the contrary is true. "Arousal" is not a psychological term (belonging to "mind language") but a physiological one (belonging to "brain language"), which indicates only short-lasting phasic on/off- reactions. Furthermore, **subvigil stage B** is associated with a paradoxical reaction to sensorial stimulation. Hand clapping or eye-opening on command will be followed by a temporary appearance of Alpha activity representing a raise of the EEG-vigilance level towards stage A.

- ***State* dependent low voltage EEG** generally gives place to a more continuous Alpha activity under (forced) hyperventilation, which is rather unusual with *trait* **dependent low voltage**.
- Low voltage EEG is clearly proved as ***state*-dependent** when it retrospectively shows up as a reversible characteristic.

Several authors have reported a correlation between age and a shifting of the Alpha amplitude maximum from the posterior towards anterior (frontal or temporo-anterior) regions (e.g., Breslau et al., 1989; Dierks et al. 1991; Gaches, 1960; Obrist & Busse, 1965, Oken et al. 1989; Ulrich, 1994). The visual impression of Dynamic Rigidity (**DR**) is due to a recording of the time independent persistence of the subvigil EEG-substage A2. With respect to dynamic variability, **DR** represents complements **DL**. The pronounced **DR**, the sensorial reactivity and recording time dependent transitions into subvigil activity patterns will less likely be present. When observed with elderly people, Bente (1981) proposed to take it as a hint to an incipient involutional process. **DR** indicated to him a **Dissolution via A-Stage,** which he contrasted with **DL** as **Dissolution via B Stage** (see 4.0). With the former, no EEG-vigilance stabilizing counterregulatory mechanism seems to be at work. Both ways of dissolution lead to the common end-path of a generally slow Diffuse Dysrhythmic EEG (**DD**). We do not know the factors that determine the choice of the mode of incipient dissolution. A working hypothesis might be that the controller's lability that characterizes the dissolution via B stage goes along with *compensatory capacity* (*brain reserve*) rather than the lagging control to be observed with dissolution via stage

A. Moreover, we do not know the mechanisms, which are responsible for the lacking of a lawfully directed succession of visually distinguishable spatio-temporal EEG patterns observed in a minority (about 10%) of healthy adults. One may speculate that visually unobservable phase relationships may also embody different levels of integrative neuronal mass organization (between full alertness and falling asleep).

In spite of enormous efforts, Alzheimer research has made relatively small progress during the past two decades. The hitherto disappointing results with quantitative EEG have contributed to a shifting of interest to brain imaging.
Knopman's (1998) statement according to which clinically apparent DAT, however mild, represents end stage disease equivalent to pathophysiological late diagnosis, has heralded a new research paradigm. Whereas the structure-function-performance equivalence has been quite self-evident, recently, a new goal of research was formulated:

" ..*to detect in the living brain the lesions, that until now have only be detected by histological analysis; to detect them quantitatively, so that the amount of rate of change of the lesions, can be used to guide the development of therapeutics, and to guide their use.*"

Moreover, the author stated:

"*The critical issue is to develop technologies that will enable us not simply diagnose Alzheimer's disease once it is already established but to predict with accuracy those individuals who are at risk for developing clinical symptoms*" (Hyman, 2004, p. 25 - 30)

Interestingly, non of the the authors in Hyman's book who all demanded the development of suitable technologies, mentioned EEG, though by its nature, it should be the ideal tool for the assessment of global neuronal mass activity. In contrast today all progress is being expected by neuroimaging. The new research paradigm implies the propagation of longitudinal instead of the cross sectional studies, which were obligatory up to now (Fox et al. 2000; Fox et al., 2001; Bradley et al., 2002; Hyman, 2004; Jack, 2004; Scahill et al., 2003;). This is remarkable especially due to the fact that longitudinal studies are to be viewed as equivalent to the single case studies being strictly proscribed till now:

"*As is evident to all clinicians, single case demonstrations – even when data are consistent across repetitions and are non-artifactual - cannot be used to prove the value of a laboratory procedure*" (Duffy, 1989, p. 379 - 384).

Absolutely unambiguous is the statement of Thompson et al. (2004):

"A more recent trend in dementia research has become to move from cross-sectional to dynamic measures. Serial MRI scans ... can provide much greater power to detect pathological atrophy, as they provide a baseline reference point to calculate change. A key limitation with single time-point measures is their poor power to detect incipient process" (p. 87 – 112).

The proponents of "dynamic studies" being based on serial MRI scans are quite aware of the inherent methodical limitations, as indicated by the additional demanded *"appropriate complex mathematical framework"* (Bradley et al., 2002). The indispensability of the EEG in realizing "dynamic studies" has been brilliantly clarified by Freeman and Skarda (1991):

"... to break with the reductionistic view that the behaviour of a system can be explained in terms of the properties and relationships between individual components that constitute the system ...information that is related with behaviour exists in the cooperative activity of many millions of neurons ... neurons are involved constantly in widespread activity with other neurons, some at great distances, constant, ceaseless, ever fluctuating activity of masses of nerve cells that start talking and never stop" (112 -125).

As already mentioned (Hyman, 2004), far-reaching consensus addresses the importance of assessing the neuropathological onset of the disease compared to the early diagnosis of clinical DAT symptoms. A purposeful prevention, as well as pharmacotherapy, presupposes a minimum amount of fully functional neurons. This can be excluded by and large with the occurrence of performance deficits:

"The optimal subjects in whom to intervene therapeutically are those who are destined but not yet manifest." (Jack, 2004, 75-83).

A reliable indicator of the "pathological functional change" (*Pathologischer Funktionswandel*) that would be suitable for mass screening is needed. Our working hypothesis rests upon the EEG, conceived as a highly integrated indicator of brain-electric mass activity. In addition to the already mentioned arguments, the EEG satisfies another important methodological requirement. It enables a valid distinction between "healthy aging" and the pathological dissolution process (4.4). The EEG shows indeed statistically age-**correlated** changes.

However, this does not mean that they are also **caused** by age. Such a distinction is fostered by the recent finding that in contrast to the DAT process, the process of healthy aging is not accompanied by a marked neuronal rarefication. Subject who died at an old age without signs of dementia always show a certain degree of cortical atrophy, but as a rule no distinct neuronal loss. This supports dehydration, which proceeds with a rate of about 1% per annum beyond the 65th year of life as the main causal factor of the atrophy. (Aizenstein et al., 2005; Beyreuther et al.,1993; Fox et al. 1999; Godbolt et al., 2004; Gomez-Islan et al. 1997; Morrison & Hof, 1997; Pakkenberg et al., 2003; Scahill et al., 2003; Schott et al., 2003; Smith et al., 2007; Terry et al. 1987; Weinberger & McClure, 2002; West et al. 1994).

The hitherto overwhelmingly negative results obtained by the EEG in Alzheimer research might have been expected for several reasons. The main reason is that the research has been "data driven" rather than theory driven. In section 3.4, we presented 8 essentials, which have been not been accounted by mainstream research. If one accepts that no "normal" EEG exists even in healthy subjects (3.3.1), statistical group comparisons are to be dropped as are computer softwares based on "Normative Data Bases". As a consequence, only the wrongly discredited single case studies and more precise quantitative comparisons between lagged EEG records remain. More than a decade ago, we have begun to develop a quantitative procedure, which tries to account for the aforementioned 8 essentials. The procedure aims to express numerically an increase or decrease in the level of Cerebral Global Function (**CGF**). This procedure is exemplified by a longitudinal case study with a patient diagnosed as clear **DAT** (7.3.1). Overall, we found:

- The deterioration to be expected with DAT was confirmed by measurement intervals of 12 weeks.
- The elected parameters changed more or less uniformly with respect to clinical deterioration.
- The numerically expressed deterioration was always found in agreement with the clinical deterioration assessed by the MMSE.
- Slight to moderate changes of the total difference score could not be foreshadowed visually.
- A therapeutic effect of AChE inhibitors (as indicated by the MMSE-Score) could be made probable –if at all- by a transitory delay of the EEG deterioration.

Whether this quantitative procedure, called Ipsative Trend Assessment (**ITA**, see 7.2; 7.3.1), is suitable for the early recognition of the incipient pathophysiological DAT- process or even a mass screening depends on the results of a great number of further studies of this kind.

4.7 DEPRESSED SYNDROMES AND DISTURBED DYNAMICS OF EEG-VIGILANCE

As we have already discussed in detail, today's predominant opinion about the lack of conclusive results from the EEG in psychiatric syndromes is based on the unsuccessful proof of "abnormal" or "specific" features. Even more than in involutional and exogenous psychoses, this conventional premise turns out to be a severe impediment to research on endogenous psychoses. Nonetheless, the literature contains substantial findings that, for the aforementioned reasons, find little recognition. This is especially true in the field of affective psychoses guided by concept of Blanc and Lairy (1960). Considering topographical as well as dynamic aspects, the authors defined two main opposing types. The first type that was overly represented in periodically occurring melancholias was a well pronounced continuous, rather monotonous-appearing alpha-rhythm with a tendency for spreading towards the frontal regions. The second type, related to neurotic-reactive depressions, showed a more or less discontinuous alpha-activity of changing topographical accentuation. The first type can easily be associated with a **DR** and the second with a **DL**. In a number of publications, Bente (1965, 1975, 1976) confirmed and fine-tuned Blanc and Lairy's (1960) distinction. Nevertheless, isolated singular features continued to be the focal point of all research activity, especially the frequency variables assessed by spectral analysis.

Today, a well-pronounced and - in comparison to control persons - slightly slowed alpha-activity is considered to be a feature of phasic depressions (John et al., 1988; Nyström et al., 1986; Pollock & Schneider, 1989; Prichep, 1986; Schaffer et al., 1983; Shagass et al., 1982; von Knorring et al., 1983;). Furthermore, all authors who included the topographical aspect reported an alpha-anteriorization that was more pronounced in populations with phasic depressions than in control persons (Pollock & Schneider, 1989; Prichep, 1987; Shagass et al., 1982;). A decreased variability or increased uniformity of the amplitudes can be considered a third quantitatively assessed feature of phasic depression (d'Elia & Perris, 1973; Goldstein, 1975; Marjerrison et al., 1974; Swartzburg & Chowdreys, 1977).

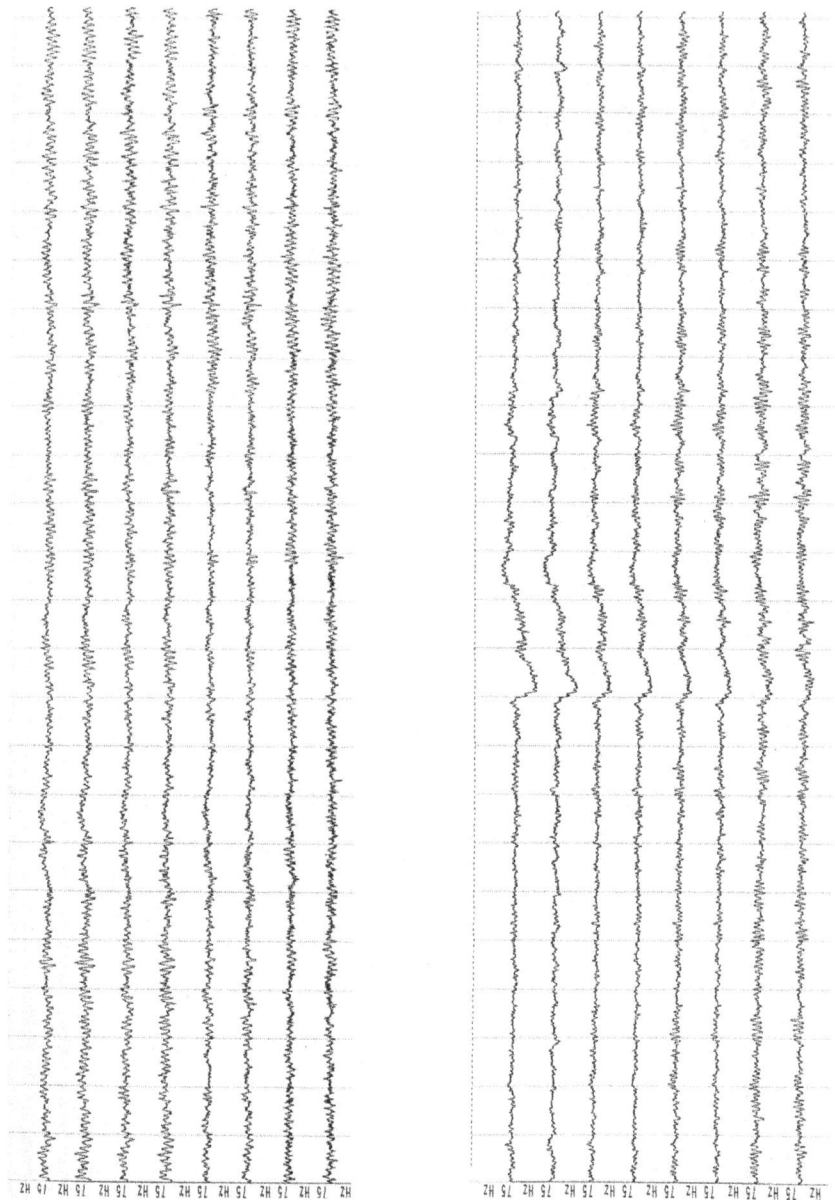

Figure 86. <u>Above</u>: 24 1-second epochs (24 seconds segment) of continuously anteriorized alpha-activity (**DR**) of about 9/s recorded at admittance because of "retarded depression"; 75mg/d clomipramine. Complaints presented about "mental block" for months but no other symptoms typical for depression. <u>Below</u>: 24 1-second epochs (24 second segment) of largely physiomorph dynamics (**PM**) with posterior-accentuated and faster alpha-activity than anteriorly; 125 mg/d clomipramine. The recording was performed after the patient had reported the sudden disappearance of her "mental block" after the second night of sleep deprivation. No improvement under the preceding 12-week clomipramine-treatment ((A.M., 43 y., f., EEG-nr. 204/92 and EEG-nr. 508/92). Figs. 85-92 identical montages.

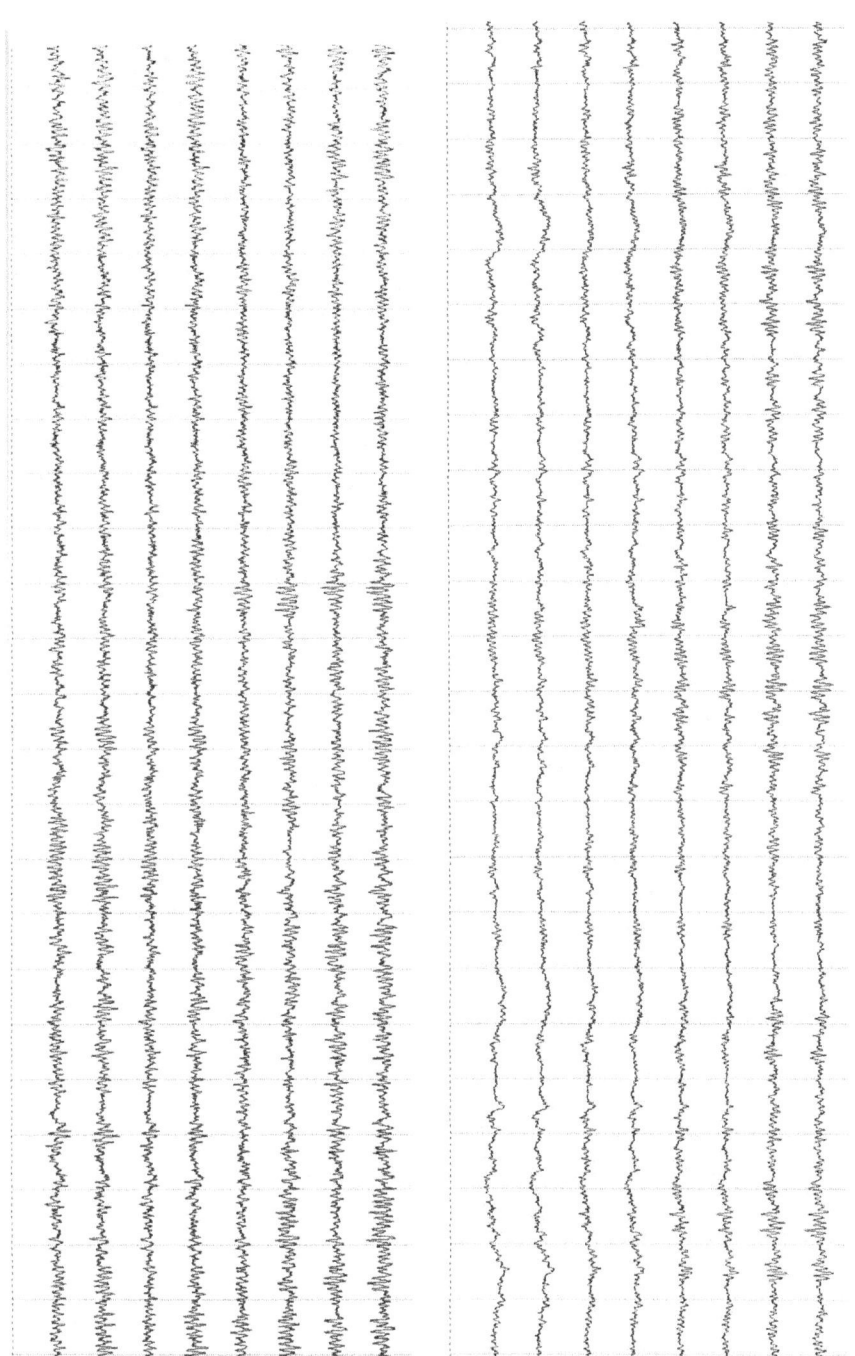

Figure 87. Patient same as in Fig.86 (unchanged electrode montages). <u>Above</u>: Recurring **DR** at readmittance 5 months later because of recidivism (compare to Fig. 86 (above). Complaints again about "mental block" (EEG-nr. 1033/92). <u>Below</u>: Essentially physiomorphic EEG (compare to Fig. 86, below) as correlate of another remission under combined sleep deprivation and clomipramine treatment (EEG-nr. 27/93).

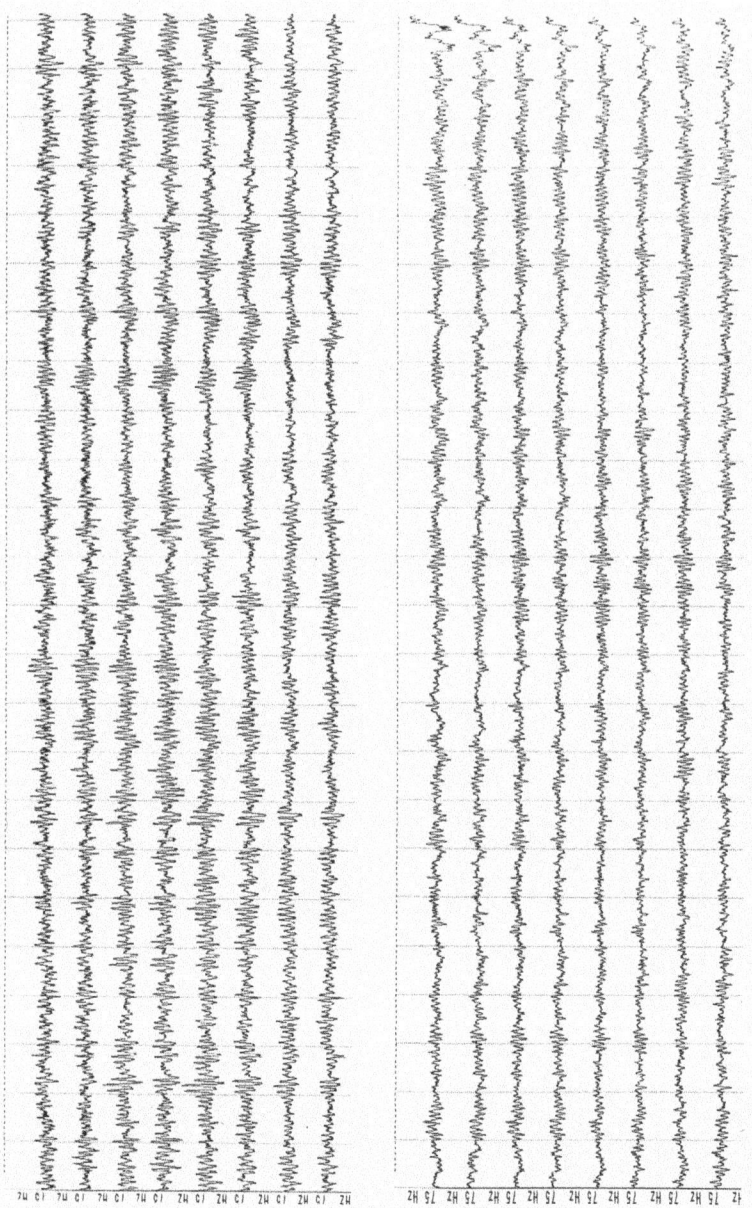

Figure 88. <u>Above</u>: 24 1-s epochs (24 second segment); continuous anteriorization of a high-amplitude and monomorph activity of about 8.5/s; picture of a **DR**; depressive syndrome with pronounced psychomotor retardation; for one week 75 mg/d imipramine, lithium-level: 0.52mmol/l (I. K., 65 y., f., EEG-nr. 614/92). <u>Below</u>: 24 1-s epochs (24 seconds segment); continuing **DR** (at best a partial regression) despite far-reaching clinical remission after 6 weeks of combined treatment with imipramine and lithium (EEG-nr. 650/92).

No comparable research exists for the non-phasic forms of depression, also called neurotic-reactive. Our retrospective study (Ulrich & Brand, 1993) aimed at a systematization of the EEG-morphodynamics of inpatients with depressive syndromes. We considered the resting EEGs recorded routinely during the first week. All patients who were treated during a 3 year period were included in the study. Excluded were patients with diffuse dysrhythmia (**DD**) following electro-convulsive treatment and those who were treated with lithium.

AMDP-Item			EEG DR no	EEG DR yes	p
affective rigidity	≦ 51 y.	yes no	22 80	19 31	0,05
	> 51 y.	yes no	26 79	21 34	0,10
inhibited thinking	≦ 51 y.	yes no	23 79	19 31	0,06
	> 51 y.	yes no	25 82	21 34	0,07
retarded thinking	≦ 51 y.	yes no	36 58	28 30	n. s.
	> 51 y.	yes no	42 68	29 23	0,04
off drive	≦ 51 y.	yes no	56 46	37 13	0,03
	> 51 y.	yes no	60 47	40 15	0,04
disturbed memorization	≦ 51 y.	yes no	18 82	17 35	0,07
	> 51 y.	yes no	22 87	16 37	n. s.

Table 7. Bivariate frequency distribution of 14 inpatients with depressive syndromes divided according to the presence (yes) or non-presence (no) of a **DR** in the EEG on the one hand and specific AMDP-features on the other hand (the degree of intensity was not considered). An additional classification occurred based on the median age (x = 51 y.) calculated for the entire sample. p: Fisher-test, two-sided.

In about one-third of the patients (total n = 314), the EEG showed a **DR**. This **DR** was found significantly more often in the patients classified as endogenous (in 42%) than in patients classified as non-endogenous (in 20%; RDC-criteria, Spitzer et al., 1982). Furthermore, the **DR** appeared closely related to the psychomotorial axis symptom of retardation. The correlation of **DR** and endogeneity as well as of **DR** and psychomotor retardation appeared to be independent of age.

The definite answer to the important question of whether the **DR** observable in acutely depressive patients is state-dependent or state-independent must be based on a sufficient number of longitudinal observations. Such observations, however, are not yet available to us. Based on unsystematic opinion forming, as well as considering certain remarks in literature (Pollock & Schneider, 1989), we find both a state-dependence and a state-independence worth pondering. This means the **DR** could be a vulnerability indicator, already observable in the euthymic state ("trait marker"), of the manifestation of psychomotor-retarded endomorphic depressive symptoms. On the other hand, we could assume a phase-related accentuation of **DR** ("state marker"). The finding that (only or at least) half of the psychopathologically relative homogenous subgroups with an endomorphic clinical picture showed a **DR**, which again illustrated that a sample that is homogenous from the diagnostic point of view does not have to be homogenous from the pathophysiological point of view. We consider this an empirical proof for the "pathobiological heterogeneity" of psychopathologically homogenous samples postulated by Wexler (1991). The psychomotor retardation does indeed indicate a pathophysiological entity delimitated in several respects, as reflected by the favorable, though only temporary reaction of syndromes with psychomotor retardation to L-dopa (Goodwin et al., 1970; van Praag et al., 1975) or to dopamine-agonists (Post et al., 1978; Silberstein et al., 1981; Waehrens & Gerlach, 1981). When Diehl and Gershon (1992) viewed the depression characterized by psychomotor retardation as an "understudied depressive subtype" and pointed out the enormous theoretical significance of this finding, a renewed interest of the neurochemically oriented psychiatry in the aspect of retardation becomes evident (s.a., Bron & Lehman, 1990). The required clinical research certainly could advance considerably if we succeeded in finding the pathophysiological correlate of "psychomotor retardation" using a more refined operational definition of the clinical item. We regard the EEG-phenomenon of **DR** as a correlate that may also be expressed quantitatively. The EEG could be particularly useful for therapy planning in all those cases where the diagnosis of melancholia seems doubtful because of the relatively slight degree of observable depressiveness - depressio sine depressione (Schneider, 1959).

About one-third of the patients with depressive syndromes in a sample tested by van Praag (1962) called themselves not-depressed. Such patients, although not particularly because of low scores on the customary depression scales, easily remain undiagnosed and classified falsely as neurotic-reactive and thus receive inadequate treatment. The psychomotor retardation typically present in these cases usually manifests itself quite clearly in the non-verbal behavior. However, we must also expect to encounter cases where the retardation affects for the most part thinking; therefore, cannot be directly observed (Ebert, 1990). The discovery of a **DR** in the EEG can improve especially those cases. Our patient A.S. (Figs. 86, 87), in whom the triad of grief, anxiety, and guilt that are regarded typical for depression was hardly present, is an exemplary case.

A phase-related mental block was perceived as particularly worrysome. A personality disturbance as a differential diagnosis could be rejected thanks to the phase- and symptom-relatedness of the **DR** rather than the EEG. A **DR**, as state-related electroencephalographic manifestation of a pathological functional change (*Funktionswandel*), can also be associated with a pathological performance change (*Leistungswandel*). There is no doubt that such a pathological performance change, at least in the phasic cases, does indeed exist, as clearly objectivated in several studies (f. i., Cornell et al., 1984; Silberman et al., 1983;). This allows the formulation of the easily testable working hypothesis proposing that the intraindividually determined degree of a **DR** corresponds to the degree of the cognitive impairment or, in other words, is its objectivly measurable indicator. In other cases, a partial regression of the **DR** accompanies the clinical improvement (Fig. 87). However, in some patients, a change of the **DR** is not recognizable, at least in a visual evaluation, despite obvious clinical remission (Fig. 88). In an attempt to explain such inconsistencies, we must remember that a clinical improvement might just as well be the manifestation of a suppression of symptoms through medication as a naturally occuring remission of the depressive phase. This distinction is important because we cannot yet determine whether a dissolution of the **DR**, as documented in Figs. 86 and 87, is associated with the suppression of symptoms through medication or with the remission of the phase. Figs. 90 and 91 document the regression of a pronounced **DR** in a moderately retarded-depressive state during successful electro-convulsive therapy. As during pharmacological and sleep deprivation therapy, the success of the treatment manifests itself in only a number of the patients through an obvious regression of the **DR**. Additionally, number of patients whose EEG does not evidence any **DR** (in our sample about half of the patients) suffer clinically from endomorph depression and also show symptoms of retardation.

During electro-convulsive treatment, the EEG-changes usually do not occur after the first or second convulsion but only after entire treatment series. The degree of change can vary considerably from patient to patient, even with identical treatment, ranging from only a minor slowing of the dominant alpha-frequency to massive diffuse dysrhythmias of several weeks' duration. Without the assumption of a dispositional factor, which cannot be deduced from the preexisting baseline EEG, it is impossible to explain such variations.

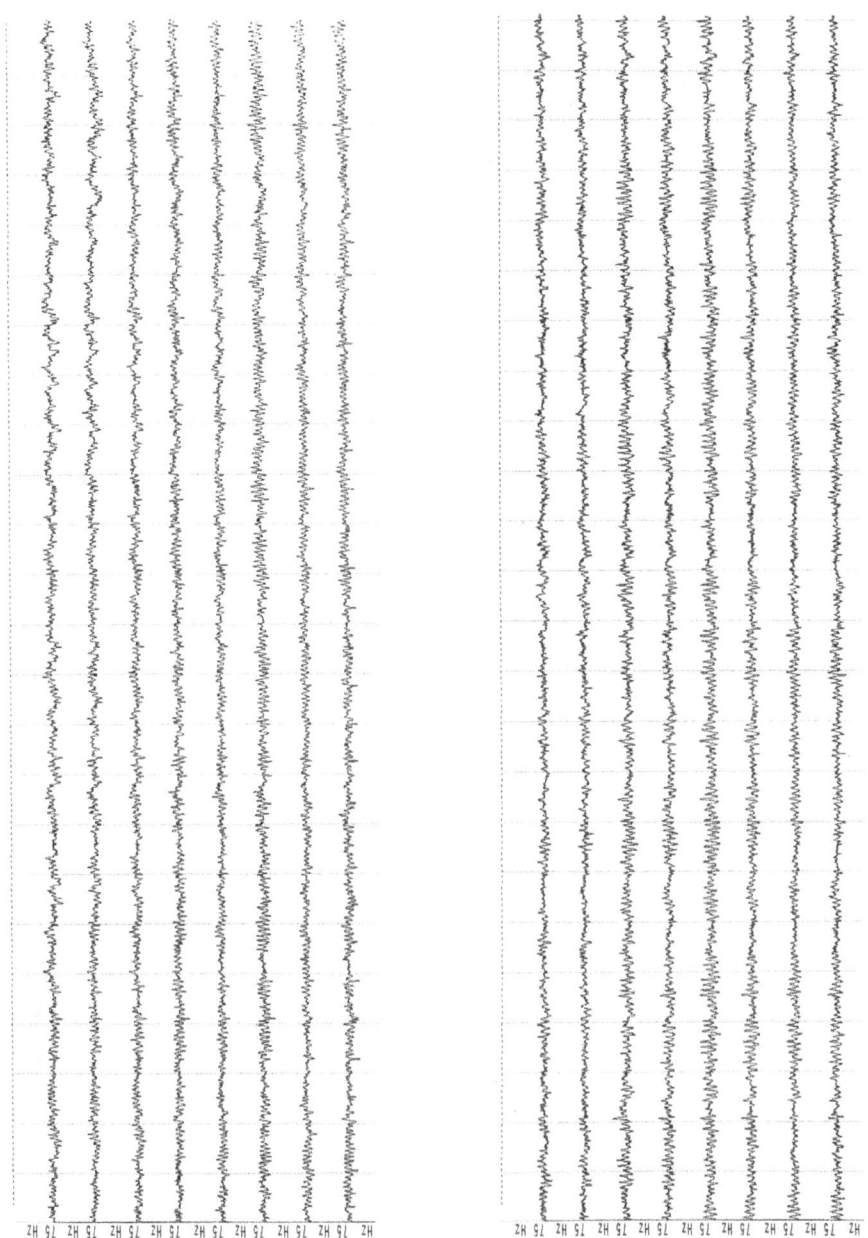

Figure 89. <u>Above</u>: 24 1-s epochs (24 seconds segment) medium degree anteriorized 10.5/s activity. Dynamic rigidity (**DR**). Retarded-depressive syndrom in bipolar affective psychosis - recorded at admittance with 75 mg/d amitriptyline. <u>Below</u>: 24 1-s epochs (24 seconds segment), no significant change in the degree of **DR** despite clinical remission after 8 weeks of antidepressive medication (in the end 150 mg/d clomipramine) (K. W., 54 y., m., EEG-nr. 87/92; EEG-nr. 157/92).

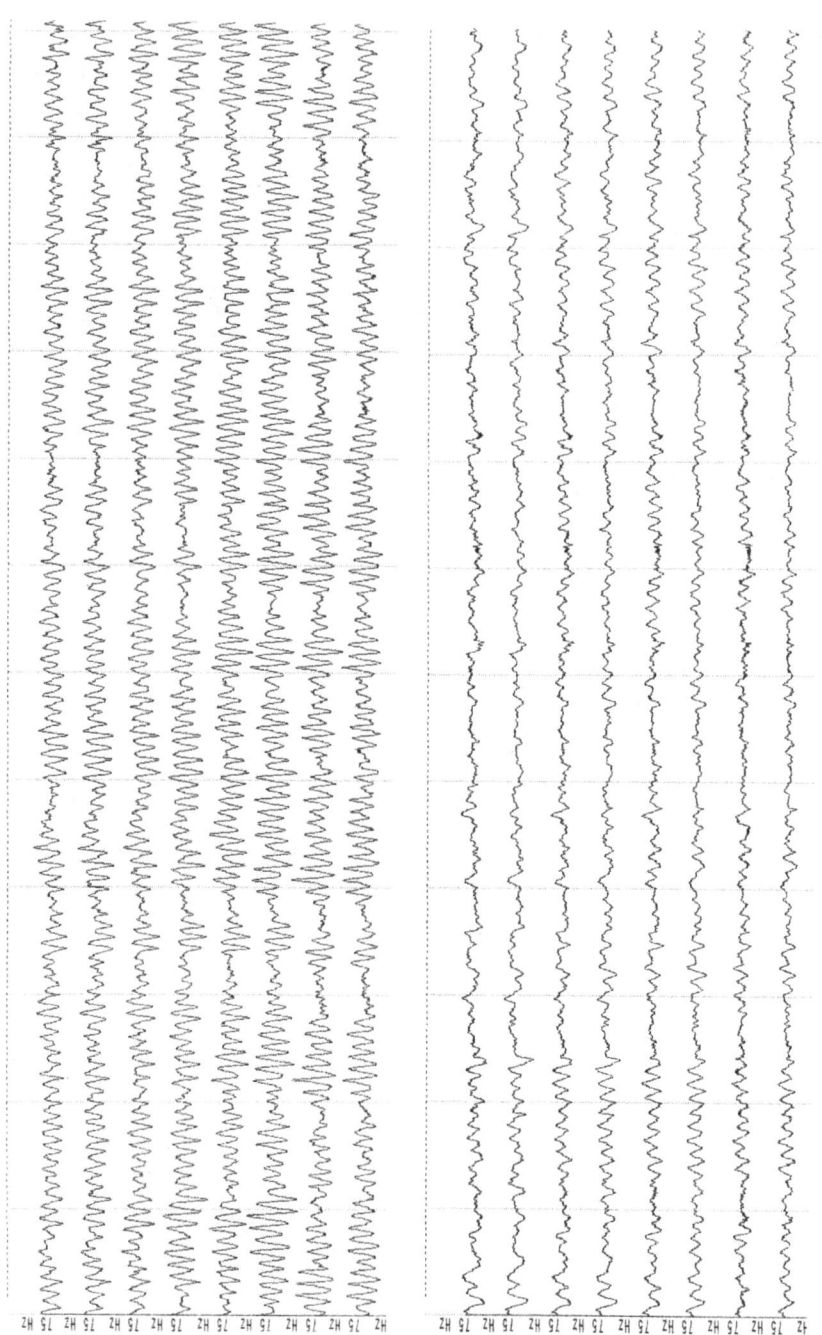

Figure 90. <u>Above</u>: 24 1-s epochs (24 second segment); continuous anteriorization of an obviously slightly slowed and monomorph 8.5/s activity; distinct **DR**; depressive syndrome (thymoleptics-resistent). <u>Below</u>: 24 1-s epochs (24 second segment); EEG after 5 electro-convulsive treatments, predominantly Diffuse Dysrhythmia (**DD**). Slight recovery from the depressive syndrome with discrete signs of an *exogenous reaction type* (mnestic disturbances) (T. K., 58 y., f., EEG-nr. 302/92; EEG-nr. 390/92).

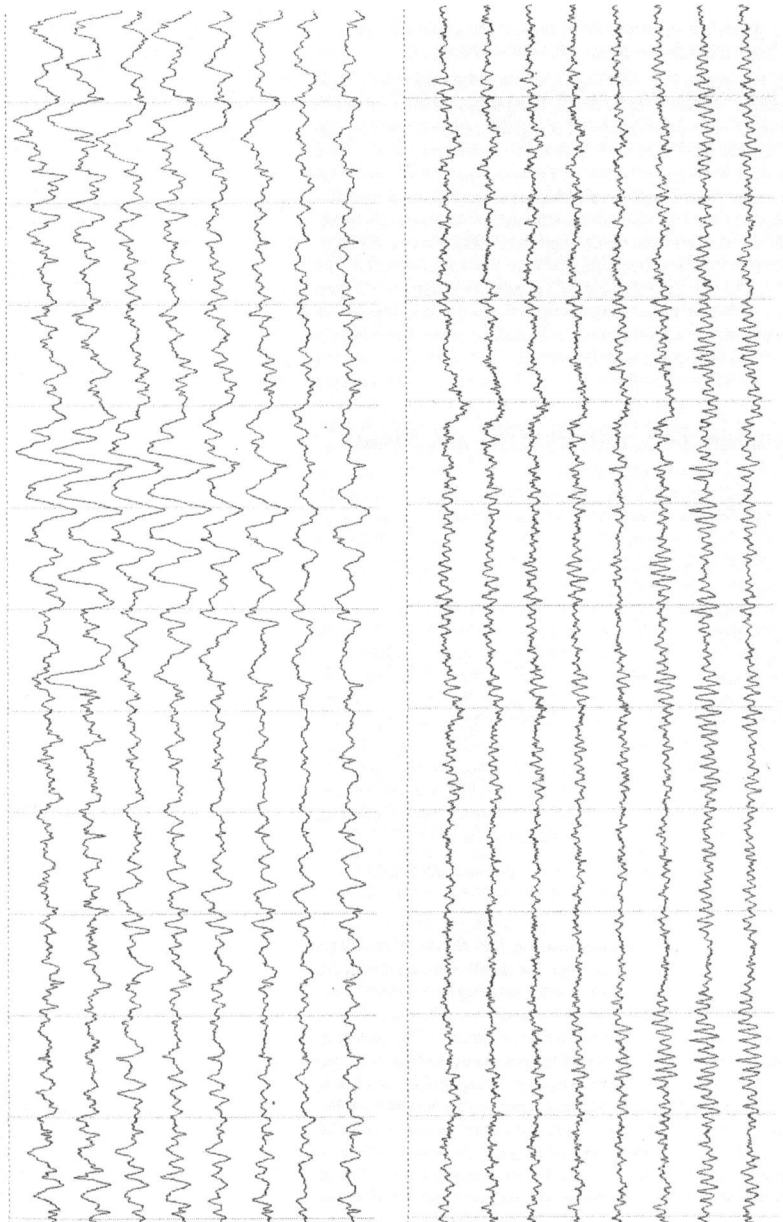

Figure 91. The same patient as in Fig. 90. Above: Distictly increased **DD** after 5 additional electro-convulsive treatments; continuing recovery of the depressive syndrome and increase of the mnestic disturbances; EEG-nr. 443/92). Below: 8 weeks after the termination of the electro-convulsive treatment under 75 mg/d clomipramine predominantly physiomorphic EEG with a posterior-accentuated alpha-activity of about 10.5/s; clinically essentially remitted, still some mnestic impairment (EEG-nr. 693/92).

It goes without saying that such case studies cannot replace statistically backed prospective studies as well as appropriate quantitative analyses. However, considering the situation of the psychiatric EEG today, it would help if these discussions inspired future researchers to trust their own eyes again and start paying attention to the phenomenon of the **DR** in connection with depressive syndromes. **DR,** with its close relation to the axis syndrome of psychomotor retardation, can be regarded as exemplary for the kind of EEG-phenomena to be expected with psychiatric disturbances. Far from being "disease-specific," such deviant EEG-"pictures" may also be observed in healthy persons, but generally with far less distinctiveness.

4. 8 Manic Syndromes and Lowered EEG-Vigilance

According to Perris (1980), we may find "*a higher incidence of unspecific abnormalities*" in maniacs. Such meaningless statements about the relationship between characteristics of the qualitatively assessed EEG and psychiatric syndromes can be viewed as representative -of today's state of knowledge. In addition, one may show a disregard for or even an ignorance of the existing few studies on the topic. Instead, we repeatedly encounter certain individual case studies and methodically questionable reports of earlier authors (for instance Harding et al., 1966; Hes, 1960; Hurst & Mundy-Castle, 1954;). The unreflected reproduction of incomplete quotes, for instance, the statement attributed to Davis (1940) that manias are characterized by frequency accelerations (Künkel, 1980), obviously without source study, may have promoted the proliferation of certain erroneous beliefs. For instance, the statement attributed to Davis (1940) that manias are characterized by frequency accelerations is incorrect (Künkel, 1980). Davis actually only pointed out the occurrence of faster frequency components in some of his patients during the transition from a depressive to a manic phase.

Judging from the description, this occurrence most likely corresponds to the "subvigil" beta-activity facultatively associated with the B1-stage. In contrast, not one contribution found in handbooks mentions that Davis (1940; 1941) emphasized manic syndromes in which EEG-correlate is a grouped, irregular, slow activity. Equally neglected were the findings by Greenblatt et al. (1944) that manias can be distinguished from depressions by a higher proportion of slow and a lower proportion of faster frequencies. The first systematic study by Liberson (1944) has remained widely unknown. Among all psychiatric patient groups, the maniacs had at 70% the highest proportion of EEGs with "drowsiness patterns". *Drowsiness patterns*, according to LIBERSON, are groups and sequences of irregular theta- and delta-activity. He also pointed out that in the EEG typical for manias, the *drowsiness patterns* already appeared at the beginning of the recording, contrary to the EEG of a healthy person under sleep deprivation. It took 16 years before Bonnet and Bonnet (1960) reevaluated and confirmed Liberson's findings. The majority of their patients in a state of acute mania evidenced frequent and abrupt transitions into phases of lower voltage of 5-10 seconds duration with embedded irregular waves, thus, in our terminology, a dynamic lability (**DL**).

During the phases of slow activity, the patients appeared quiet, but definitely not asleep. Upon the reappearance of the alpha-rhythm, as a rule, they showed signs of restlessness. After the treatment with neuroleptics over several days, the clinical recovery was paralleled by an increase in the continuity of the alpha-activity.

The authors thought it paradoxical that the untreated sleepless and acutely manic patients showed signs of drowsiness in the EEG, whereas the EEG recorded under high dosages of neuroleptics seemed to indicate a relatively higher degree of alertness. The objection that this is only the manifestation of the neuroleptics effect was countered by the observation that the subvigil activity phases were most pronounced in patients who received comparatively lower doses of neuroleptics. The interpretation that the subvigil activity is a manifestation of exhaustion in manic restlessness seems equally contestable to the authors.

Contrary to what would be expected in exhausted persons with a tendency to fall asleep, none of the maniacs fell asleep during the recording. Thus, the authors concluded that a mania or at least an important subtype, is associated with a disturbance of maintaining the physiological state of alertness. With this, they referred to Ey (1954) who rejected the popular opinion that the manic is lucid or even hyperlucid. According to Ey, acute mania is a "sommeil incomplet et épuisant, etalé a longeur de journée" (an interrupted and exhaustive sleep equivalent which spreads out the whole day) without the patient being able to find a deep and refreshing sleep. The mnestic deficits after complete remission indicated a disturbed consciousness during the acute manic phase.

The authors thought that the number of cases was insufficient to answer the interesting question whether manic syndromes with slow EEG-activity differ from those without.

Obviously ignorant of the work of Liberson (1944) and Bonnet and Bonnet (1960), Van Sweden (1980) reported two patients with acute mania in whose medication-free resting EEG beta-spindles, corresponding to the light sleep stage C, could be observed shortly after the beginning of the recording. The author emphasized that the patients had not felt tired, let alone fallen asleep. Despite high doses of neuroleptics, the EEG became normal after the completion of the clinical recovery. In our experience, EEGs with phases of slow activity in manics are, if not the rule, at least remarkably frequent.

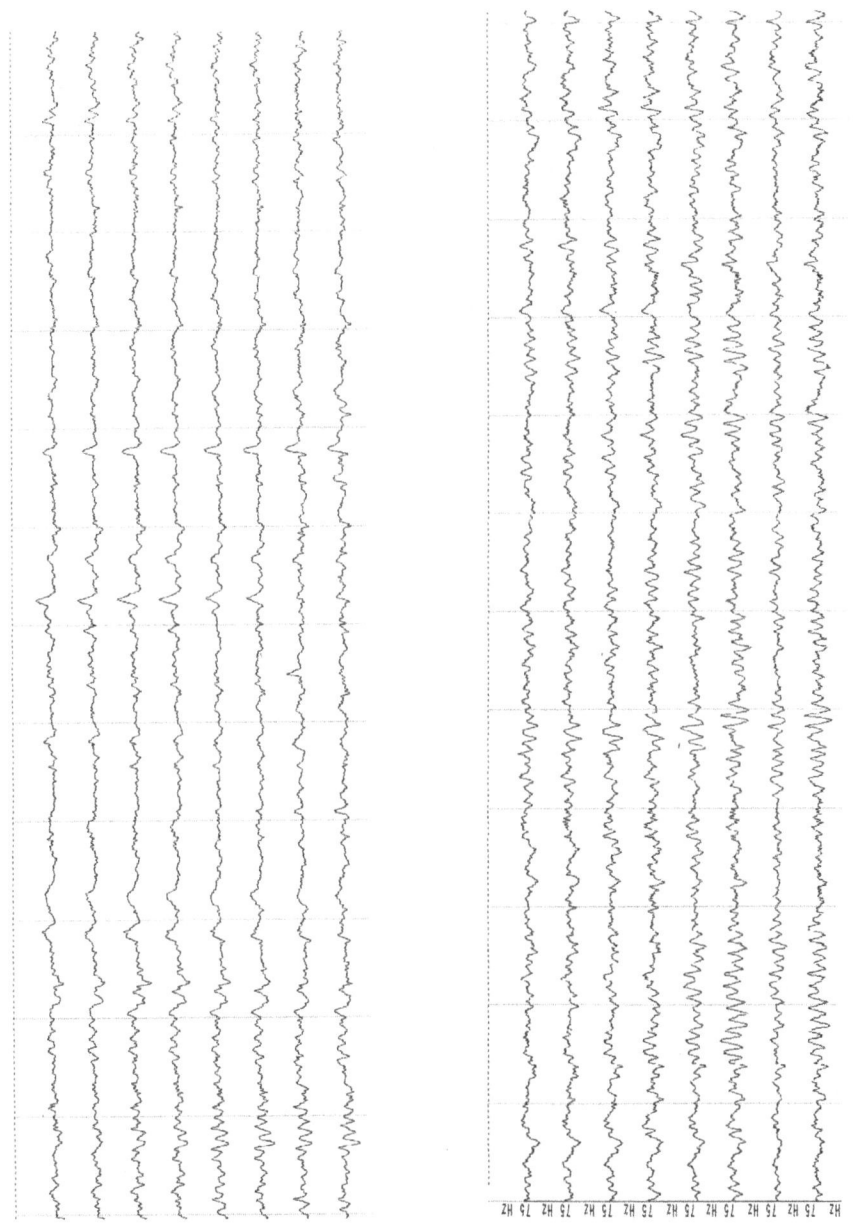

Figure 92. Manic syndrome in bipolar affective psychosis. 12 2-s-epochs (24 second segment. <u>Above</u>: Recording on the 3rd day after admission under 400 mg/d perazin; Dynamic lability (**DL**): abrupt transitions between A- and mid- to late B-stages until stage C; the sample was taken from the first recording minute. <u>Below</u>: regression of **DL** after 6 weeks of therapy (600 mg/d perazin and 600 mg/d carbamazepine, lithium-plasma level: 0.78 mmol/l; electrode placement: F3-A1, F4-A2, C3-A1, C4-A2, P3-A1, P4-A2, O1-A1, O2-A2) (G. S., 48 y., m., EEG-nr. 911/92; EEG-nr. 1090/92).

It is difficult to understand that a phenomenon as frequent and conspicuous has received so little attention thus far. One of the reasons is possibly that it cannot be observed in all manic syndromes and therefore cannot be called "specific." Nosologically unspecific phenomena, however, were and still are erroneously considered irrelevant and therefore ignored. Moreover, defining subvigil activity as mania-typical does not conform to the popular prejudice held by many psychiatrists that manic overactivity must correspond to a vigilance increase. To expand what doubtlessly remains far too narrow an empirical, we decided that the topics of EEG and mania would also benefit from a retrospective study of a greater number of patients (Ulrich & Sylla, 1993).

Included were all persons treated as inpatients in our hospital during a 5-year period whowere diagnosed with a manic syndrome at discharge and who also fulfilled the RDC-criteria of a mania (Spitzer et al., 1982). The few patients for whom no EEG was available and patients for whom more than a week had passed between the documentation of a clinical record and the recording of the EEG were excluded. As a control group, we chose sex-, age-, and medication-matched (chlorpromazine equivalent) patients with a dismissal diagnosis of paranoid-hallucinatory psychosis. The EEGs stored on microfiche were rendered anonymous by assistants and then, based on a catalogue of criteria, assigned by two interpreters independently to one of 5 categories (0 = no DL, 1 = minor DL, 2 = moderate DL, 3 = obvious DL, 4 = pronounced DL with lowered average vigilance level). The interrater reliability test resulted in a kappa = 0.91 ($p < 0.01$), which means that our evaluation mode is appropriate.

Table 8. Frequency distribution of the EEGs with non-present, minor and moderate DL (categories 0, 1, 2) as well as with obvious or pronounced DL (categories 3, 4) in a group comparison between maniacs (n = 101) and schizophrenics (n = 101) with and without indication of sex.

		Maniacs	Schizophrenics	
♀ + ♂	DL 0, 1, 2	79	90	$p < 0{,}03$
	DL 3, 4	22	11	
♂	DL 0, 1, 2	32	42	$p < 0{,}01$
	DL 3, 4	15	5	
♀	DL 0, 1, 2	47	48	n. s.
	DL 3, 4	7	6	

Our sample included 101 patients, 60 of whom suffered from a mania related to an affective psychosis and 41 from a mania related to a schizo-affective psychosis. Of the 101 patients included in our sample, 54 were female (average age = 37, ± 9.2 years) and 47 male (average age 36 ± 8.7 years). To test the hypothesis that **DL**, especially together with a lowered mean vigilance level, is a mania-typical phenomenon, we arranged our frequency data in a table (Table 7). For this purpose we grouped together EEG-categories 0, 1, and 2 (no, minor and moderate **DL**) on the one hand and 3 and 4 (obvious and pronounced **DL** associated with lowered average vigilance level) on the other hand.

As shown in Table 6, the more pronounced forms of **DL** (categories 3 and 4) are overrepresented in the manics compared to the schizophrenics, as claimed in our hypothesis (Fisher-test, $p < 0.03$, one-sided). To our surprise, however, we discovered after considering the distribution by sex that the manic males were solely responsible for the group differences. While the manic men presented more pronounced forms of **DL** (categories 3 and 4) considerably more often compared to the schizophrenic men ($p < 0.01$), the manic women did not differ from the schizophrenic women.

4.9 Schizophrenic Psychoses

"The hope to find the physiopathological substrate of the schizophrenic process and the passion to search for it should not falter because of the multitude of failures" (Conrad, 1958, p. 140, transl. from German).

The actuality of this demand, marked by a genuine desire to learn and discover, has not faded since. However, the study of medical literature increasingly conveys the impression that the methodically ever more diversified research runs the risk of losing its original, psychopathologically determined topic. However what could evoke the passion for research demanded by Conrad if not this topic, which can be experienced with the senses and defined through differentiated psychopathological efforts? The method-centered way of doing things for the sake of doing things, which is accompanied by a contempt for methodological-conceptual aspects, has provided, particularly in electroencephalographic schizophrenia research, a plentitude of useless and uninterpretable data. Those who try to gain a quick overview of the present state of knowledge through some summary are confronted with lists of findings collected in a primarily quantitative way from groups of schizophrenic patients who were diagnosed following only a certain schema. The target variables have been, for approximately two decades and nearly exclusively, frequency band parameters obtained through spectral analysis and averaged across the entire recording time and across all patients. Such findings are, for a number of reasons still to be discussed, of only limited value. The following quote exemplifies this:

"Schizophrenics reveal more delta, theta, and fast beta activity, and less fast alpha and slow beta waves than normals ..." (ITIL et al. 1972).

Such a statement suggests that a disease called schizophrenia exists also as an pathophysiologically defined entity and that the power-spectral characteristic is **specific** to it. Most writings do not mention the interindividual variability of psychopathological pictures at different times of recording. In most cases, we are also kept in the dark as to whether the findings are considered *state-* or *trait-*features, let alone what they actually mean. The absolute methodological low is reached, in our opinion, in recent work where the colorful topographical depiction of spectral parameters - so-called EEG-mapping - averaged across the total recording time and the total patient sample is considered a contribution to scientific knowledge.

In findings obtained by spectral analysis, only a beta-power increase in comparison to healthy people seems worth discussing, since quite a number of researchers agree on this point (f. i., Bernstein et al., 1981;Giannitrapani & Kayton, 1974; Itil et al., 1972; Itil, 1977; Kemali et al., 1981; Vacca et al., 1980). An attempt for interpretation requires, in our view, a decision about whether we are dealing with a *state-* characteristic indicative of the acuity of the disorder or with a *trait*-characteristic that exists independent thereof, thus possibly indicating a certain disposition for the disease. As far as we can see, this question has not yet been answered. Regardless, the beta-increase has been interpreted as a manifestation of "hyperarousal" (Itil et al., 1977) as well as of "hypoarousal" (Giannitrapani & Kayton, 1974). The objection that the data do not justify such interpretations was raised correctly (Künkel, 1975; Koukkou-Lehmann, 1987). If we tried to reconstruct the quantitatively measured increased beta-power visuo-morphologically, we immediately think of the picture of a low-voltage desynchronized EEG with variably pronounced fast activity (**DL**). Davis (1939;1942) regarded such organizational type - which she called *choppy activity* (Fig. 40) - as typical for schizophrenia more than half a century ago. She viewed *choppy activity* prognostically as a rather unfavourable and *state*-related sign of *overstimulation or irritation* of the cortex.

Agreeing with the neurophysiological interpretation, Davis et al. (1975) considered "*choppy activity*" or "*low voltage desynchronized fast EEG pattern*" a *trait*-feature that revealed a disposition for schizophrenia. They speculated that it should be possible to prevent the manifestation of schizophrenia in predisposed individuals by using neuroleptics to reduce the hyperarousal corresponding to an alpha-activation. Furthermore, a widely confirmed finding suggests a decreased variability of the voltage values as determined by successive time intervals being integrated over the total frequency spectrum (Goldstein et al., 1963, 1965; Goldstein & Sugarman, 1969; Lifshitz & Gradijan, 1972; Marjerrison et al., 1967; Shagass, 1976; Shagass et al., 1982; Sugarman et al., 1964). Regarding available clinical data, this was typically found with chronic schizophrenics. With the increased beta-power, the question about *state* and *trait* cannot be answered here clearly, either. Here, too, a hypoarousal interpretation confronts the hyperarousal interpretation defended by the majority (Lifshitz & Gradijan, 1972). According to Goldstein (1983), the hypovariability of the voltage integral constitutes a *trait*-feature, since repeated measuring after weeks or months showed a high stability of this feature, as opposed to those without hypovariability. This evaluation, however, appears to contradict earlier findings by the same working group claiming that the variability of the voltage integral increases with clinical recovery

(Goldstein et al., 1965; Sugarman et al., 1964). Interestingly, a clear decrease in variability was found in healthy persons on amphetamines (Murphee et al., 1962) or LSD (Goldstein et al., 1963; Sugarman et al., 1973). In chronic schizophrenics, on the other hand, LSD led to an increase in variability (Goldstein et al., 1963).

While the limitations of the then available methods can easily explain the failure of psychophysiological schizophrenia research mentioned by Conrad (1958; 1959), the failure today paradoxically occurs from the almost unlimited availability of technologies continuously developed at dazzling speed. The failure is the logical consequence of the undisputable fact that the research conducted today is centered around methods instead of being guided by a theory. We refer to this repeatedly mentioned deplorable state of affairs again, among other reasons, to make it quite clear the EEG as a research tool of supposedly little value cannot be blamed for the scarceness of the results gathered after half a century of costly research. Electroencephalographic schizophrenia research today requires, even more than all other areas of the psychiatric EEG, a reevaluation of the methodological preconditions for a meaningful use of the available technological potential. Resuming our arguments from the chapter on EEG and Psychiatry (3.4.8), we would like to define the only methodological framework within which EEG studies seem meaningful using the following premises:

- The different psychopathological pictures termed schizophrenic correspond to a "Pathologischer Leistungswandel" (pathological change of performance), which corresponds more or less to a "Pathologischer Funktionswandel" (pathological change of function).

- Spontaneous Resting-EEG reveals a uniform pathophysiological disintegrative process, which proceeds in a lawful manner and is potentially reversible.

- Within this pathophysiological process, electroencephalographically characterized dissolution stages can be deliminated.

- The process shows, with regard to its dynamics, a great inter- and intraindividual variability and can, at each level, come to a standstill, persist or more or less remit.

Since every sample, even under strict observance of the usual operational clinical inclusion criteria, must always be pathophysiologically heterogeneous due to the dynamic character of the schizophrenic process, the customary, primarily group-statistical research designs are of only dubious value. A possible alternative could be, as Huber (1974) already demanded, individual longitudinal analyses. Regularities will only be deduceable from a sufficiently large number of single case studies. That this alternative research strategy still causes so many problems cannot be explained merely by force of habit. Another reason is possibly that the biological variability, in our view the proper topic of research, is viewed from a purely statistical point of view as some kind of variance by errors of measurement whose effect can be minimized by choosing the largest possible sample.

Demanding individual longitudinal analyses, however, makes sense only if there is a clear concept about which variables are relevant from the perspective of both psychopathology and EEG. We are faced here with the task of not just accepting in toto the usual standardized listing of features, but also examining critically whether the listed features actually have any bearing on the specific problem. We certainly cannot be satisfied with a collective description by means of a catalogue agreed upon by convention. A distinction according to their pathophysiological meaning as indicators for specific dissolution stages of the schizophrenic process can only be accomplished from a higher point of view, i.e., through a theory. We would like to add to Koukkou-Lehmann's (1987) suggestion to correlate syndromes or symptoms instead of nosological terms with the EEG by stating that each kind of correlation needs to be guided by theory. Since we are dealing here with the correlation of two logically incommensurable description levels, theories that only apply to one of the two domains are inadequate. Required instead is a superimposed biological theory of higher general validity that encompasses both areas and allows a logical basis for correlating psychopathology and EEG. We refer here especially to chapter 3.4.3.

From a biometrical point of view, it is absolutely necessary to limit the number of features to be correlated; the psychopathological records of the AMDP-documentation includes no less than 100 items. The adjustment of the significance level required by multiple testing promotes the risk of false-negative results.

A discussion of the methodological conditions also clarified the boundaries of what is possible. First, we will have to accept that there hardly ever will be a premorbid EEG available for comparison. An EEG recorded during the remission stage is an insufficient substitute because there, generally, a more or less pronounced residual functional deficit must be assumed. The second unavoidable restriction results from the often mandatory treatment with psychotropic drugs. Since that which can be expected from the EEG is the result of a dynamic interaction between the effect of psychotropic drugs and the psychopathological process, we can draw only indirect conclusions about the process dynamics we are actually interested in. This also clarifies, which questions can be answered and therefore can logically be asked. Since recently, the opinion that there exist no "schizophrenia-specific" EEG-phenomena seems to gather wide support. Overall, we need to consider essentially three problem areas:

- Are there any correlations between changes in the psychopathology and changes in the EEG during the course of the disease and if so, what are they?
- Does the EEG recorded from a medication-free patient at the beginning of the treatment or the EEG derived after administering a test dose of neuroleptics give any indications about the prognosis or the response to neuroleptics?
- Can any state-unrelated features be defined that could be considered vulnerability indicators (*trait*-features)?

The findings available to address the first problem area date back to the 1960s and 1970s. According to Huber and Penin (1968), untreated schizophrenics with psychopathological signs of a process activity showed a higher number of so-called *parenrhythmias* (Table 2), corresponding to our pathomorphic variants of the A-stage, which we related to a pathological functional change (**IBA**, 4.1). As signs of a process activity, they considered disturbed coenaesthesia, delusional mood, and hallucinations. In remitted schizophrenics, i.e., in those without process activity on the other hand, the EEG was mostly normal. Huber and Penin's findings were confirmed to a certain degree by Iserman (1973) whoemphasized, without touching on the question of acuity, that the bilateral synchronous theta- and delta-groups to which her referred to as *paroxysmal dysrhythmias* are a "disease-specific" phenomenon and are not caused by neuroleptics. The *paroxysmal dysrhythmia* was also the core of interest in a study by Helmchen (1968). *Paroxysmal dysrhythmia* and *parenrhythmia* seemed to have the same meaning for Helmchen. Contrary to Huber and Penin and to Isermann who focused only on the EEG recorded at the beginning of the treatment, Helmchen conducted systematic longitudinal studies under largely standardized neuroleptics medication. To our knowledge, this study wsa the only one to comply with this methodological desideratum. Helmchen found that an accumulation of more or less rhythmic slow waves of high amplitude, corresponding to our IBA-phenomenon according to the and curve examples, accompanies and follows closely the disappearing of delusional mood/delusional perceptions.

Concerning Conrad's (1958) subtle gestalt analysis of the development of schizophrenic delusion, comprising delusional mood and delusional perceptions, as done by Helmchen, seems worth pondering. "Delusional mood" (*Wahnstimmung*) in the sense of Jaspers' (1946) definition is only a prodrome of developing delusion, according to Conrad. Pathognostically, however, this phase, also called *trema*, is very ambiguous. One can talk about a schizophrenic process only after the onset of an initially still diffuse abnormal sense of the meaning of things. Concrete delusional perceptions in the proper sense would be typical for an even later stage. Thus, *delusional mood* and *delusional perceptions* are also likely to mark pathophysiologically distinguished phases of the disease. This should be taken into account in replication studies.

A similar, though less close relationship, was found between the subsidence of hallucinations and the appearance of **IBA**. However, no relationship between the item *delusion* and the EEG was observed. As Helmchen (1968) emphasized, no relationship with the EEG could be found without considering the clinical longitudinal profile. Helmchen came close in his interpretation to Baeyer (1951) who, in order to explain the therapeutic electro-shock effect, coined the formulation of "not-be-available- any- longer" (*Nicht-Mehr-Haben-Können*) of the psychosis because of the induced massive brain-organic functional disturbance. In a later work, however, (Helmchen, 1975) considered a "temporary functional disturbance" as the correlate of an acute psychosis. The contradiction that the subsidence of the psychosis at one time is associated with a "pathologization" (Helmchen, 1968) and the next time with a "normalization" (Huber & Penin, 1968) of the EEG, which Helmchen (1975) believed was unresolved, seems to us quite solvable. First, we want to state that the findings collected by Huber and Penin (1968) in medication-free patients fully agree with our theoretical premises. On the one hand, these findings support the concept of psychiatry in which the various clinical pictures are associated with various mental dissolution levels. On the other hand, *parenrhythmias* or *paroxysmal dysrhythmias*, as pathomorphic variants of the A-stage (**IBA**) indicate a very specific disintegration level of the global brain function CGF (see Fig. 43) that apparently can be reached or passed during an acute schizophrenic episode. Under the plausible assumption of cyclic process dynamics governed by their own laws, **IBA** marks the turning point from the disintegrative to the reintegrative phase. From Selbach's (1976) regulation-theoretical point of view, we could postulate that reaching a certain desintegration level, as indicated by **IBA**, constitutes the precondition for an initiation of the spontaneous remission. Therefore, **IBA** is an indicator of a currently existing, relatively advanced schizophrenic disintegration as well as of an imminent remission.

The observation that the EEG-phenomenon is very often accompanied by clinical pictures of catatonic behavior supports that **IBA** indeed constitutes the correlate of a far progressed disintegration (Rowntree, 1952; Hill, 1957). As supported by all studies, **IBA** is a fleeting, usually only briefly observable phenomenon. Therefore, it would be difficult, if not impossible, to offer a psychopathologically exact picture of the transition from the disintegrative to the reintegrative phase. This methodological problem supplies a plausible explanation for the seemingly contradictory findings by Helmchen (1968) on the one hand and Huber and Penin (1968) on the other. Helmchen's findings were confirmed in a study by Koshino et al. (1993). Apparently unaware of the findings obtained 25 years earlier, the authors reported a significant decrease in the distinctiveness of schizophrenic symptomatology at the occurrence of FIRDA (s.a. Table 2), a phenomenon subsumed under **IBA**.

Therefore, in cases where this specific disintegration level is not reached because of only minor process dynamics, the precondition for a spontaneous remission is also lacking. Instead, we must expect the development of a chronic state, which is exactly what everyday clinical practice teaches us. The antipsychotic effect of neuroleptics therefore could be that, because of their central-disintegrative ("dampening") effect, they create the precondition for a spontaneous rebound-like reorganization (Bente, 1963). This would be true for all cases in which the critical disintegration level, as indicated by **IBA**, is not reached spontaneously. In our opinion, the assumption that a lowering of the central-nervous functional level is the precondition for a spontaneously occurring functional reorganization is supported, not in the last place, by the passing character of the EEG-phenomena, since generally no further evidence for **IBA** exists after remission. Based on the individually existing spontaneous dynamics of the pathophysiological process, we can postulate a continuum that starts with the rather rare patients who after the highest possible clinical acuity (catatonia!) experience a relatively speedy and complete remission even without neuroleptics, which then continues with most frequent occurring cases who recover with the help of neuroleptics within a few weeks, and finally concludes with patients who even after long-term and high-dose medication seem to be neuroleptics non-responders. We must assume that the patients in the middle category were responsible for the results in Helmchen's study. This interpretation also conforms to the often-confirmed impression that a neuroleptics-induced pathologization of the EEG represents a clinically favorable sign (f. i., Bente, 1963; Dasberg & Robinson, 1971; Koukkou-Lehmann et al., 1979, 1983). That in Helmchen's study disturbed thinking and delusion appeared to be independent from a pathologization of the EEG is not surprising, since these features are signs of chronicity rather than acuity.

The assumed differences in the spontaneous dynamics of the pathophysiological process lead to our second problem area. It has long been known that the medication-free recorded EEG provides some prognostic clues. A well-pronounced, continuous, monomorphic alpha-background activity, possibly even spreading to the frontal regions, - according to the descriptions corresponding to the picture of our dynamic rigidity (**DR**) - is generally considered a negative sign. On the other hand, an essentially low-voltage EEG with only discontinuously occurring short alpha-groups and a more or less distinct higher proportion of fast subvigil Beta waves (see above, Davis' *'choppy activity'*), corresponding to the picture of Dynamic Lability (**DL**), is considered a positive sign (Bente, 1963; Helmchen & Künkel, 1964; Igert & Lairy, 1962; Itil et al., 1966, 1975; Small & Stern, 1965).

We pointed out earlier that the EEG-phenomena of dynamic rigidity (**DR**), dynamic lability (**DL**), and the pathomorph variants of the A-stage (**IBA/ILA**) associated with a pathological functional change can also be observed in healthy persons. The same is true for patients in remission. In that case, we talk about constitution-related variants that remind us of a functional brain maturation deficit. We must remember here that such variants of course also vary according to the spontaneous cycle dynamics, i.e., they manifest themselves only during a spontaneous or pharmacologic lowering of the vigilance level. When we say state-unrelated, we mean a relative unrelatedness from the psychopathological state. However, strictly spoken, this definition, too, is rather weak, since in most cases, the comparison with the premorbid state is impossible. Moreover, once a psychosis has been diagnosed, the assessment of a psychosis-free interval is shaky. A stable remission phase indicates a minor process activity. Since each outburst encounters a changed structure, there is also no remission or residual state that is identical to a previous one. Therefore, difficulties with the interpretation do not arise only for the above-mentioned peculiarities, but also for a seemingly ideally typical patient-EEG with, for instance, a continuous posterior-dominated 9/s background activity. Such an EEG can very well be the manifestation of a low-level functional change, like in the case of a premorbid frequency of the background activity of 11/s.

As for the rest it seems to be obvious that the *choppy activity* (or beta-increase) considered typical for schizophrenics results from a higher proportion of subjects with constitution-related dynamic lability (**DL**). It certainly is a serious flaw that we know next to nothing about the different composition that can be assumed for samples of schizophrenics on the one hand and of healthy persons on the other hand with regard to constitution-related EEG-variants (Table 3). Such knowledge, however, would be one of several indispensible conditions to justify the effort and expense usually associated with group-statistical comparisons between schizophrenics and healthy persons. Since this has not been clarified, it is possible that the discovered differences between groups of psychiatric patients or specific psychiatric groupings and healthy persons are not the result of a disease-specific pathophysiology but of group differences with regard to the proportion of constitution-related EEG-variants. On the contrary, this has to be considered as rather probable.

4.10 Epileptic Psychoses

The psychological disturbances accompanying epilepsy presented a specific challenge for neurology and psychiatry from the beginning. The symptomatology of these syndromes playing in different colors and thereby obscuring the artificially erected boundaries between the organic and the endogenous has always been an inspiration for psychiatric theory formulation. An enormous leap in knowledge is owed to the use of the EEG. On the other hand, the institutional separation of neurology and psychiatry was an impediment. The psychosyndromes under discussion raise differential-diagnostic difficulties that can only be conquered by subtle psychopathological analysis. Epileptology has established itself unequivocally as a neurological discipline.

However, for some of today's psychiatric clinicians, epileptic psychoses that they see only rarely are a sealed book. This is evidenced also by the helplessness in defining concrete problem areas to be addressed during the EEG-examination. An always vividly discussed question of particular interest for the psychiatrist is whether an epileptic psychosis can be diagnosed even if there has never been any evidence of epileptic seizures. Generally, we must answer affirmatively (Bash, 1969; Firnhaber & Ardjomandi, 1968; Gruhle, 1936; Kraepelin, 1919; Wagner, 1969; Wolf 1976). However, due to the risk of an uncritical expansion of the diagnosis of "epileptic equivalents", we must here apply the strictest criteria. Of particular importance is that the decision is under no circumstances left alone to the collegue who is responsible for EEG assessments. She/he ideally may be an experienced physician but will as a rule not have contact with the patient when assessing his EEG.

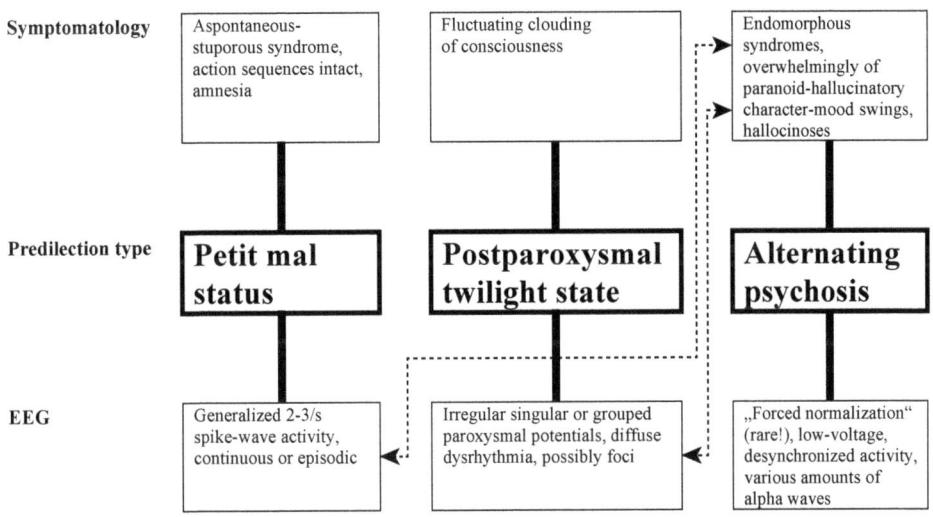

Figure 93. Clinical- and EEG-criteria for the definition of the main types of epileptic psychoses

Since a one-on-one association of syndrome-typical - and of EEG - characteristics does not exist, a diagnosis based solely on the EEG is impossible.

To immediately counter any objections expected here, we hasten to point to the rule-confirming exception, the petit mal status. In the case of continuous generalized regular 2-3/s spike- and slow-wave activity, a clinical diagnosis can indeed be formulated based on the EEG with a high degree of certainty. However, one and the same EEG-picture can be associated with rather different levels of severity of the syndrome (Dongier, 1967). As with each classification of psychiatric syndromes, here, too, we cannot arrive at a sharp delineation of clearly defined units. Such classifications can only be justified by virtue of their categorizing, order-creating function.

The form of acute epileptic psychoses in all likelihood most frequently takes the form of the postparoxysmal twilight state, typically after a grand mal status.

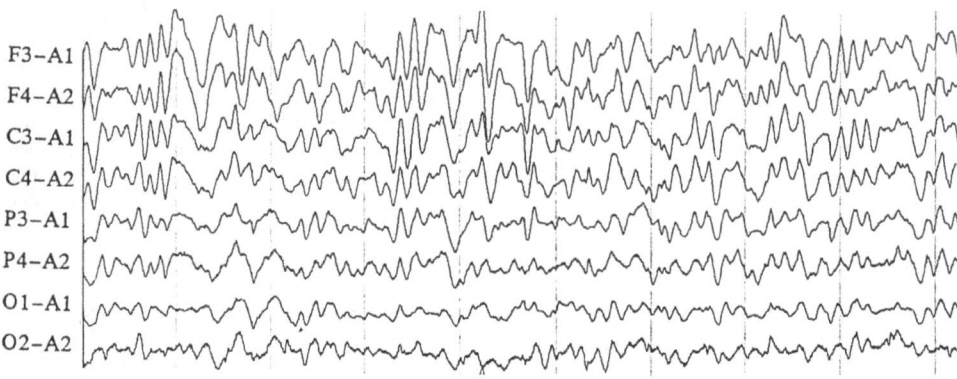

Figure 94. Diffuse-dysrhythmic EEG with anterior-accentuated sharp waves in connection with slower ones during the postparoxysmal twilight state. Recording approximately 6 hours after a nocturnal grand mal (K. K., 67 y., m., EEG-nr. 227/89).

Wolf (1976) associated a generally observed frequency decrease with the availability of increasingly more powerful anti-epileptic medication. As a rule of thumb, we can assume that the severity of the postparoxysmal twilight states corresponds to the severity and frequency of the previously suffered seizures. Clinically, a pronounced brain-organic symptomatology is often prominent. Frequently, it is accompanied by motor phenomena, such as abortive actions and stereotypical movements. The spontaneous remission occurs over a period of 2-3 weeks. The EEG typically shows a diffuse, mostly anterior-dominated dysrhythmia in connection with "postparoxysmal after-discharges" (Fig. 94). Although the patients normally evidence the axis symptom of disturbed orientation, forms with predominant paranoid-hallucinatory symptomatology also exist. Sometimes, lucid phases alternate with twilight states (De Haas & Magnus, 1958; Dongier, 1959; Ey, 1963; Helmchen, 1975; Janzarik, 1955; Kraepelink, 1919; Landolt, 1960). However, there is no evidence that the EEG shows the alternating per se or the actual severity level of the psychosis. On the other hand, EEGs with massive changes of the described kind without a clinically definable twilight state of whatever kind also exist. If there have been no seizures in the recent past and yet the EEG shows very distinct changes, we must consider a possible intoxication with anti-epileptic medicaton. Recent literature suggests the possibility that an acute postictal psychosis, which is clearly distinguishable in its appearance from the postparoxysmal twilight state, exists (Logsdail & Toone, 1988; So et al., 1990). In clear sensorium patients, a schizophreniform syndrome with symptoms of delusion and hallucinations manifests itself after a symptom-free interval following the seizures. In most cases, this picture lasts only a few days but in rare instances, it can be observed over several weeks. A typical EEG-correlate has temporal spikes. From the differential-diagnostic point of view, we must consider especially a state of complex-partial seizures (status psychomotoricus). The most distinctive difference is the lack of a clouded consciousness. Whether the "autochthonous twilight states", i.e., those that are unrelated to a seizure time-wise and are not caused by intoxication, which are occasionally discussed in a forensic-psychiatric context, actually exist seems rather doubtful. If we are faced with a clinically evident twilight state while the EEG does not indicate any changes, we must consider an "alternative psychosis" (see below). The differential-diagnostic significance of the EEG is, as previously remarked, greatest for the petit mal status or the Lennox-syndrome.

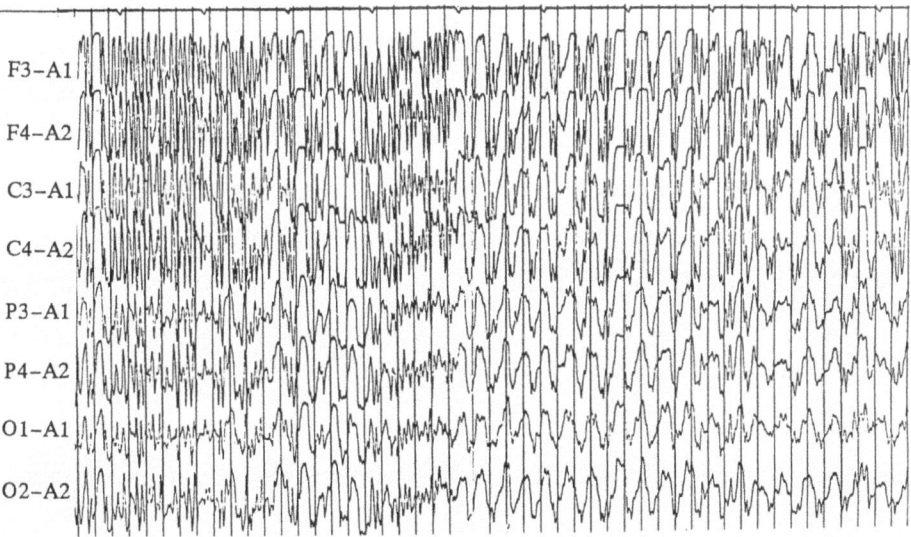

Figure 95. Continuous and generalized spike-wave activity of variable frequency in a petit mal status since 3 h; finally terminated by clonazepam injection (H. J., 41 y., m., EEG-nr. 115/88)

Clinically, this is a aspontaneous-stuporous picture with mostly massive impairment of cognitive-adaptive or communicative performances. This is contrasted by a largely maintained ability to perform automatic actions. An activity that starts before seizure onset, even reading and writing, is continued in a more or less meaningful way. At the same time, the patients are unable to give reasonable answers to questions. It has been pointed out on several occasions that there also are states without recognizable psychic changes that can clearly be diagnosed electroencephalographically (Dongier, 1967; Landolt, 1955). Petit mal status with a prevailing paranoid-hallucinatory picture is extremely rare (Andermann & Robb, 1972; Prüll, 1976). Nevertheless, we mention them because these cases confirm once more the impossibility of a complete reduction of the psychopathology to the EEG and vice versa. A petit mal status can continue for hours, days, even weeks. Besides the prototypical continuous generalized rhythmic spike and slow-wave activity discussed previously, we also find discontinuous sequences of such activities in the EEG. A psychiatrist should be familiar with the clinical and electroencephalographic indicators of a petit mal status not just because this often is the only form of manifestation of an epilepsy, but because he might be the first one to be confronted with such patients.

The third main group, that of the "schizophreniform psychoses," *alternative psychoses* or also chronic interictal psychoses is clinically characterized by a paranoid-hallucinatory symptomatology without major intellectual deficits. These, too, may last for days or weeks. A hebephrenic or catatonic symptomatology is considered absolutely atypical (Janz, 1969; Köhler, 1975; Slater et al., 1963; Tellenbach, 1966). A feature difference with endogenous schizophrenia is that the patient can at all times report in a distanced way his or her delusional experiences. This ability of "double-sided accounting" ("doppelte Buchführung", Janzarik, 1955), which implies that the patients can literally be talked out of their delusions and that a systematization of the madness usually does not occur, can be considered as almost pathognomonic. With regard to Conrad's (1958) gestalt analysis of the development of schizophrenic delusion, we can state that contrary to endogenous schizophrenias, the delusion here remains related to the environment. Since the inner world or the EGO is not touched, *anastrophé* does not occur. This parallels the early stage or the minor forms of the developing endogenous-schizophrenic delusion during which the possibility of the reflective crossing from not-EGO to EGO and thus of a distancing from the delusion is also maintained. Since the patient does not go through the subsequent *apophenic* (*apophäne*) stage, he also does not reach the *apocalyptic* stage characterized by catatonic symptomatology. The initiation of the actual psychosis by a phenomenologically similar preliminary syndrome is common to both the endogenous and epileptic syndromes. In both cases, we find a delusional mood in the sense that "something threatening is in the air" (Janzarik, 1955).

Landolt (1955) was the first one to point out that the pre-existing paroxysmal potentials occurring during seizure-intervals as well as dysrhythmias disappear during psychoses of this kind. He coined the term *forced normalization* of the EEG to label this phenomenon. Today, after extensive research, we can assume that although *forced normalization* does exist, it is the exception rather than the rule (f. i., Rodin, 1970; Köhler, 1975).

According to Rodin (1970), "schizophreniform" psychoses can be associated far more frequently with a low-voltage desynchronized EEG than with an alpha-typical one, as postulated by Landolt (1957). The numerous observations that "schizophreniform" psychoses are possible also if a "pathological" EEG exists (f. i., Firnhaber & Ardjomandi, 1968; Grüneberg & Helmchen, 1969; Köhler, 1975) further revitalize Landolt's concept. However, the existence of a reciprocal relationship between the EEG and psychopathology, i.e., between seizures and psychosis was confirmed without any reservation. Tellenbach (1965) called these *alternative psychoses* instead of seizure occurring syndromes. It takes on average 14 years before an *alternative psychosis* occurs after the first manifestation of epilepsy - usually of the primarily generalized type . From the manifold observations that mood swings in epileptics frequently have an EEG-correlate, it becomes evident that the principle of reciprocity between "pathological" changes of the EEG on the one hand and behavior/experience on the other hand has a general importance that reaches beyond the topic of *alternative psychoses* becomes evident.

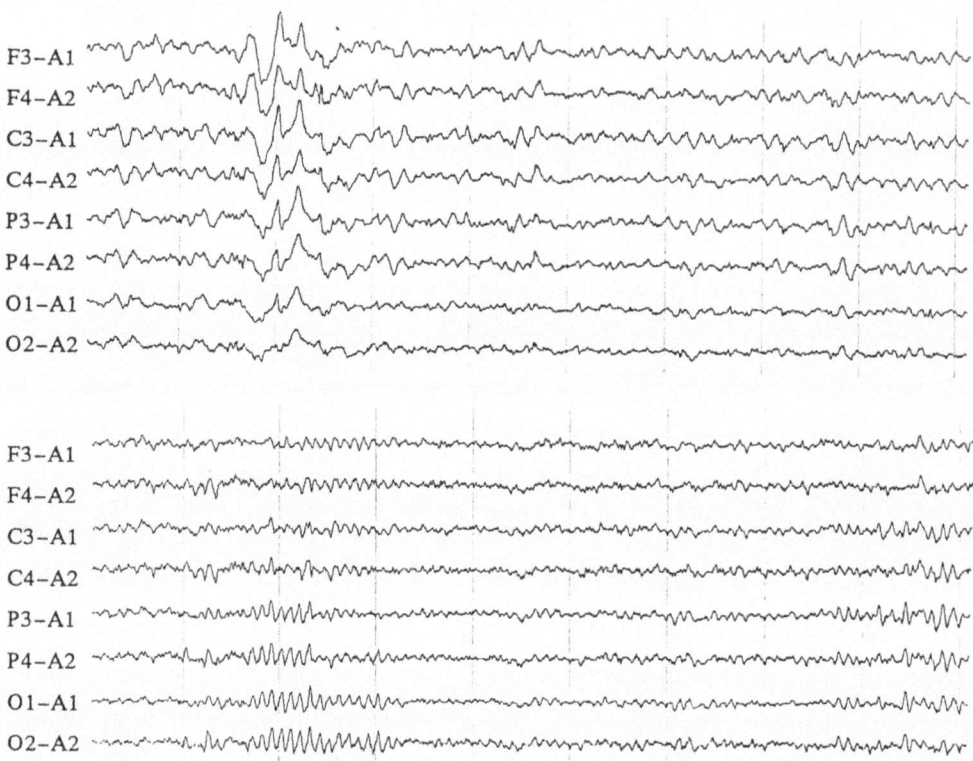

Figure 96. <u>Above</u>: Predominantly diffuse-dysrhythmic EEG with irregular 5-7/s-activity and interspersed sharper to steep elements in a psychopathologically inconspicuous patient under treatment with phenytoin and carbamazepine because of genuine epilepsy (K. B., 51 y., m., EEG-nr. 942/88).
<u>Below</u>: Extensive regularization (*forced normalization*) of the EEG with manifestation of an acute paranoid-hallucinatory syndrome after ending the phenytoin treatment because of adverse reactions (EEG-nr. 1008/88).

The rule of thumb is that a subjective sense of well-being more likely corresponds to a "pathological" EEG while dysthymia, irritability, and affective lability are reflected by a "normalized" one. This has been observed in episodic parathymic conditions (Köhler, 1975) as well as in preparoxysmal states (Schorsch & Hedenström, 1975). The preictal flattening as typical aura-correlate was related to a *forced normalization,* as reported by Landolt (1963). The knowledge of such psycho-physiological relationships causes the physician to request systematic repetitive recordings. However, the EEG-interpreter can rightfully expect that he will not just receive general instructions to record an EEG every day, for example, but that the question will be rephrased at each request based on the actual clinical situation. While we know today that *alternative psychoses* occur in the first place in primarily generalized epilepsies, in the past, it was assumed that there existed a special relationship with "temporal lobe epilepsy" (Bingley, 1958; Flor-Henry, 1973; Gastaut et al., 1956; Glaser et al., 1963; Herrington, 1960;Lorentz De Haas & Magnus, 1958;). The neuroanatomic speculations surrounding the temporal lobe, the limbic cortex, and and the midbrain can in retrospect be called erroneous. The creation of a temporal lobe mythology was promoted by an inappropriate EEG-interpretation. Phenomena that were confined to specific regions were without further ado considered to be manifestations of topographically, i.e., neuroanatomically, corresponding damages. Consequently, bilateral symmetrical changes were also interpreted in the same sense, i.e., as a manifestation of bilateral focal damage. Based on our own observations and on a critical evaluation of the case studies found in literature, we think that the unitemporal and bitemporal foci described as typical for "temporal lobe epilepsies" are generally phenomena like the ones subsumed by us under **ILA/IBA**. However, since these patterns can typically be observed in interictal EEGs with a totally inconspicuous behavior/experience, this probably is much less a manifestation of pathological functional changes than of constitution-related phenomena indicating a maturational deficit. This interpretation must, however, take into account the typically observed disappearance of the phenomenon at the onset of the psychosis. A number of authors postulated an active mechanism for this alternation (Bente, 1969a; Glaser, 1964; Hess, 1955; Hess et al., 1971; Köhler, 1975; Wolf, 1973).

Wolf (1973) discussed a "change in the propagation mode" or an expansion of the paroxysmal activity into other functional areas. He also raised the question of whether such a shift in exitation is associated with the regular anti-epileptic mechanism of action or whether a special predisposition of the simultaneously excited systems is necessary.

The fact that *alternative psychoses* occur only with a certain latency after the first manifestation of the epilepsy, that only a relatively small number of epileptics develops *alternative psychoses,* and finally that the supposed *trait*-quality of the temporo-anterior projecting EEG-patterns (**ILA/IBA**) seem to be clear indications of the significance of predisposing factors. Although the *forced normalization,* which is not as important for the practice as originally thought, has inspired far-reaching speculations (Landolt, 1957; Penin & Huber, 1968; Penin, 1971). Landolt adopted the view held by Hess (1955) that a "hyperactivity" of the formatio reticularis is the underlying reason for the *forced normalization.* This "hyperactivity" manifests itself in the twilight states being charcterized by a peculiar agitation component. Those "orderly" twilight states without any agitation symptoms, which are known to us also as *alternative psychoses,* defy such an interpretation. Pharmaco-electroencephalography seems to be opening the way to a more promising interpretation. We know from experiments with LSD (Bente, 1958) that this substance causes a characteristic dissociation of experience/behavior and EEG. After pretreatment with LSD, sleep occurred during intravenous barbiturate administration just as well as without pretreatment, although the associated sleep patterns in the EEG did not present themselves. Similar observations were made during intravenous administration of chlorpromazine. As Bente (1958) proved with impressive curve examples, a *forced normalization* of diffuse-dysrhythmic EEGs of patients with genuine grand mal epilepsy occurs under the influence of LSD. This drug-induced *forced normalization* reached its maximum, manifested in an almost ideal-typical alpha-EEG about one hour after the intravenous administration of LSD. The patient felt sleepy at that point of time. Besides a bilateral frequency acceleration, Korein and Musacchio (1968) observed a more or less complete disappearance of the foci under the influence of LSD in neurological patients with unilateral focal injuries. According to them, the EEG appeared to be "less abnormal" along with an intensified hemisymptomatology. However, the authors failed to make the almost obvious connection between this LSD-effect and the then already well-known *forced normalization* in epileptics. On the other hand, Landolt (1963) discussed the possibility of a mechanism related to *forced normalization,* evidently without knowledge of the EEG-effect of LSD and based solely on the psychotogenic features of this substance. As far as we can see today, this problem area, by no means scientifically exhausted, no longer receives specific attention.

The rarely diagnosed but in reality not so rare status psychomotoricus is also worth mentioning (Engel et al., 1978; Medalia et al., 1988; Bauer et al., 1992; Ritaccio & March, 1993). Since the clinical picture is multifarious and the EEG is not as typical as for the petit mal status, the diagnosis is easily missed.

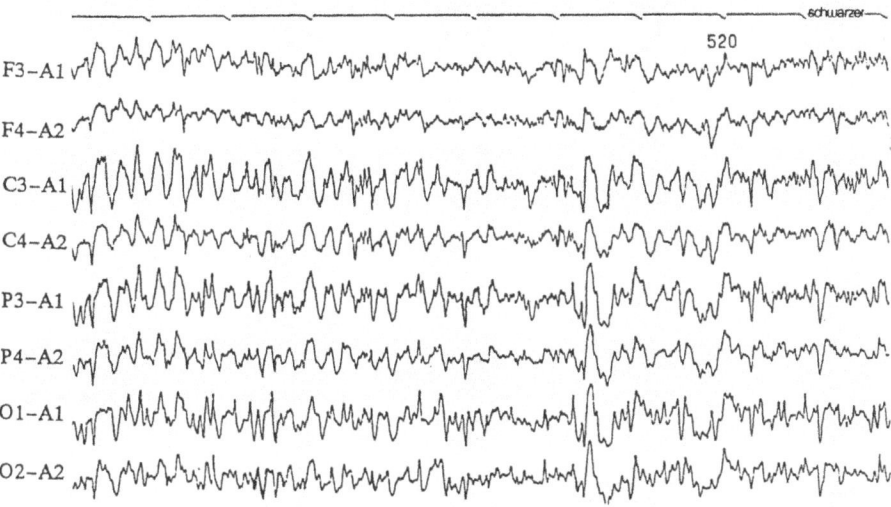

Figure 97. Paroxysmal-dysrhythmic EEG with intermittent left temporo-anterior accentuation of a slow high-amplitude and sharper rhythmic activity during a status of complex-partial seizures with right-side perioral myoclonus, verbigeration, and clouding of consciousness. Fading of the status after approximately 48 hours under the treatment with clonazepam and phenytoin (R. S., 29 y., m., EEG-nr. 707/87).

In contrast to *alternative psychoses*, such persistent temporal region-projected paroxysmal activity represents the immediate pathophysiological correlate of the psychosis (Dreyer, 1965; Gastaut et al., 1956; Hedenström & Schorsch, 1959;). For a safeguarding of diagnosis, a comparison of ictal and interictal EEG is one of the decisive aspects. The most common form of an episodic epileptic parathymic condition can be more or less regularly observed, prior to the actual seizure, as so-called aura. In our opinion, the term "preparoxysmal twilight state" is an unfortunate choice, since it suggests a non-existent proximity of the syndrome to the postparoxysmal twilight state. Mostly, we are dealing with bland displeasure. Auras also present themselves as paranoid-hallucinatory syndromes, as states of elation or even ecstasy, as states of compulsive restlessness and infrequently, as dipsomania or poriomania. The EEG-correlates of these states vary. Several authors esteem a decrease in voltage accompanying desynchronization as typical . Landolt (1963) considered this as a form of *forced normalization*. A rather infrequent phenomenon is the aura-status or the aura continua. Clinically, these are mainly rising and ebbing and sometimes also persistent, intense sensations of diverse provenance. Here, too, the EEG often is uncharacteristically or not at all changed (Wolf, 1980).

Only for the sake of completeness, we also want to mention adversive seizures, which are typically accompanied by visual hallucinations (Helmchen et al., 1969; Lugaresi et al., 1971; Palem et al., 1970). Sometimes, only an isolated hallucinosis exists. As in the equally infrequent isolated hallucinoses associated with alcoholism, one usually finds an alpha-typical or low-voltage EEG rather than a paroxysmal EEG-activity during these epileptic equivalents.

The polymorphism of epileptic psychoses, confusing with regard to the clinical appearance and the associated EEG-phenomena, prompts speculations regarding a conceptual framework that could create some order. Thus, Landolt (1961) considered the petit mal status and the psychoses related to *forced normalization* as "extreme states of a dynamics continuum." Penin (1973) added the aspect of process activity and contrasted the *absence* as a kind of "time-accelerated" psychosis with "peractive" EEG and schizophreniform psychoses with "subactive" EEG. Wolf (1973) endorsed this model, saying that in both cases, we are dealing with a psychosis that originates from a pre-syndrome and is terminated by a grand mal. He explained further that in both cases, an epileptic process documented by the EEG corresponds to the psychosis. While a polar antagonism of petit mal status and psychoses related to *forced normalization* has clinically and electroencephalographically been established beyond doubt, no empirical proof exists to justify the assumption of a continuum of intermediary forms. EEG-changes associated with the petit mal status (Fig. 95) cannot be classified under our model of the pathological functional change (Fig. 43). The petit mal pattern represents a special modus of brain-functional disorganization that belongs in the field of epileptic pathophysiology. The same is true for the *forced-normalized* EEG that does not reveal its underlying pathological events. Contrary to all other modi of functional dissolution, the disorganization manifests itself here in a regularization of a "normally pathological" EEG (transl. from German: "normalerweise pathologisch", Landolt, 1975) . The disappearance of dysrhythmia, paroxysmal potentials, and focal changes should not fool us about the pathological character of the *forced normalization*. We are reminded of it not least by the obviously totally analogous gestalt change under LSD-influence (see above). To be consistent, one should have mentioned here an exogenously induced *forced normalization*. The fact that the *forced normalization* corresponds to a pathological event fosters the expectation that, contrary to the first impression, characteristic differences to the physiomorphic EEG can be found using the appropriate analytical methods. We are primarily thinking here of a disturbance of the morphodynamics, i.e., of the "Verlaufsgestalt" or "Zeitgestalt" (time course pattern) or also of the chaos-theoretical correlation dimension D2 (see there). Such primary quantifying analyses, which qualify without negating our methodological premises of the electroencephalography as a primarily visuo-morphological discipline, are worth investigating with respect to possible relationships to the schizophrenias.

A working hypothesis could be formulated that the mechanism of forced *normalization* also plays an important role in the endogenous schizophrenic syndromes. Such a working hypothesis implies that schizophrenics present a "pathological" EEG before the outbreak of the disease, like an increased proportion of interspersed irregular slow waves and/or paroxysmal activity, and that these peculiarities disappear or alternate with the occurrence of the psychosis. Thus, Landolt (1957) indeed reported that non-catatonic schizophrenics, before the outbreak of the disease or between acute psychotic episodes, had shown "temporal seizure potentials" or "generalized or focal dysrhythmias." During the acute psychotic episode, a more or less complete normalization of the EEG occurred. However, this information, has a more anecdotal rather than systematic character. Finally, we want to emphasize once more that also with epileptic psychoses, the association of pathological pictures with certain EEG-changes is the exception rather than the rule. Wolf (1976), who discussed this matter of association in depth, pointed to the possibility of a complete decoupling of psychosis and epilepsy based on case studies. We agree with Wolf when he firmly rejects the idea that a psychosis is nothing but an epiphenomenon of a pathophysiological process. We also have to consider here that once a psychosis has started, it follows its own rules.

4. 11 THE EEG IN MEDITATION

An overview of the literature shows that EEG-changes observed under meditation vary too much to talk about **the meditation EEG.** However, many studies from various research groups agree about the existence of a triad of amplitude increase, background alpha-frequency decrease, and the occurrence of a theta-activity. An alpha-anteriorization has also been mentioned (Anand et al. 1961; Banquet, 1972; 1973; Etson et al., 1977; Hebert & Lehmann, 1977; Hirai,1960; Kasamatsu et al., 1957; Kasamatsu & Hirai, 1966; Lehrer et al., 1980; Wallace,1970; Wallace et al., 1971; Wallance & Benson, 1972). Especially instructive is the study by Kasamatsu and Hirai (1966), because it contains a number of curve examples (their illustrations 4-8) that very impressively document the existence of a **DR**. Only 50 minutes after the beginnng of a Zen-meditation, an increase in the alpha-amplitudes in connection with an anteriorization can be observed. After 8 1/2 minutes, a stable stage of A2 to A3 as a correlate of the desired psychic condition is reached. Interestingly, the EEG-change extends beyond the end of the meditation for at least a few minutes in slightly less pronounced form. From the morphodynamic point of view, these changes can be associated with a pathological gestalt/functional change as typical for a dissolution via the A-stage (**DR**, s.a. Fig. 43). Several authors also pointed out the occurrence of frontal rhythmic sub-alpha- and theta-groups (Hebert & Lehmann, 1977; Kasamatsu & Hirai, 1966; Wallace & Benson, 1972). The provided curve examples allow an association of these changes with the dissolution via the pathomorph variants of the A-stage (**ILA/IBA**, s.a. Fig. 43). However, it would be wrong to talk about a pathological gestalt/functional change in the case of such meditation correlations since we are dealing with a deliberately induced state that uses physiological mechanisms that can be terminated at any time and that, of course, has no relationship to any disease. As experiential correlate of the discussed EEG-changes, a very pleasant state of floating between wakefulness and sleep is mentioned. The fact that these peculiarities cannot be deduced from the gestalt/functional changes of the EEG is another empirical confirmation of the principle excluding a one-on-one association beween EEG and behavior/experience.

4. 12 Multiple Sclerosis

Multiple sclerosis is a syndrome, which is particularly important not only in neurologic but also psychiatric practice because it is observed in a high percentage of cases with various degrees of disturbances of the waking-sleeping regulation (Clark et al., 1992; Freal et al., 1984; Weinschenker et al., 1992) as well as with affective disorders. As can already be observed in visual routine diagnosis, EEGs from such patients surprisingly often show Dynamic Lability (**DL**), whereas we hardly ever find **DR**. In a study involving 23 patients, we tried to objectify this impression quantitatively. Moreover, we were interested whether the dynamics of the disease course is reflected through changes in the EEG-dynamics (Bräu & Ulrich, 1990). The data were collected at the time of clinical admission and after four weeks of treatment. As an indicator of the severity of the disease, we chose the clinical sum scores introduced by Kurtzke (1983). Besides a 10-minute EEG-recording at rest, a visuo-motor tracking test was performed. As expected, the Kurtzke-scores indicated a statistically significant group improvement after 4 weeks. Equally as expected, this improvement was not reflected in the conventional average power spectra (s. a. Colon et al. 1981; Gibbs & Becka, 1968; Rieger et al. 1970). However, the improvement was evidenced in the quantitatively assessed vigilance dynamics.

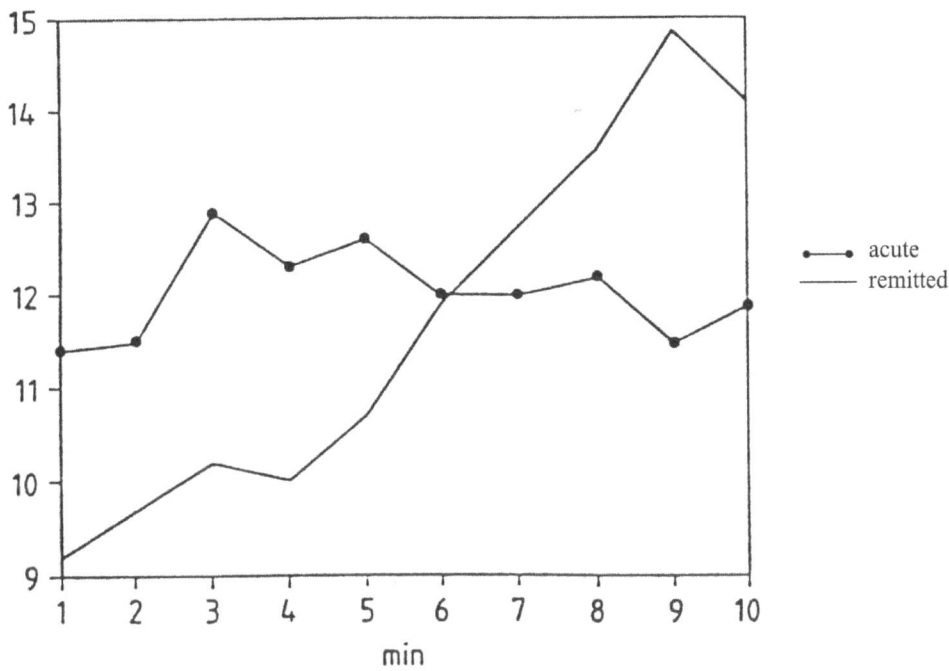

Figure 98. Time course of the rate of the non-A-segments (23 patients suffering from Multiple sclerosis; group averages, n=23); 10-minute recording at rest; with a time window of 2 seconds for the analysis, a maximum of 30 non-A-epochs are possible per minute

Fig. 98 shows the rate of successive subvigil non-A-epochs (time window: 2 seconds) observed for each single minute of the 10-minute recording at rest (see chapter 7.2 for more details about the methodology of quantitatively assessing non-A epochs). While the rate of the non-A-epochs in the first EEG, i.e., during the acute stage of the disease, is completely independent from the duration of the recording, the group average per minute of recording is approximately 12 non-A-epochs of the 30 possible ones. Four weeks later, we find the time-dependent frequency increase, which is also characteristic for groups of young and healthy probands. This physiomorph behavior (**PM**) is characterized by the relatively high stability of the non-A-rates during the first 5 recording minutes, followed by a steady increase in frequency. No differences are evident when comparing the total of non-A-epoch frequencies before and after treatment. Of the 300 possible non-A-epochs (corresponding to 600 seconds of recording time), 121 were found as a group average before treatment and 117 non-A-epochs after 4 weeks of treatment. Through an inspection of the original printouts, we could also convince ourselves that these quantitative difference resulted from a **DL**. The time course of epoch frequencies in Fig. 98 shows highly significant differences (examination time x non-A-rates per recording minute: $F_{9,198}$ = 3.28, $p < 0.001$. Thus the clinical improvement is not reflected, as we originally expected, in decreased **DL** but in a normalization of the EEG dynamics towards **PM**. Moreover, a positive correlation between this normalization and a performance improvement during visuo-motor tracking was found.

These results can be of interest far beyond the narrow frame of the examined patient group. First, they demonstrate once again the limitations of primary quantification that has sacrificed the morphodynamics of the original time function and thus the most important source of information.

Further studies will be necessary to determine whether the prevalence of the B-dissolution (**DL**) typical for our sample can also be found in other samples. If this proves to be the case, we have to ask what could cause this special relationship between multiple sclerosis and the kind of pathological gestalt change observed in the EEG. Since multiple sclerosis is a primary degeneration of the white matter of the brain, we could speculate that primarily subcortically attacking processes lead to B-dissolution (**DL**) while primarily cortically attacking processes lead to A-dissolution (**DR**) instead. Furthermore, we will have to examine - in differently diagnosed populations - whether the time structure determining the course for the resting EEG possibly represents a particularly sensitive indicator of the pathological functional change (*Pathologischer Funktionswandel*).

CHAPTER 5
Changes in the EEG Induced by Psychotropic Substances: The Basics

The investigation of the effects of psychoactive drugs on the EEG was an important field of research within psychiatry about half a century ago. With the general availability of the Power-Spectral analysis by means of the Fast-Fourier algorithm, the Pharmaco-EEG gained a central position within psychiatric electroencephalography, which was largely due to commercial interests. Eventually, this development influenced largely proper psychiatric EEG-research. Within the last two decades, the interest in the Pharmaco-EEG has faded away for reasons discussed in the following sections.

Methodically, the Pharmaco-EEG rests on three pillars. As we will attempt to prove, serious doubts about the soundness of these pillars are permitted, as they are largley unfounded theoretical and empirical presumptions.

1. A similarity in the EEG-effects of various substances indicates a similarity in the clinical-therapeutical effects.
2. The so-called power spectra obtained by means of spectral analysis of short-time epochs being averaged across the entire recording time represent the only relevant information.
3. Healthy young male probands on the one hand and psychiatric patients on the other hand generally show similar pharmaco-electroencephalographic effects.

The first-mentioned presumption was certainly necessary as a working hypothesis to initiate research after all. However, instead of modifying the initially necessarily undifferentiated working hypothesis by means of the obtained findings, one concentrated on the compatible findings and ignored the incompatible ones. The formula claiming that similar EEG-effects allow us to expect similar therapeutic effects therefore soon became dogma (Itil,

1974; Fink, 1975). The difficulty resides not only in the fact that substances, which must be distinguished based on their clinical action profile, can present similar EEG-effects, but also that different EEG-effects can be associated with the same clinical action. We must also consider that practically every psychotropic substance does not have only one clinically defined effect but a whole spectrum of effects. Which effect takes predominance depends both on the person and on the kind of substance.

It is evident that a Pharmaco-EEG, which claims the ability to predict the clinical action of a substance from the EEG-effects, must be of the highest interest to everybody involved in the development of new psychiatric pharmaceuticals. In retrospect, however, we notice that the original optimism quickly evaporated. Numerous findings, which did not comply with the postulated regularities, can no longer be relativized as "exceptions". The second presumption, declaring that the usual average power spectra are actually the relevant target variables, was also proclaimed as dogma. This happened even though Bente (1963), as one of the pioneers of Pharmaco-EEG, declared already three decades ago that the "form change of cortical macrorhythms" (transl. from German: "Formwandel der kortikalen Makrorhythmen") under psychoactive substances cannot be sufficiently recognized if one limits oneself to the technically easily measurable frequency and voltage variables. Instead of changes in complex structural characteristics (transl. from German: "Höhere Strukturmerkmale), i.e. changes in the spontaneous morphodynamics are to be considered. Although these statements remained unchallenged, the resonance was deplorablyinfinitesimal. The authors rarely dared to contradict the trend of primary quantification supported by the mainstream. A sheer magical significance, immune against any questioning, gained the phrase "computer-assisted EEG." The only exception was Künkel (1980), regrettably not in an original publication but in internal discussions of researchers engaged in Pharmaco-EEG. He emphasized that in order to answer the question of how far the EEG-effects of a substance A and a substance B vary, one must start with the raw EEG unaltered by transformation. Only then is it guaranteed that the information decisive for the distinction, e.g. the dynamic information, is eliminated. As already explained, two morphodynamically different EEGs can result in rather similar average power spectra.

Fink (1975) phrased the third presumption with commendable clarity:

"*The methods of cerebral electrometry or quantitative EEG depend on observations that normal male volunteers respond to psychoactive drugs indistinguishably from patients ...*"

With this, Fink ignored, in our opinion, indisputable fact that EEG-effects depend as a matter of principle on the baseline condition. Numerous findings substantiate that this dependency is not only evidenced in the degree of distinctiveness of the EEG-effect but that in certain cases, even diametrally opposite effects must be expected. Since the psychopathological disintegration of a psychiatric patient always corresponds to a brain-functional disintegration, it is logically compelling to postulate differences in the EEG-effects to psychoactive drugs. Thus far, we have confirmed such differences in all studies comparing healthy persons with patients. In this context, we would like to refer to the basic pharmacological knowledge that psychotropic substances can result in "paradoxical" clinical effects depending on the psychic baseline condition (e.g., Dimascio et al., 1968; Heimann, 1974). A particularly instructive example is the lithium-effect that manifests itself differently in groups of healthy young men rather than in patients suffering from affective psychoses (Ulrich et al., 1987; Ulrich et al., 1993). The premises we have called into question provide some reasons for Pharmaco-EEG not doing justice to the tremendous range of possible EEG-effects. It is evident that the natural variety was ignored in favor of the desire to arrive at purely pharmaco-related systematics of EEG-effects. The elimination of the annoying variance succeeds by the well known and established statistical methods. Incidentally, the problems here are similar to those encountered in the EEG of endogenous psychoses, especially schizophrenia. It has to be emphasized, however, that an empirical variety can never be annoying to the researcher. On the contrary, it is the actual source of all knowledge in research. Group-statistical designs together with case number estimates may be useful for the comparison of the effectiveness of two pharmaceuticals; however, for the investigation of psycho- or pathophysiological mechanisms they are dreadfully out of place. As we explained in detail with the example of the EEG-effects of lithium (Ulrich et al., 1993), respecting a certain sequence of steps is mandatory for an appropriate research strategy. It always has to begin with the visual analysis of the morphodynamics.

In summary, we conclude that the three pillars supporting today's pharmaco-electroencephalography prove to be rather unsound on closer inspection. This is also the ultimate explanation for the dwindling interest in this discipline for which people once had such great hopes. Its initial goal was to gain insights into the pathophysiology of endogenous psychoses through the examination of the action mechanisms of psychoactive drugs. In these early stages, biochemistry and electroencephalography mutually inspired each other. The pioneering work was in the hands of clinically experienced psychiatrists. In retrospect, however, we cannot claim that the entire psychiatric discipline was under the spell of the new research impetus. Because of their background in the humanities, many kept a reserved distance. Although we owe a multitude of insights and extremely stimulating speculations to the sixties, the entire discipline suffered from a lack of purposeful execution. Many promising approaches were, for whatever reason, abandoned along the way. The speculative element, forever in search of new insights, clearly dominated the confirmatory element striving to conserve existing knowledge. Thus, many of the hopes initially entertained remained unfulfilled.

This was especially true for the high expectations and demands for results being immediately applicable to daily practice. The disappointed hopes led to a loss of prestige for the EEG in psychiatry. Since the early seventies, the most current technology has been applied to compensate for this loss of prestige. When a growing disproportion between technological costs and benefits began to manifest itself in the mid-seventies, psychiatry quickly discovered other, supposedly more promising methods, such as the event-correlated potentials. The finishing touch was added by the true fetish of "funded projects" as a decisive criterion for evaluating the quality of research. Due to this development, it goes almost without saying that methods rather than theory guide psychiatric research today. Pharmaco-EEG developed a life of its own, essentially supported by the pharmaceutical industry while being ignored by the psychiatry. The original intent of exploring the pathophysiology of endogenous psychoses via the Pharmaco-EEG has completely disappeared from view.

Nevertheless, the study of pharmacon effects still holds a central position in our efforts for the revival of the EEG as a psychiatric research tool. However, clinical trials comparing the effects of substance A to those of substance B or correlating clinical parameters with EEG-variables of dubious meaning are of little help, if not downright counterproductive. Our criticism of today's practices implies a number of conclusions. The most elementary conclusion is that an unequivocal taxonomy of the EEG-effects of the various psychotropic substances has not been rendered prosperous up to now. The "classifications" of psychotropic substances based on the homogenized samples of healthy young men (Herrmann, 1982; Itil, 1982) can always apply only to those very samples. They tell nothing concrete about the effect in a specific individual. We must be constantly aware that the effect of a substance is always the result of its interaction with an organism and that organisms, despite all attempts of homogenization, will always differ. Consequently, the EEG-effects of psychotropic substances can be described only relationally to a defined state of the central nervous system. Therefore, it does not make any sense to associate a specific EEG-effect with a specific psychotropic substance without mentioning the baseline situation. However, it would also be meaningless to use a group-statistically calculated average baseline as its basis. Occasionally, the inclusive criterion "alpha-subject" is mentioned. However, without further specification of topography, dynamics, and frequency of the alpha activity, this is far too vague. Moreover, we must consider that the real baseline can sometimes be inapparent. This follows from the observation of rather different EEG-effects despite a seemingly identical baseline EEG. In these cases, a specific initial disposition inapparent in a pharmacon-free state manifests itself only through the action of the pharmacon. Since only a relatively limited number of different baseline conditions can be defined, in the most simple case of two condicions, the possibility of arriving at a certain order by defining "reaction types" presents itself (Ulrich et al., 1993). However, such a reaction typology is basically already a schematic simplification. Strictly spoken, one deals with a medication-free baseline only in the case of the not very naturalistic acute test. The regular administration of a pharmacon, typical for the therapeutical situation, over an extended period of time implies that each new administration encounters a change relative to the previous state of the system. We can assume that after a certain time, the system state no longer changes essentially. The EEG-effect associated with this state is also termed **chronic effect**. The pharmacon **and** the organism most probably determine degree and speed of the adaptive processes. The analysis of the pharmacogenic gestalt- or functional change therefore also must be done from a **dynamic** perspective. It is obvious that the pharmacon effect determined by both the baseline condition and the dynamics of the adaptive mechanisms has a wide range of variations. This insight is incompatible with the premise criticized at the outset of the chapter that similar EEG-effects can be associated with similar clinical-therapeutic effects. Incidentally, apart from all theoretical considerations, the untenability of this premise manifests itself in daily clinical practice. A positive effect of the same pharmacon on the production of schizophrenic delusions can, for instance, be accompanied by an alpha-activation as well as desynchronization or by a diffuse dysrhtyhmia with or without paroxysmal activity. The opposite situation that psychotropic substances with different action mechanisms have rather similar EEG-effects is thus far relatively unnoticed yet important. Such different substances as diazepam, lithium, clomethiazol, or amitriptyline can cause a beta-increase, for instance. However, we must immediately ask whether these are not merely delusive similarities caused by insufficient methodical power of discrmination. Whatever the explanation, the findings support our request for a reaction-typological characterization of psychotropic substances.

As discussed in detail using the example of the EEG-effects of lithium (Ulrich et al., 1993), a suitable strategy requires a specific sequence of steps. The visual analysis of the morphodynamics must always be the first step. However, the generally practiced convenient routine procedure, i.e., restricted to a power-spectral analysis, will not create the empirical induction basis necessary for the definition of reaction types. Instead, a permanent openness of mind for new impressions and insights that seem to us just as inexhaustible as the diversity of human faces is indispensible. The second step serves to reconstruct the discovered differences quantitatively. As already Bente (1961) demanded, this quantification must be guided by the visual gestalt perception.

Like the electroencephalography of the endogenous psychosis (see below), the future Pharmaco-EEG has to start from the meticulous study of individual cases. Here, too, statements about regularities can only be formulated when a sufficient number of individual case studies is available.

The sole purpose of this quantitative reconstruction is to establish intersubjectively obligatory assertions. It would be wrong, however, to consider the quantitative parameters as a superior, condensed information. Instead, we have to consider the unavoidable loss of information caused by the quantifying data reduction during their evaluation. We assess the usefulness of quantitative parameters by determining the degree to which they can be "re-translated" into the the original visuo-morphological qualities of the time-function. It is obvious that such a re-translation from an averaged power spectrum, maybe even from a single track, cannot be accomplished without a more or less pronounced loss of information. Therefore, the usual frequency band variables are not suitable for a dynamically oriented quantitative Pharmaco-EEG. According to our concept of the EEG as a morphological discipline, the description elements required here can only be the *"formative tendencies"*, as specified by Bente.

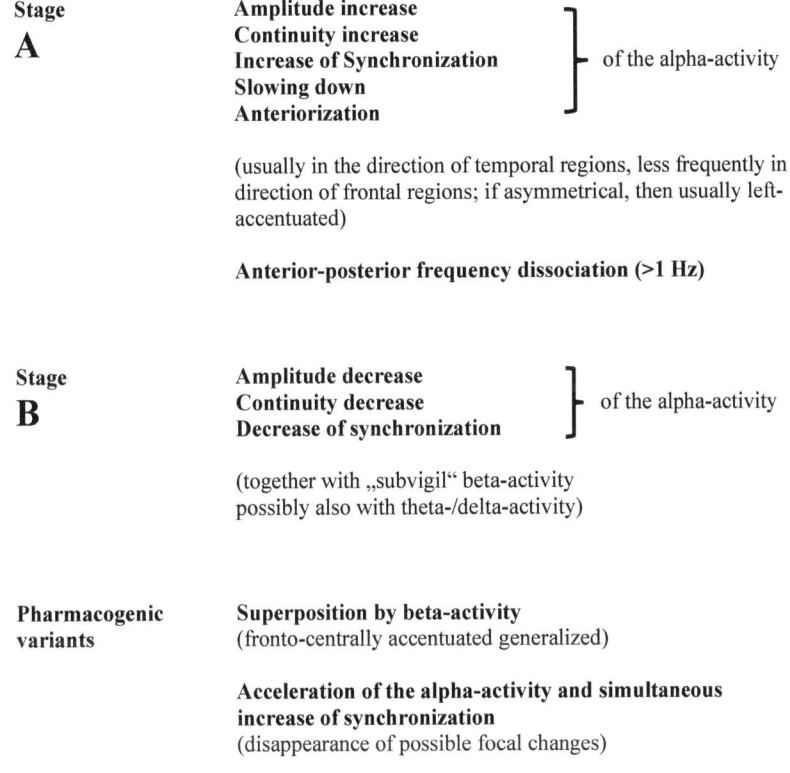

Figure 99. The formative tendencies as components of the pharmacogenic gestalt-/functional change ("Gestalt-/Funktionswandel") of the EEG.

With this, we follow Bente's (1961) concept claiming that psychoactive drugs cause a "changed proportionization" (transl. from German: "veränderte Proportionierung") of the pattern correlated with the physiological process of falling asleep. It will hardly be necessary to emphasize that this concept is incompatible with the continuous demand for "vigilance stabilizing measures", such as "alerting tasks", during the recording (Coppola & Herrmann, 1987; Fink et al., 1977; Matousek & Petersen, 1983; Salinsky et al., 1991; Sannita et al., 1980), since exactly those measures eliminate the relevant information.

As we will concretize later, the "pharmacogenic gestalt change" follows a natural course relatively independent of the respective psychotropic substance. With an alpha-typical base-EEG, the *formative tendencies* of the A-stage will prevail in the acute test and later those of the B-stage. From a certain serum concentration, the *formative tendencies* of the mid and late B-stages will already prevail from the beginning. Along with increasing recording time, the picture of a diffuse dysrythmia (**DD**) together with a loss of spontaneous cycle dynamics become increasingly dominant. This course of changes is essentially independent of the kind of the psychotropic drug.

This two - or three-phase regularity of the "Verlaufsgestalt" ("time course": transl. from German) provides the frame for a differential, reaction-type oriented Pharmaco-EEG. Within the boundaries established by the diverse baseline conditions, the various substances can be more or less distinctly delineated from each other because of the different disproportionalizations and dynamics of the *formative tendencies*. With certain substances, for instance, the initial formative tendencies of the A-stage remain inapparent because of their fleetingness, while with others, they are prominent, independent of the doses. Finally, pharmacogenic modifications, which can be viewed as accentuations of partial aspects of the subvigil intermediary stages or "pharmacogenic variants", also exist (Fig. 99). It is obvious that the dynamics of an EEG as decisive differentia specifica can be determined only by meticulous analyses of individual case studies and never primarily by group statistics.

5.1 Neuroleptics

An enhancement of the *formative tendencies* that characterize the subvigil A-stages, i.e., slowing and increase in amplitude as well as increased synchrony and anterior spreading of the Alpha-background activity, is considered typical for the **chronic** effect of the classical neuroleptics of the phenothiazine-type (BENTE, 1965a,b). Such a constellation resulting in a **DR**-like appearance can be observed in the majority of the treated patients. With **acute** medication, a two-phase effect was described as typical at the beginning of the era of psychopharmacology (Bente & Itil, 1954; 1959; 1960). An initial phase characterized by formative tendencies of the A-stage was followed, under slow intravenous administration, more or less regularlyby a desynchronization with the facultative occurrence of fast beta- and slow irregular waves corresponding to a stage B. In a psychiatric therapy that focuses on "target symptoms" (Freyhan, 1957), neuroleptics are chosen according to their diverging effects on excitement on the one hand and delusion on the other. Both properties are assumed to be interrelated in a reciprocal manner. In Fig. 100, the common "typical" neuroleptics are arranged on a continuum between the extremes of strongly sedating/slightly antipsychotic and slightly sedating/strongly antipsychotic. The phenothiazines with aliphatic lateral chain (chlorpromazine, levomepromazine, trifluopromazine) are considered to be more sedating and less antipsychotic, while the phenothiazines with piperazine ring in the lateral chain (perphenazine, fluphenazine, butyrylperazine) as well as the butyrophenones (haloperidol, benperidol, pimozide, fluspiriline) are considered to be less sedating and more antipsychotic. The phenothiazines with piperidine ring in the secondary chain (thioridazine, pericazine) and the thioxanthene-phenothiazines (chlorprothixen, flupenthixol) take an intermediary position.

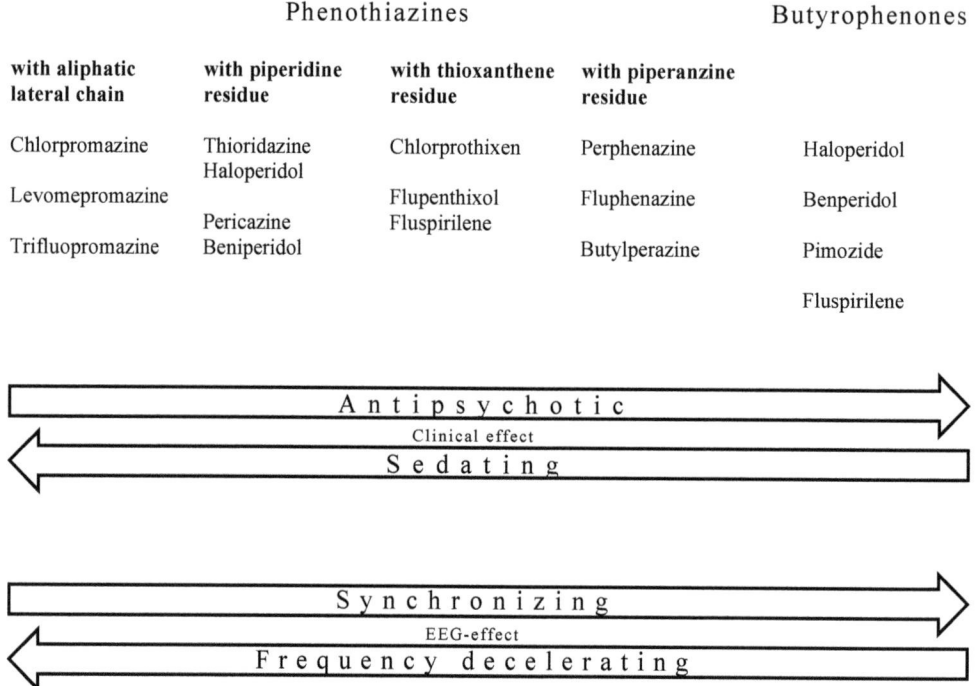

Figure 100. Clinical-electroencephalographic characterization of the "typical" or classical neuroleptics.

It has been mentioned repeatedly that the relationship between sedating and antipsychotic potentials is also expressed in the EEG. Besides a postitive correlation between synchronization and antipsychotic effect, a positive correlation between frequency deceleration and sedation has also been postulated (s. a. Fig. 100). Of course, such regularities can only be expected in the case of an alpha-typically organized baseline EEG. To the degree that the premorbid baseline EEGs of healthy young men on the one hand and schizophrenics on the other hand differ, the pharmacon effects will differ depending on the sample. In many aspects, a special position is also occupied by the chemically clearly different tricyclic dibenzdiazepine derivative **clozaril**. This neuroleptic has the strongest sedating effect, at least initially. A frequency slowing reaching into the delta-region is considered a pharmacon-typical effect (e.g., Bente et al., 1978; Isermann & Haupt, 1976; Kügler et al., 1979). Although the clozaril-modified EEG hardly shows any synchronizing effect, the substance also has outstanding antipsychotic effects. The tendency towards synchronization or even hypersynchronization, which is associated with the antipsychotic effect, is possibly reflected by the intermittently occuring clozaril-typical sharp and high-amplitude waves, whereas the EEG appears in general rather desynchronous due to the prevalence of irregular slow waves (Koukkou-Lehmann et al., 1979; Kugler et al., 1979).

Unlike diffuse dysrhythmia (DD) in encephalopathies, a clozaril-induced DD can be eliminated to a large degree by sensorial stimulation, sometimes even resulting in an alpha-typical EEG. This property has clozaril in common with carbamazepine (see below). The assertion that a "pathologization" of the EEG promises a successful treatment (e.g., Bente, 1963; Dasberg & Robinson, 1971; Helmchen, 1968) is supported by the positive correlation between the pharmacogenically induced synchronization tendency, being more distinct with clozaril than with the typical neuroleptics, and the antipsychotic effect.

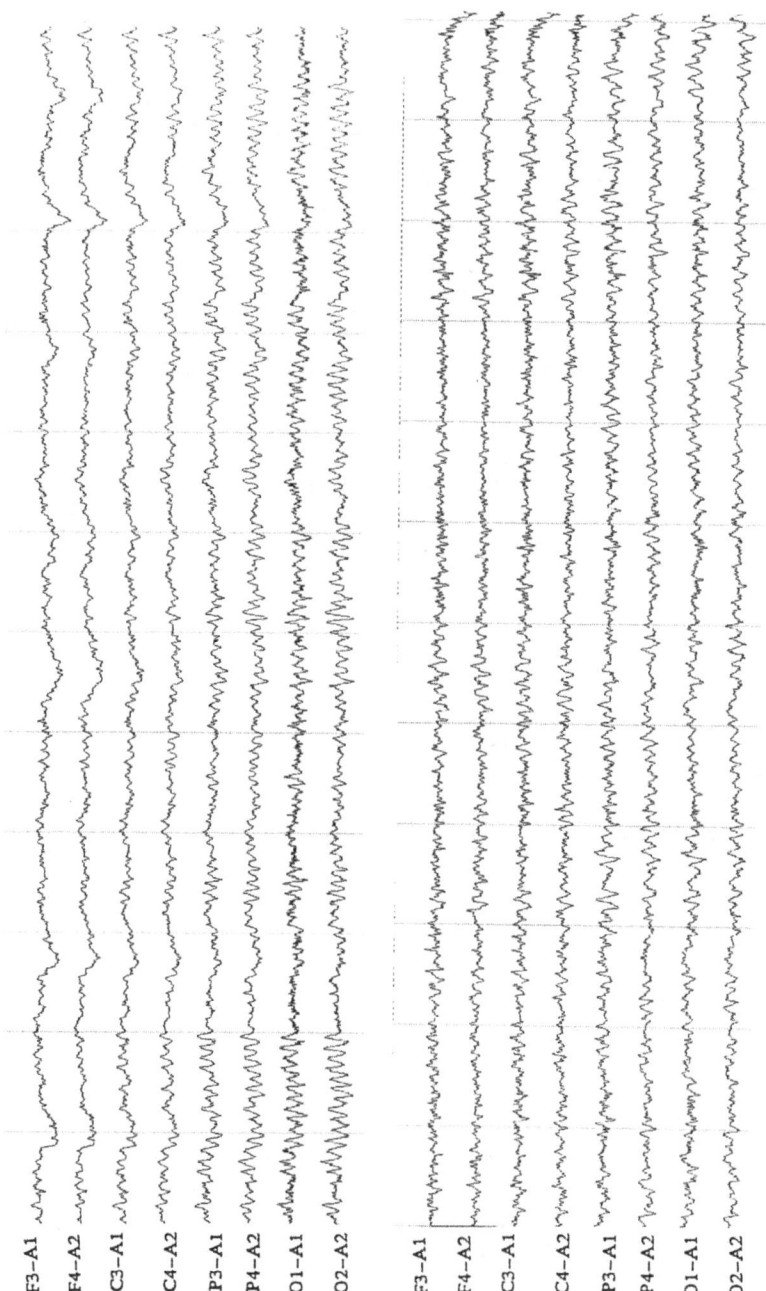

Figure 101. <u>Above</u>: Essentially physiomorph, medication-free recorded EEG with slight frequency-variable posterior-accentuated activity of approximately 9/s with acute paranoid-hallucinatory syndrome (K. H., 31 y., f., EEG-nr. 299/92).
<u>Below</u>: After 6 weeks of treatment with neuroleptics (at the time of recording 15 mg/d haldol and 150 mg/d perazine), slowing and rarefication as well as anteriorization of the background activity occurred. The change points in the direction of a diffuse dysrhythmia (EEG-nr. 401/92) (Fig. 101-112, 12 2-s epochs, 24 second segment; identical derivation schema).

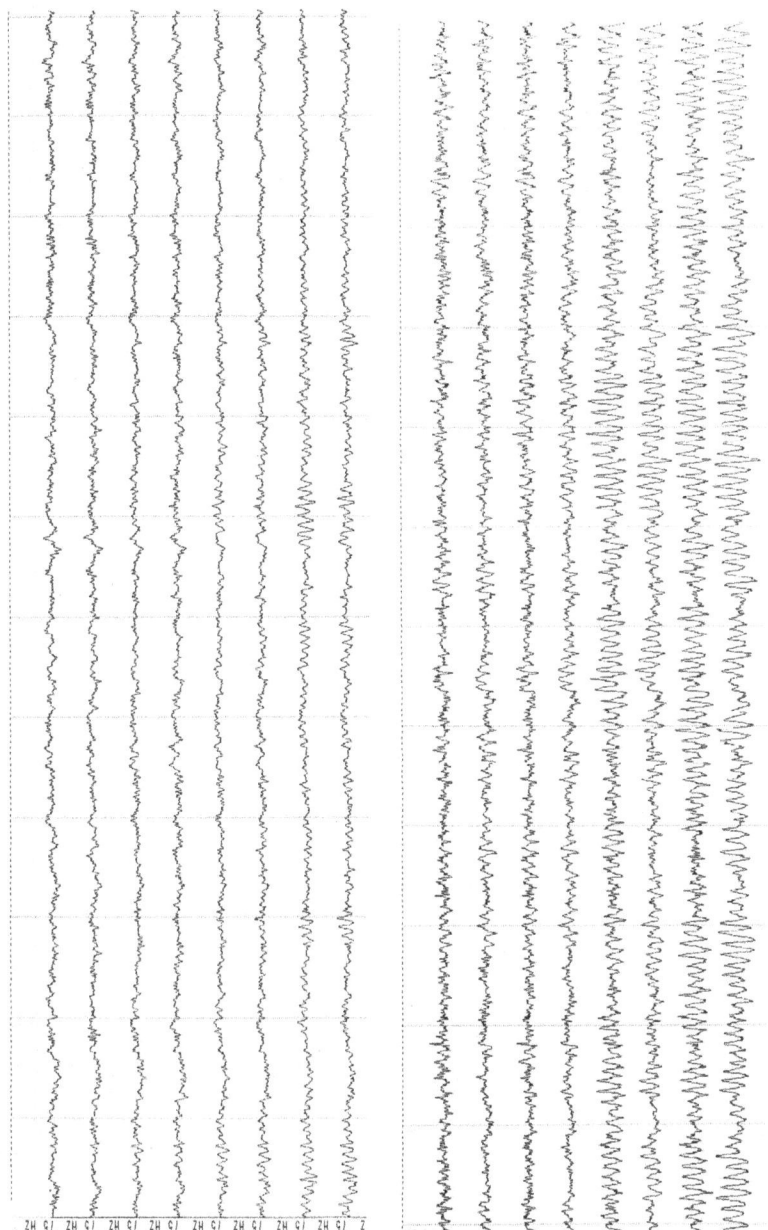

Figure 102. <u>Above</u>: Slightly discontinuous 10/s-activity with posterior dominance. Minor dynamic lability under 50 mg/d promethazine with acute paranoid-hallucinatory syndrome.
<u>Below</u>: After 4 weeks of treatment with neuroleptics (at time of recording 100 mg/d perazine and 10 mg/d haldol), increase in continuity and amplitude and frequency decrease of 1 Hz of the alpha-activity occurs (K. F., 41 y., m., EEG-nr. 203/92; EEG-nr. 304/92).

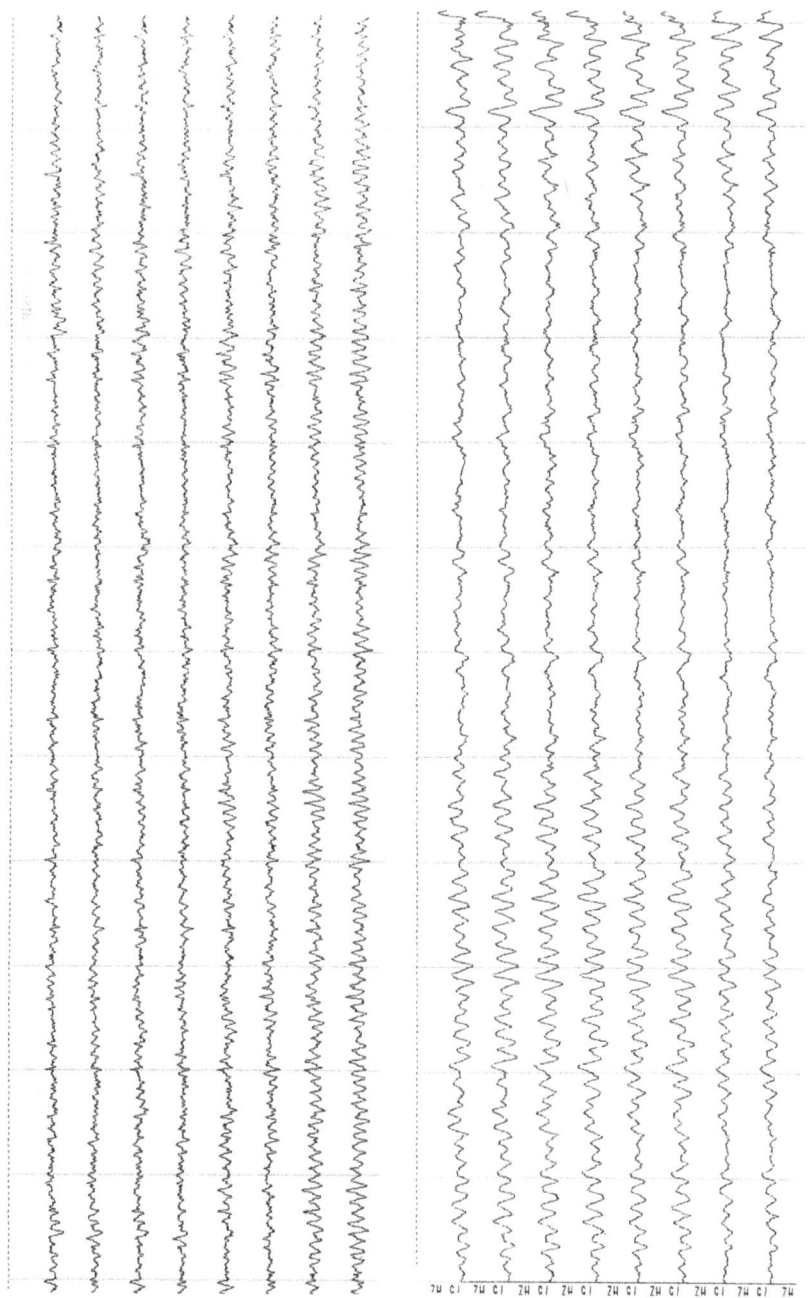

Figure 103. <u>Above</u>: Ideal-typically organized EEG with a continuous posterior-accentuated activity of approximately 9.5/s under 75 mg/d amitriptyline with chronic delusional psychosis. <u>Below</u>: After 8 weeks of treatment with neuroleptics (at time of recording 15 mg/d haldol), the dominating frequency slows down to 6.5/s with spreading to the frontal regions and frequent transitions into low-voltage phases corresponding to the stages B1 - B2 (A. L., 46 y., m., EEG-nr. 702/92; EEG-nr. 926/92).

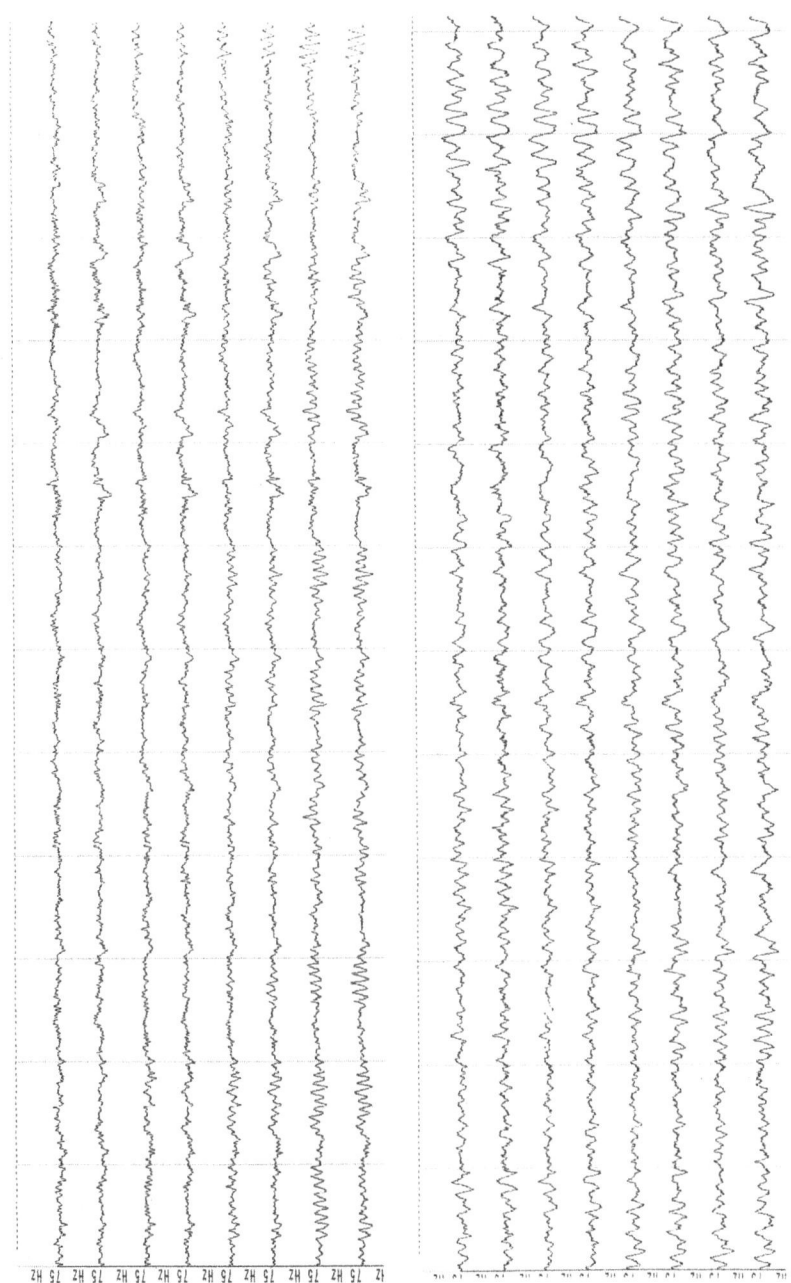

Figure 104. above: Slightly discontinuous activity of approximately 10-11/s with posterior dominance under 10 mg/d diazepam with acute paranoid-hallucinatory syndrome. Below: After 3 weeks of treatment with neuroleptics (at time of recording 300 mg perazine), diffuse-dysrhythmic EEG (DD) is dominated by an irregular theta-activity and only sporadically short alpha-groups of changing topographical accentuation (A. B., 23 y., m., EEG-nr. 601/92; EEG-nr. 1015/92).

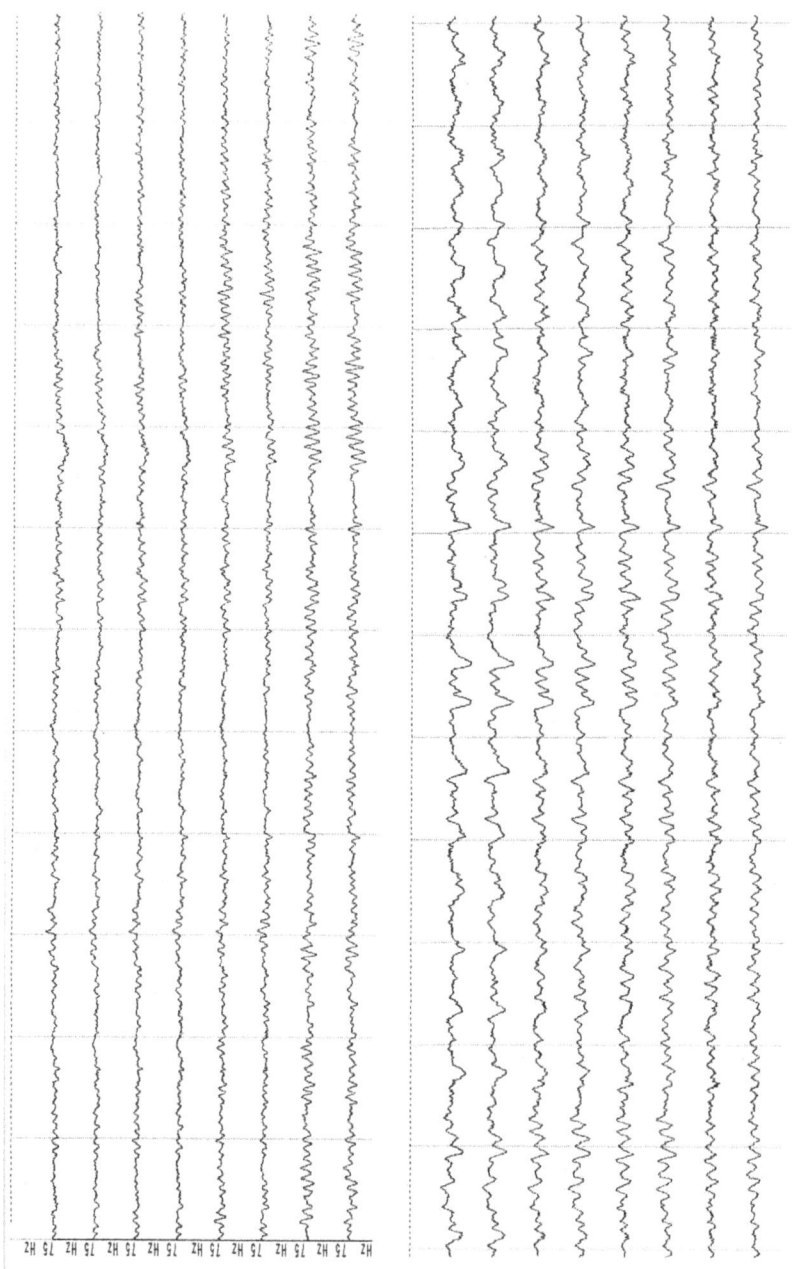

Figure 105. <u>Above</u>: Slightly discontinuous alpha-activity of approximately 10/s with minor intermittent anteriorization under 50 mg/d perazine with acute paranoid-hallucinatory syndrome. <u>Below</u>: After 6 weeks of treatment with neuroleptics (at time of recording 350 mg/d clozapine), the dominant frequency slows down to approximately 8/s with spreading to the frontal regions, and dysrhythmia caused by diffuse irregular slow activity increases (K. K., 27 y., m., EEG-nr. 104/92; EEG-nr. 286/92).

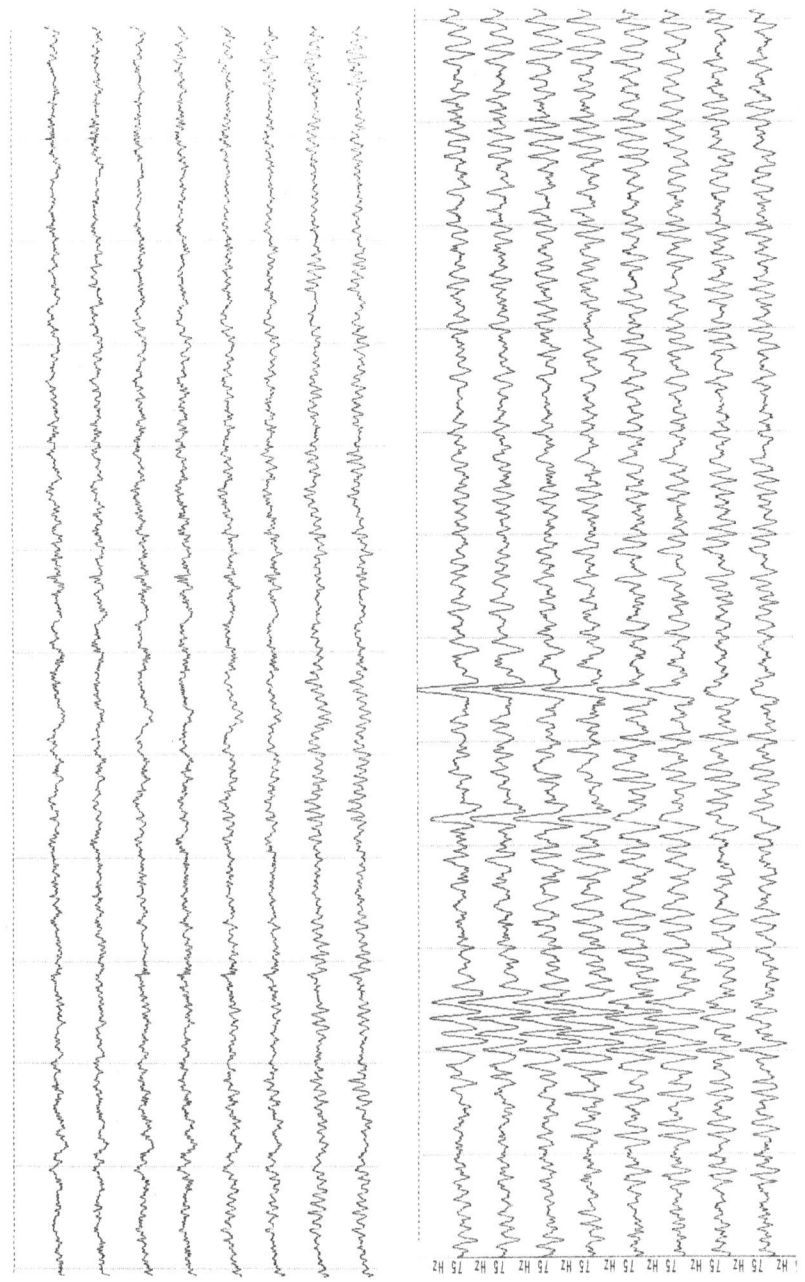

Figure 106. <u>Above</u>: Posterior-accentuated 11-12/s-activity under 50 mg/d promethazine, 500 mg/d chloraldurate, and 10 mg/d diazepam with acute hallucinatory syndrome. <u>Below</u>: After 3 weeks of treatment with neuroleptics (in the end 150 mg/d clozaril), the dominant frequency slows down to 7-8/s with anterior spreading and singular as well as grouped more or less sharp waves that increase in frequency (R. S., 41 y., f., EEG-nr 800/92; EEG-nr. 870/92).

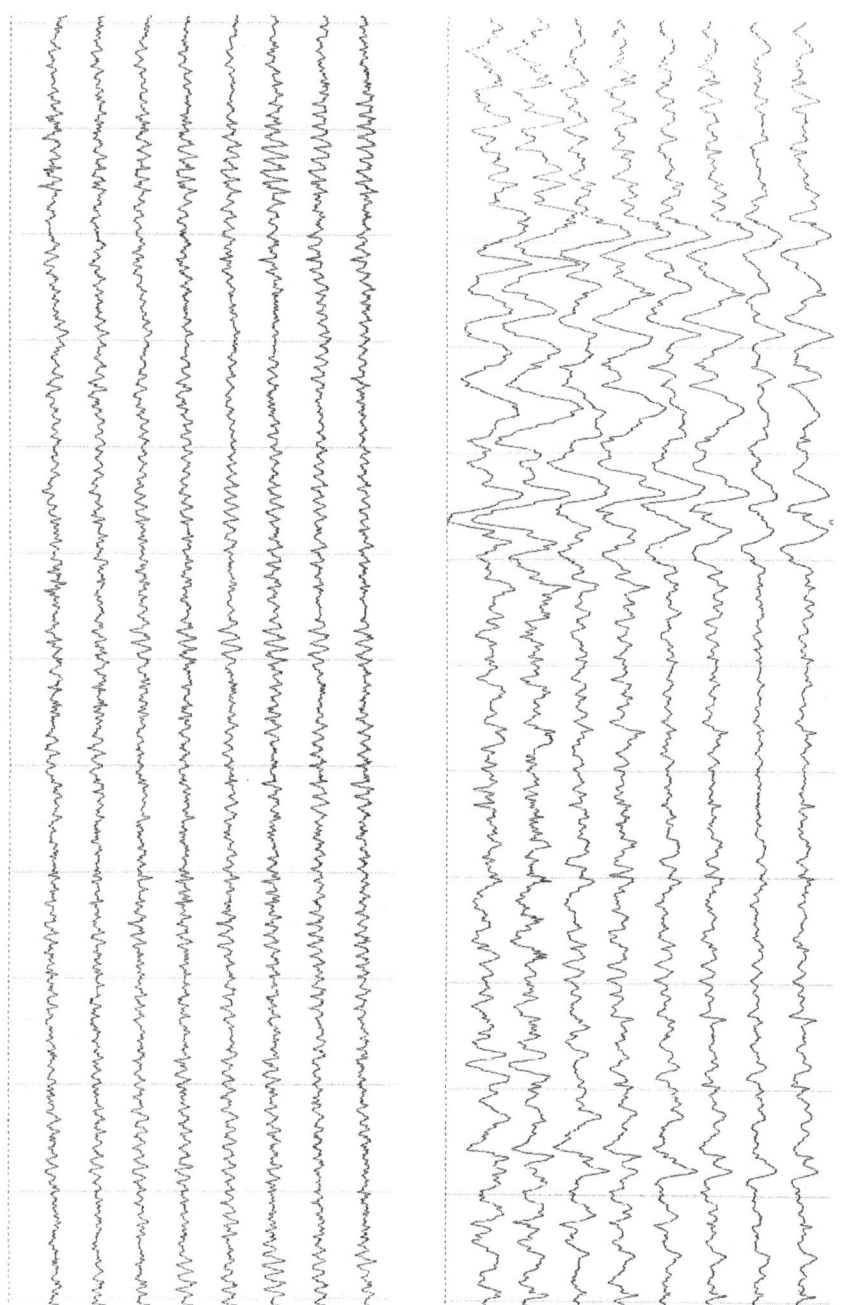

Figure 107. <u>Above:</u> Frequency-variable activity of approximately 9/s with changing topographical accentuation under 100 mg/d perazine and 5 mg/d haldol with acute paranoid-hallucinatory syndrome. <u>Below:</u> After 2 weeks of treatment with neuroleptics (at the end 250/mg/d clozaril diffuse-dysrhythmic EEG. (K. L., 56 y., f., EEG-nr. 158/92; EEG-nr. 219/92).

The authors understood "pathologization" primarily as a phenomenon based on synchronization that can be associated with our **IBA/ILA**-phenomenon (see above). These phenomenon includes the anterior-accentuated rhythmic waves, occasionally in connection with more or less sharp and sometimes also irregular slow waves. However, this could also be the pharmacogenic revelation of an otherwise latent constitution-related *trait*-feature. Flügel and Bente (1950) were the first to consider the question of a possible neuroleptics-induced behavioral and cognitive change (*pharmakogener leistungswandel*). They coined the term *akinetisch-abulisches syndrom* (akinetic-abulic syndrome, transl. from German) in order to subsume a decrease in spontaneous motor behavior, drive, interest, somatic, and emotional irritability in the presence of undisturbed consciousness. With clozapine, such an *akinetic-abulic syndrome*, regarded typical for phenothiazine, neuroleptics cannot be found. Thus, the original assumption of a causal connection between such a syndrome and the antipsychotic effect cannot be upheld.

As discussed earlier, a clozaril-induced paroxysmal activity does not allow us to assume an increased seizure-risk in individual cases. However, a number of studies revealed significantly higher risk for seizures under clozaril than under a medication with phenothiazines or butyrophenones (e.g., Povlsen et al., 1985; Haller & Binder, 1990). The daily dose seems to be the determining but in the discussion often neglected factor seems. According to Ereshefsky et al. (1989), only 1.4% of the patients treated with daily doses up to 600 mg have epileptic seizures compared to 14% of those treated with daily doses between 600 and 900 mg. Devinsky et al. (1991) found an incidence of 2.7% for doses up to 600 mg/d. These numbers must be viewed against the background of seizure risks in psychiatric patients under medication in general, which falls between 0.5 and 1% (Itil & Soldatos, 1980). The seizure risk also increases considerably if clozaril is combined with another neuroleptic (Liukkonen et al., 1992). Clozaril-induced seizures usually do not occur at the beginning of the therapy but only after weeks or months, i.e., in the chronic medication phase, and thus unexpectedly. A seizure occurring under clozaril is by no means a reason to terminate the treatment. In most cases, dosage reduction is sufficient to prevent further seizures. Additional administration of an anti-epileptic, such as phenytoin, is also possible. Especially younger clinical colleagues have to be reminded repeatedly that decisions about a clozaril therapy cannot be delegated to the EEG-interpreter.

The insufficiency of the conventional Pharmaco-EEG being content with a simple Power-Spectralanalysis became especially conspicuous from the few publications dealing with the newer atypical neuroleptics. The expectation that the chemically novel compounds would influence likewise novel EEG effects was thoroughly disappointing. Each one of the recently intoduced atypical neuroleptics (including the older clozaril), such as olanzapine, risperidone, amisulprid, quetiapine, and the like, showed a general slowing down of frequencies and particularly an increase in the theta- and delta-components (Pillman et al., 2000; Schuld et al., 2000; Steinert et al., 2011; Wichniak et al., 2006; Yamada et al., 2004; Yoshimura et al., 2006). Apart from its intensity, this effect was essentially the same as the one observed with the conventional typical neuroleptics. It goes without saying that the EEG-effects of any kind of neuroleptics are dose-dependent. Few studies focused on distinguishing neuroleptics according to their "risk" to produce "EEG abnormalities", as for instance the amount of irregular slow wave activity and epileptiform activity (Centorrino et al., 2002). As to be expected, Clozapine was the lonesome leader of such a "risk ranking", followed by olanzapine and risperidone. considering the dose dependence of such "abnormalities" on the one hand and the superior antipsychotic efficacy of those drugs that are especially prone to produce "EEG abnormalities", such studies do not make much sense. The only clinically relevant remarkable finding seems to be that with comparable therapeutic doses of olanzapine and clozapine, the former seems to produce less epileptiform activity compared to the latter whereas no difference exists with regard to the amount of irregular slowing. In appreciating the occurrence of paroxysms of hypersynchronic or epileptiform activity, we always have to bear in mind that such features does not necessarily imply a heightend seizure risk (see also Koukkou et al., 1979; Pillay et al.,1996; Stevens, 1995; Wilson, 1995).

5. 2. THYMOLEPTICS

Compared to the effects of phenothiazines, the effects of the thymoleptics are much more complex. This is caused by the simultaneity of formative tendencies of the A- and B-stage typical for thymoleptics. Bente et al. (1965a) termed the complexity of the thymoleptic EEG-effects as "polyrhythmic frequency dissolution" ("*polyrhythmischer Frequenzzerfall*" in German). The authors used this term to describe a pronounced frequency-variable EEG with an only moderately marked, more or less discontinuous alpha-activity, continuous superposition with Beta activity and an increased diffuse dysrhythmia due to diffusely subseding irregular theta-activity. There is some indication that the picture of "polyrhythmic frequency dissolution" depends less on a specific chemical structure than on the thymoleptic effects of a substance. Thus, a "polyrhythmic frequency dissolution" was observed not only under tricyclic antidepressives, such as imipramine and amitriptyline, but also under the chemically completely different tetrahydroisochinoline derivation nomifensine. As Bente et al. (1976) proved, such a picture occurs in healthy persons after approximately two hours of a single oral administration of 100 mg. In contrast to the placebo-group, an initial accentuation of *formative tendencies* of the A-stage was observed, i.e., an increase in the alpha-activity in connection with a minor slowing of the dominating alpha-frequency. After a few minutes, there was a progressive increase of *formative tendencies* of the B-stage, such as voltage decrease, desynchronization, and increase in beta- and irregular theta-activity, finally resulting in the typical picture of a" polyrhythmic frequency dissolution".

These findings also support our suspicion of a regular two-phase character of the EEG-effect of psychotropic substances. Naturally, because of the general dependency of all EEG-effects on the baseline condition, totally different reactions can occur in individual cases. Thus, the initial increase in the alpha-activity under nomifensine has been observed only in persons with average and especially underaverage alpha-dominance in the baseline EEG whereas persons with above-average alpha-dominance showed an initial alpha-decrease (Bente, 1973). Lehmann and Hopes (1978) reported similar observations for imipramine. It certainly would be worthwhile to distinguish whether the direction of the mostly unnoticed initial effect has any relationship to the clinical effect. It is well known, that imipramine, amitriptyline, or maprotiline have a sedating or alienating effect on healthy volunteers. With endogenous-depressive patients, in contrast, these drugs increase the drive and have an elucidative effect on mood (Bente et al., 1965a; Dimascio et al., 1968; Heimann, 1974; Ulrich et al., 1984; 1983).

Contrary to neuroleptics, thymoleptics do not decrease performance in attention-load tests in healthy test persons. However, a regular lowering of the fusion frequency of flickering light (Hartung et al., 1964) takes place. The authors explained this discrepancy, termed "dissociative vigilance shift" (*dissoziative Vigilanzverschiebung*, in German), with a simultaneity of dampening and stimulating effects, where the latter become particularly important in attention-load tests and thus compensate for the dampening effects.

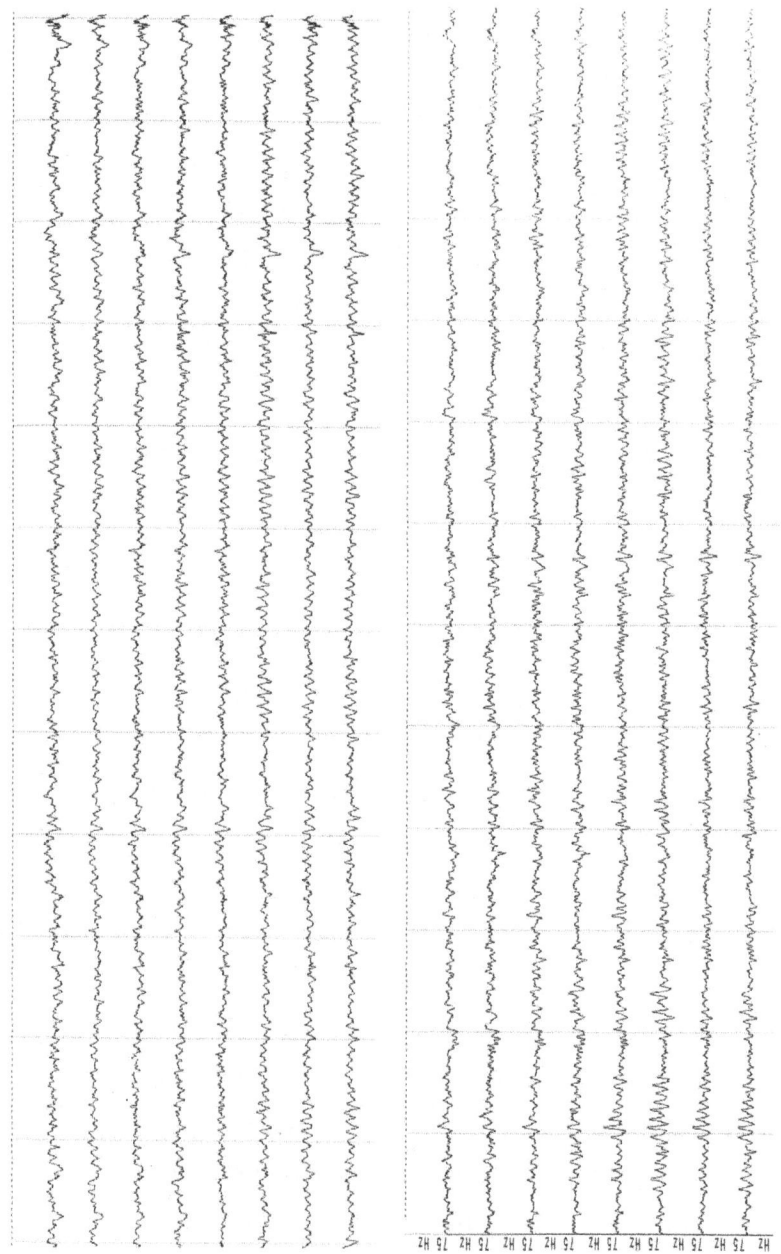

Figure 108. <u>Above</u>: Continuously anteriorized 10/s-activity. Dynamic rigidity (DR) - recorded medication-free during a depressive state of a bipolar affective psychosis.
<u>Below</u>: After 6 weeks of treatment with thymoleptics (in the end with 150 mg/d clomipramine), the picture of a "polyrhythmic frequency dissolution" dominates with only sporadic alpha-groups dominated by desynchronized activity with higher beta-proportion and interspersed irregular theta-activity (K. A., 36 y., f., EEG-nr. 13/92; EEG-nr. 192/92).

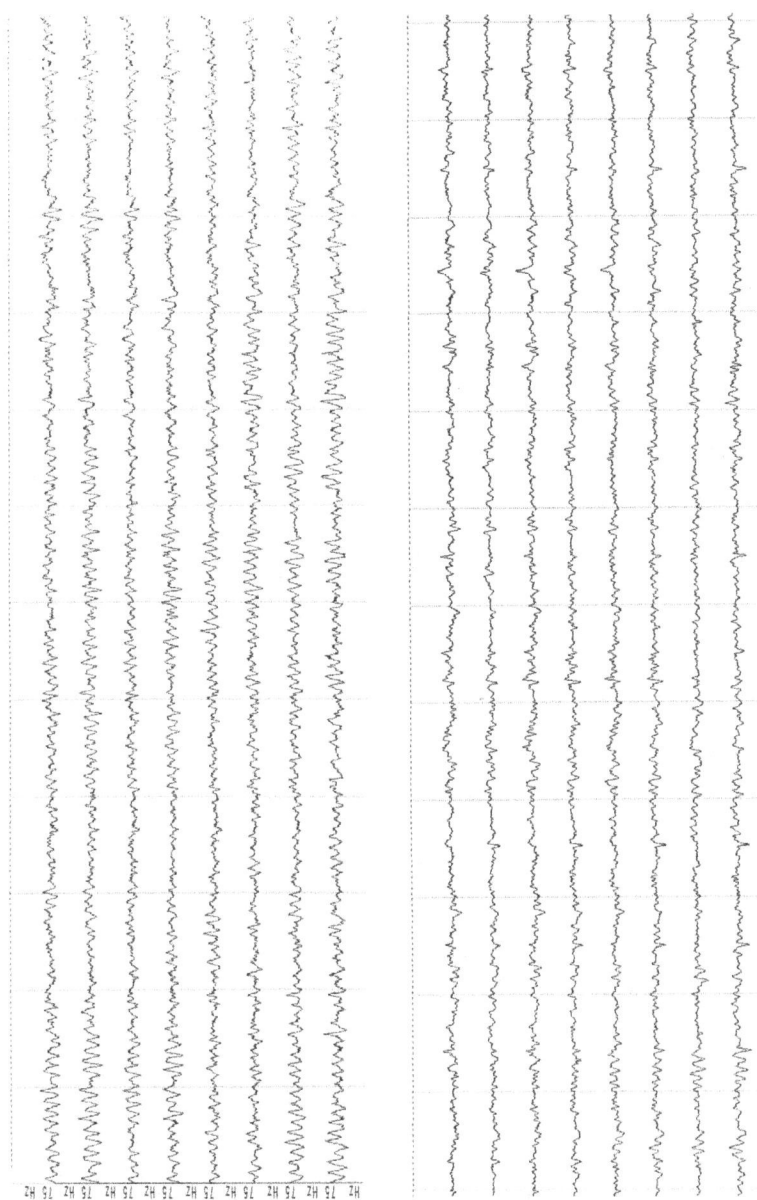

Fig. 109 <u>Above</u>: Discontinuous 8-9/s-activity with intermittent anteriorization under 75 mg/d of perazine with depressive syndrome. <u>Below</u>: After 3 weeks of treatment with thymoleptics (in the end with 150 mg/d imipramine), the picture of a "polyrhythmic frequency dissolution" dominates, corresponding to Fig. 91, below (L. L., 48 y., m., EEG-nr. 26/92; EEG-nr. 115/92).

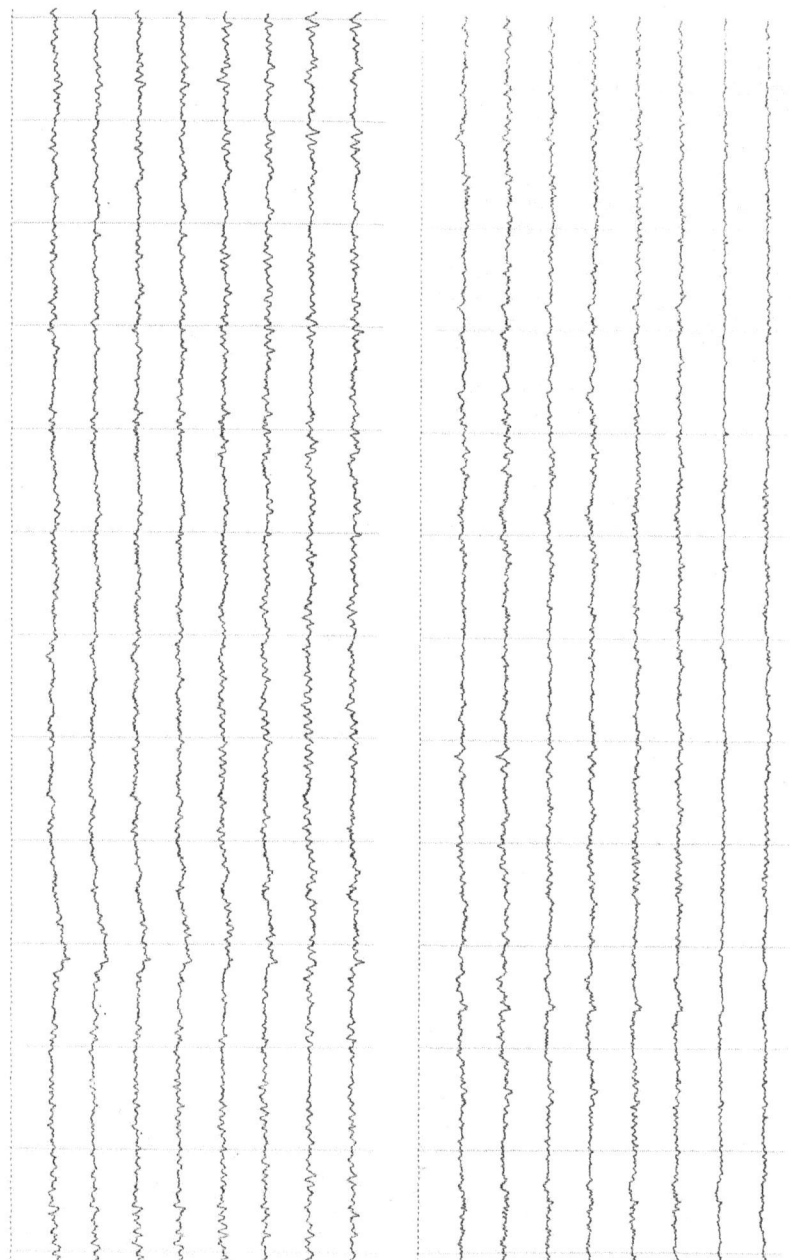

Fig. 110 <u>Above</u>: Slightly discontinuous posterior-accentuated 10/s-activity with depressive syndrome (bipolar affective psychosis) recorded medication-free. <u>Below</u>: After 6 weeks of treatment with thymoleptics (in the end with 150 mg/d clomipramine), picture of a "polyrhythmic frequency dissolution" corresponds to illustration 91, below (A. A., 33 y., f., 127/93; EEG-nr. 310/93).

The different clinical effects observed in healthy probands and depressive patients should correspond to equally different EEG-effects. Based on the findings that suggest differences in the electroencephalographic baseline condition, this indeed seems to be the case. According to Bente (1975; 1976), who tried to overcome the conventional hypotheses about action mechanisms that concentrate on just one particular biochemical partial effect of a systemic concept independent from the method, thymoleptics are able to resolve the syndrome-correlated dynamic restriction of central-nervous regulating mechanisms (Bente et al., 1965a). Such a resolution was probably connected to the simultaneity of sedating and stimulating partial effects.

The formulation of theories about the action mechanisms of thymoleptics can be traced back to research with centrally active anticholinergics conducted in the early sixties with healthy persons and for exploratory reasons also with psychiatric patients. It was found that substances, such as atropine, scopolamine, as well as various synthetic anti-parkinson drugs show a characteristic common reaction pattern coined by *formative tendencies* of the B-stage. The initial activation of *formative tendencies* of the A-stage typical for most other psychotropic substances seems to be missing for the centrally active anticholinergics (Heimann, 1952; Bente et al., 1964; Itil & Fink, 1968). As a behavior/experience correlate of the "pharmacogenic gestalt/functional change," these authors described an "amential-delirious desintegration of consciousness" (*amentiell-deliranter Bewußtseinszerfall*) or a "hyponoic-hypobulic syndrome with intentional weakness, Korsakoff-like mnestic deficits as well as disorientation with regard to time and place" ("hyponoisch-hypobulisches Syndrom mit intentionaler Schwäche, korsakow-artigen mnestischen Defiziten sowie zeitlicher und örtlicher Desorientiertheit;" (Bente et al., 1964). With the fading of the psychic and brain-electric changes, a "centrally stimulating, drive-enhancing, and displeasure-relieving effect" was observed in patients with depressive syndromes (Flügel & Bente, 1961). Analogous to the supposed indicator function of the neuroleptics-induced "abulic-akinetic syndrome," Bente (1961) considered the "anticholinergic-deliriogenic potency" of centrally active anticholinergics as a measure of the degree of their antidepressive efficacy. The fact that all tricyclic antidepressives known at that time had a more or less pronounced anticholinergic effect lent certain plausibility to this speculation. In the meantime, the discovery of substances with non-anticholinergic and yet thymoleptic effects does not mean that the authors erred. This situation is similar to the neuroleptic-antipsychotic effect thatis not related to the causation of an "akinetic-abulic or extrapyramidal-motor syndrome," as assumed previously. This is not surprising and almost to be expected, as it is in agreement with our premise that excludes a one-on-one association of physiological and psychological facts. As with neuroleptics, we also have to expect a statistically increased seizure risk with thymoleptics, as a matter of fact,, even higher risk than with neuroleptics. By far, the greatest seizure risk exists when thymoleptics are combined with more sedating and thus less antipsychotic neuroleptics. The paroxysmal, often spike-like outbursts, constitute, different from the clozapine-induced outbursts, typically slower high-amplitude transients or sharp- and slow-wave complexes, that is, a warning signal.

Last, but not least, the EEG characteristics or effects of a relatively new substance group with a favourable profile of adverse effects and superior antidepressant efficacy, namely the serotonergic compounds (SSRI), have to be considered. Disappointingly, the literature on this topic is lacking. We may cite two older articles concerning the 5HT reuptake inhibitor fluvoxamin (Saletu, 1982; Saletu et al. 1983) in which 10 healthy voluteers were given a single oral dose a single oral dose of fluvoxamin. The authors obtained a "typical thymoleptic pharmaco-EEG profile". Under "typical-thymoleptic", they understood imipramin - or amitriptyline-like profile. Since the chances of gaining new insights were meager, it is all but amazing that further studies with SSRI remained undone.

Nevertheless, the finding deserves attention, as it supports Bente's firm conviction that the "EEG picture" depends far less on a specific chemical structure than on the clinical effect. Eventually, it can be stated that Pharmaco-EEG does not seem to be based on simple spectralanalysis any longer, i.e., the Fast Fourier Transform. Instead, a kind of EEG topography (LORETA = Low resolution electro-magnetic tomography) is being propagated (Saletu et al., 2006).

5.3 LITHIUM

The inadmissibility of drawing conclusions about the EEG-effects in patients with the EEG of healthy persons became particularly evident to us by investigating patients under lithium therapy. As we also could prove quantitatively (Ulrich et al. 1987; 1990), a lithium treatment of 2 weeks caused an increase in the *formative tendencies of the A-stage*, i.e., a change towards dynamic rigidity (**DR**), in the vast majority of young healthy male volunteers with an "Alpha-typical" baseline-EEG. In a minority of the probands, however, an opposite effect has to be expected, that is, a dissolution of the alpha-activity dominated by *formative tendencies of the B-stage* occurs, i.e., a change towards dynamic lability (**DL**).

Contrary to the healthy probands, the effect was extremely inconsistent in patients with phase-prophylactic lithium treatment (Ulrich et al., 1983; 1987).

EEG-dynamics under lithium prophylaxis in euthymic state	Relapses (hospitalizations) within an observation period of 4 years	
	no	yes
DR	1	8
DL	6	3
PM	14	3

Table 9. Frequency distribution of patients with bipolar affective psychoses, classified according to the spontaneous dynamics of the EEG-vigilance (**DR** = dynamic rigidity, **DL** - dynamic lability, **PM** = physiomorphic) depending on the phase-prophylactic effect.

If we asked for the reasons for the different effects in healthy persons and in patients, we must first think about differences in the pre-medication baseline condition (Ulrich et al., 1993). Definite clarification would require a patient study of prospective nature where the baseline EEG and lithium EEG would have to be recorded in a medication-free as well as psychopathologically inconspicuous phase. A retrospective study (Ulrich & Müler, 1993) allowed us to confirm the suspected relationship between the EEG-dynamics under chronic lithium medication and the phase-prophylactic effectiveness.

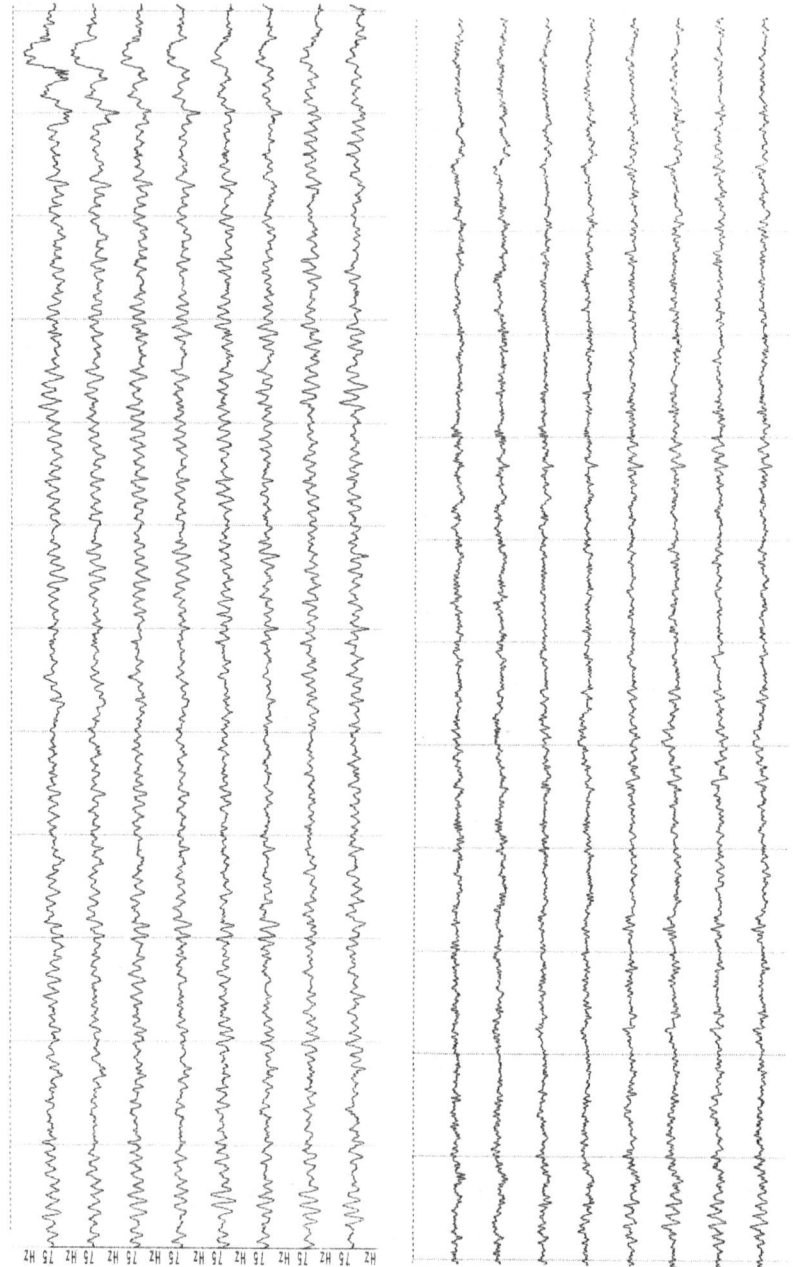

Figure 111. <u>Above</u>: Frequency-variable activity of approximately 9/s with continuous spreading to the frontal regions (DR); medication-free record in the euthymic interval with a patient with bipolar affective psychosis). <u>Below</u>: The effect of a chronic (prophylactic) lithium medication with a plasma level of 0.76 mmol/l: dominating are low-voltage desynchronized activity phases corresponding to a stage B1 with fast beta-activity and only sporadic alpha-groups; patient unchanged euthymic (K.B., 63 y., f., EEG-nr 701/93; EEG-nr. 902/93).

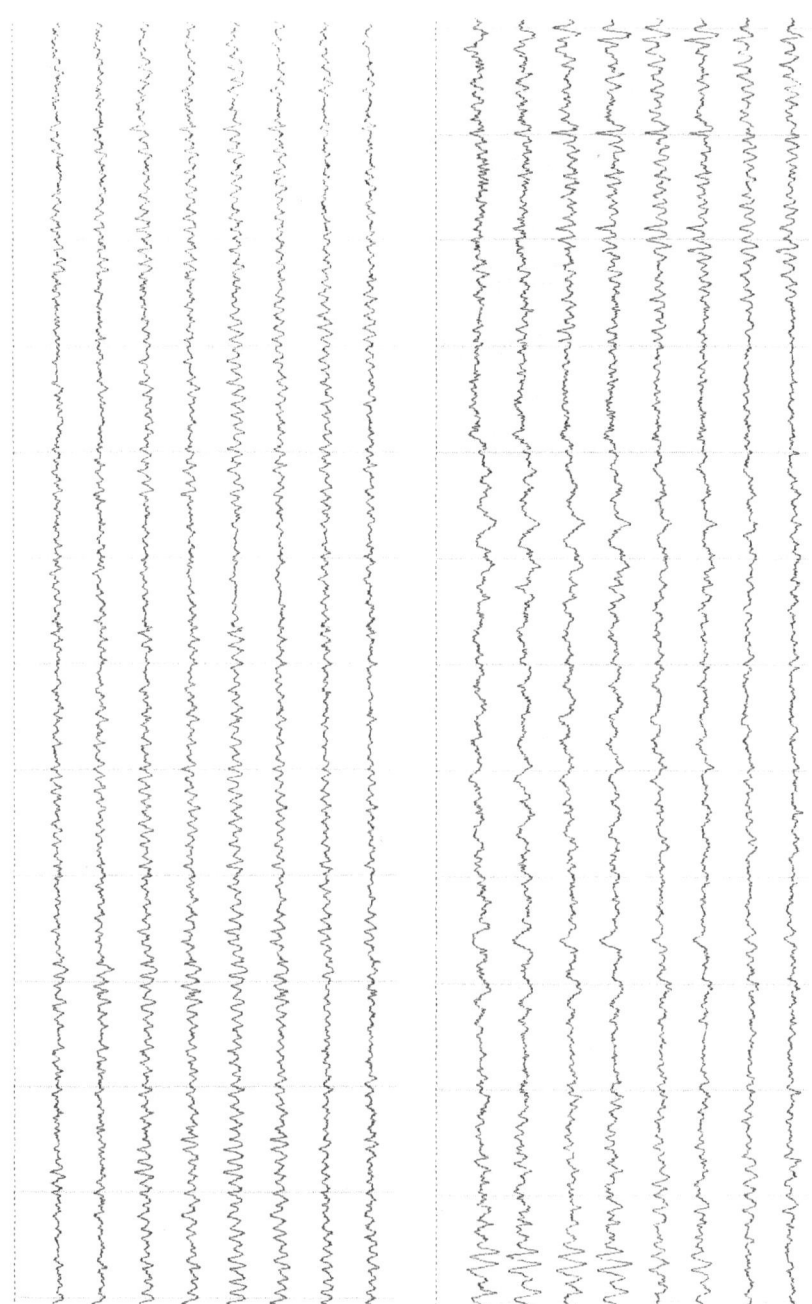

Fig. 112. Above: Medium-degree anteriorized 9/s-activity (**DR**) - recorded in the euthymic interval and medication-free from a patient with bipolar affective psychosis. Below: The effect of a chronic (prophylactic) lithium medication with a plasma level of 0.61 mmol/l; pronounced dynamic lability (**DL**) with abrupt transitions from A- to mid- and late B-stages. Patient remained euthymic (R. R., 56 y., f., EEG-nr. 127/93; EEG-nr. 1010/43).

The relationships presented in Table 9 were observed for 35 patients of our lithium ambulatory with a diagnosis of a bipolar affective psychosis who were treated phase-prophylactically for at least 4 years (26 female, 9 male, age average: 55.7 ± 13 years, mean plasma level: 0.70 ± 0.14 mmol/l). Paired comparisons (FISHER-test, double-sided) indicated that **DR** can be linked to a rather unfavorable phase-prophylactic effect. Differences between relapse rates, **DR** versus **PM** ($p < 0.001$) and **DR** versus **DL** ($p < 0.05$), were statistically significant. Only a minor statistically insignificant difference was found between **PM** and **DL**. Because of the retrospective nature of the study, we cannot answer the question of which EEG-dynamics in the baseline EEG allow the prediction of a phase-prophylactic effect. Regarding our earlier findings obtained from healthy persons as well as patients, we cannot exclude any theoretical possibilities. Clarification can come only from a study of prospective nature. The most plausible explanation seems to us that **DR**, which is overrepresented in patients with melancholia, predicts a favourable response. With preexisting **DR** - be it a *trait* or a *state* feature - lithium works towards a **DL** (Ulrich et al., 1993). Therefore, physiomorph dynamics (**PM**), which correlates positively with a favorable clinical effectiveness, could represent the pharmacogenic modifications of a preexisting dynamic rigidity (**DR**). Whether and how the lithium effect can be delineated from the neuroleptics effect has, to our knowledge, never been investigated systematically. Thus, clarification would entirely hinge on the strict observance of their dependency from the baseline condition. Special attention should be given to the different effects lithium and neuroleptics have on the same person. However, the usual group comparisons certainly will not help shed further light. We suspect that the intermittent left-anterior foci of slow waves (**ILA**), described by many authors (Bente et al. 1982; Czernik, 1978; Helmchen & Kanowski, 1971; Itil & Akpinar, 1971; Johnson et al., 1970; Rwilly et al. 1973), are a lithium-typical feature.

In a retrospective study (Ulrich et al., 1983), we compared 70 outpatients who had been for some time under a phase-prophylactic monotherapy with lithium (average age = 45 ± 7.2 years, mean plasma level = 0.65 mol/l) with

- a group of endogenous-depressive inpatients treated with tricyclic anti-depressants (n = 34; age: 34.8 ± 7.6 years);
- a group of schizophrenic inpatients treated with neuroleptics (n = 83, age: 32.6 ± 6.1 years);
- a group of healthy male volunteers (n = 46, age: 26.5 ± 4.6 years).

Overall, 19% of the lithium-treated patients showed a left-anterior and 6% a right-hemispheral accentuation of slow waves, the latter being less distinct compared to the former. Pair-wise group comparisons showed a significantly higher rate of the left anterior foci in the lithium-treated patients. These differences were not age-related. For ethical reasons, we cannot answer the question of whether this effect of a chronic lithium medication would also occur in healthy persons or whether it requires a patient-specific disposition. Meanwhile, the long-favoured explanation of lithium foci as pharmacogenic unmasking of latent foci resulting from circumscribed brain damage has been rejected for lack of empirical proof.

As explained in the chapter about the "pathological gestalt/functional change of the EEG" (Chapter 4.1), we consider the intermittent left anterior accentuated foci (**ILA**), independent of their respective genesis, as a local manifestation of a global functional disturbance. As we further try to substantiate, (**ILA**) and the intermittent bilateral anterior groups of slow waves (**IBA**) are nothing but different phases of one and the same disintegration process. Therefore, if we combined **ILA** and **IBA** in the same category, the majority of lithium-treated patients will indeed show signs of the disintegration modus associated with this category (s.a. Fig. 43). Although **ILA** and **IBA** typically appear in the same EEG, and it would be hard to find an EEG with ILA that does not also show more or less clearly **IBA**, the "focal" changes, i.e., **ILA** drew attention as lithium-typical EEG-phenomenon. Bilateral anterior-accentuated groups of slow rhythmized waves are mentioned as lithium-typical phenomenon only in the older literature (Andreani et al., 1958; Passouant et al., 1953). We would like to remind the reader the confusing multitude of synonyms under which **ILA** appears in the literature.

5.4 CARBAMAZEPINE

Carbamazepine (CBZ), introduced in the early Sixties as an anti-epileptic, has gained importance as a psychoactive drug only in the last decade. Its current main indications within psychiatry are, as for lithium, the prophylaxis of relapses of affective psychoses as well as the acute treatment of manic syndromes. Based on many years of observations, we want to firmly reject the widely accepted opinion that CBZ has only minor EEG-effects, similar to those observed with tricyclic anti-depressants (Schmidt & Greil, 1987). Although in many cases, the EEG shows only a moderate slowing of the dominant alpha-activity (s.a.

Besser et al., 1992; Bülow, 1987; ; Halder et al., 1975), we frequently encounter diffuse-dysrhythmic EEGs without significant alpha-activity under CBZ. While Ketz (1974) blamed modified EEGs on overdosing, other authors also considered a spectral-analytically assessed increase of the theta- and delta-power as CBZ-typical for the therapeutic dosage range (Besser & Krämer, 1987; Marciani et al., 1992; Wilkus et al., 1978). In this context, we want to mention that diffuse dysrhythmias (DD), although rarely, can also be observed under therapeutic serum concentrations of the anti-epileptic phenytoin. Such changes, also related to a dispositional factor (Riehl & McIntyre, 1968; Roseman, 1961), must be separated from similar ones, which are typical for the cumulative intoxications with phenytoin (Roger et al., 1959). In case of doubt, the assessment of the plasma level will clarify the situation.

Several authors (Bente, 1975; Jeavons, 1972; Pryse & Jeavons, 1970; Rodin et al. 1974; Sachdeo &Chokroverty, 1985) emphasized that CBZ, contrary to other anti-epileptics, frequently leads to an activation of epileptiform activity patterns with simultaneous decrease in the frequency of seizures. The considerable interindividual variation range of the EEG-effects, also pointed out by Besser et al. (1992), can certainly not be explained simply by different dosages or plasma levels. Although generally visually noticeable EEG-effects can only be expected with daily doses higher than 600 mg, we see a distinctly increased degree of dysrhythmia in our clinical patients prophylactically treated for relapses already with daily doses of only between 200 to 400 mg. Thus, an individual-specific factor must play a decisive role. If we are looking for a pharmacon with a similar variation range of the EEG-effects, we encounter clozaril. As discussed already, here, too, an increase of irregular theta- and delta-activity, frequently accompanied by an activation of paroxysmal hypersynchronic potentials, is considered typical. As with CBZ, inconspicuous and highly changed EEGs can be observed under the same dosage. Another similarity is the frequently stunning synchronization of a pharmacon-induced dysrhythmia caused by psycho-sensorial stimulation.

Fig. 113a shows the resting EEG of a patient with grand mal epilepsy under 1200 mg/d CBZ. We are seeing a diffuse dysrhythmia (**DD**) because of dominating irregular theta-/delta-activity. Alpha-waves can be defined only sporadically. Fig. 113b shows the change after opening the eyes. Compared to 113a, the proportion of high-amplitude delta-waves has decreased and the alpha-proportion slightly increased. Fig.113c shows the EEG recorded with opened eyes and standing. Compared to Figs 113a and 113b, a further regularization can be noticed.

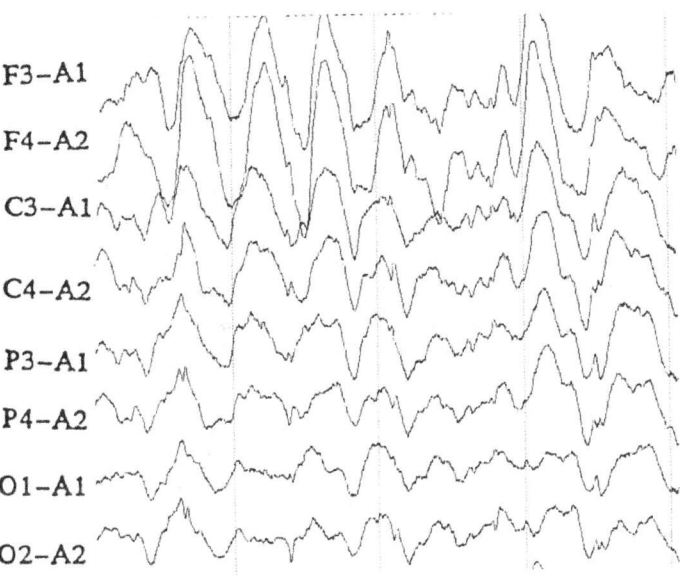

Figure 113a. Eyes closed: Diffuse delta-dysrhythmia with dominating polymorphous and high-amplitude and partially sharp waves.

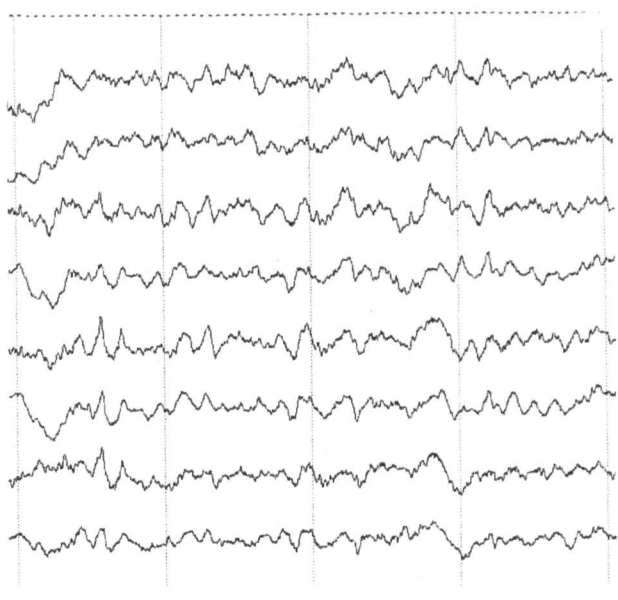

Figure 113b. Eyes open: Diffuse theta-dysrhythmia, singular alpha-waves.

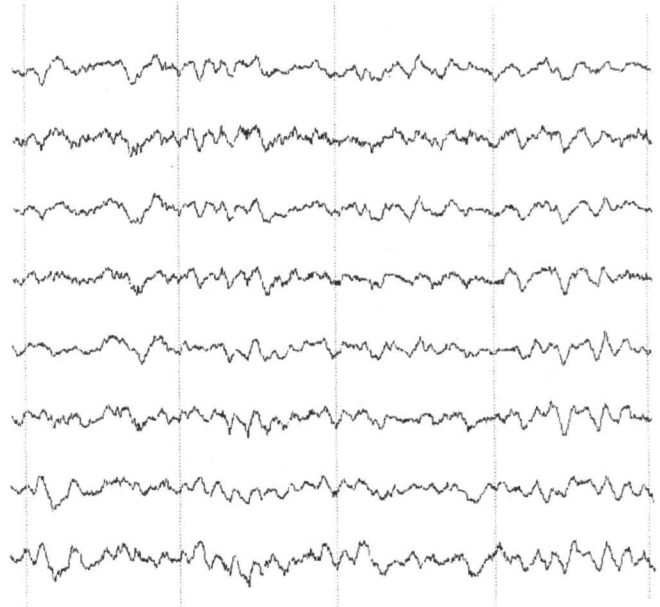

Figure 113c. Eyes open, patient standing: Increase of fast frequencies as compared to b.

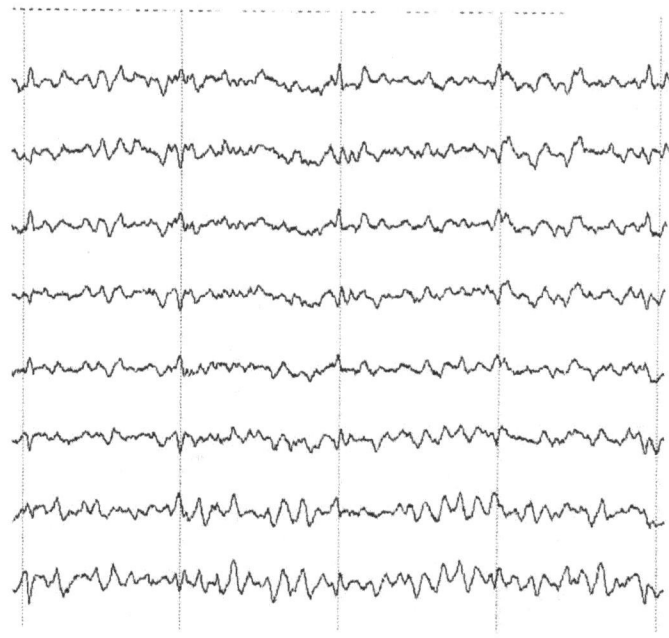

Figure 113d. Eyes open, patient stands and does calculations (serial addition of single-digit numbers): Further regularization compared to b and c, dominating is a posterior-accentuated alpha-rhythm.

Figures 113, a, b, c, d: Carbamazepine effect under various recording conditions.

The maximum attainable effect is shown in Fig.113d. This EEG was recorded under the conditions "eyes open" + "standing" + "calculation" (serial addition of single-digit numbers). The results of a more recent study of primarily spectra-analytical nature conducted with epileptics also confirmed a pharmacon-typical effect (Marciani et al., 1992). Under various degrees of sensorial-cognitive load, a significant decrease in the theta- and delta-power was found compared to the resting EEG. Incidentally, the pharmacogenic diffuse dysrhythmia (DD) convincingly illustrates the inappropriateness of the German term "Allgemeinveränderung". The user of this term will also have to describe carbamazepine and clozaril effects as an "Allgemeinveränderung" of medium to severe degree. This, however, promotes erroneous conclusions or misunderstandings, since this term can hardly be separated from its associated connotation of a pathological performance change ("pathologischer Leistungswandel").

The therapeutically used psychotropic effect that points in the direction of a mood-improvement obviously occurs with very low dosages (Clarenbach et al., 1981; Janke et al., 1983) and does not seem to be dependent on a more massive pharmacogenic gestalt change of the EEG.

Even massive delta-dysrhythmias, as we find them in epileptics under daily doses of 1600-2400 mg of carbamazepine, usually do not have a behavior correlate. We must remember here that such changes are for the most part associated with the "resting" conditions, i.e., an artifical lab situation. Morphodynamically, the CBZ-induced dysrhythmia under resting conditions can be compared to an EEG of the sleep stages D and E. However, since our patients did not sleep and in most cases did not even feel tired, we are faced with another example of the unfeasibility of a one-on-one association between EEG and behavior/experience phenomena. While these relationships, even under normal circumstances, are more or less vague, we see here a systematic dissociation of the two description levels. Whether the phenomenon described here constitutes a starting point for the explanation of the action mechanism remains to be discussed.

5.5 Tranquilizers, Hypnotics, Narcotics

An increase in the beta-portion is considered typical for a multitude of psychoactive drugs with different main indications that have a sedating and sleep-inducing effect in common. A prominent position among these substances is occupied today by the

benzodiazpines that could not be missing any more from any medical discipline. The **barbiturates**, formerly widely used as hypnotics are today applied largely as anti-epileptics in a combination with analgesic products. Here, phenobarbital and primidon still maintain their established position. A typical beta-superposition is also caused by **mephenytoin,** which distinguishes it from the clinically similarly working phenytoin. Because of its therapeutic importance especially in the detoxification treatment, we mention **clomethiazol** here and, without claiming to be complete, the tranquilizier **meprobamat**. All **inhalation narcotics,** as for instance the halogenized hydrocarbons, chloroform, and nitrous oxyde have the same effect as above mentioned substances on the EEG.

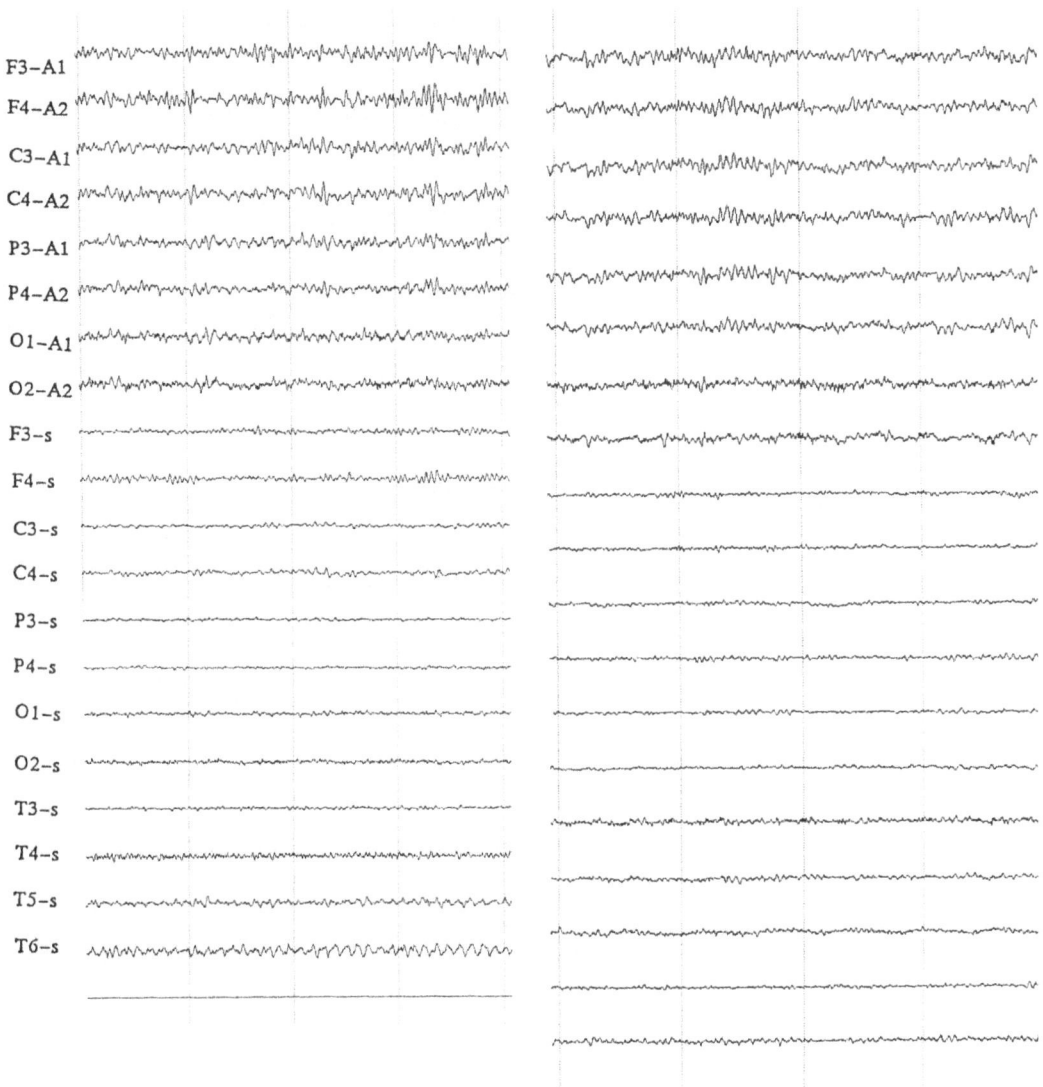

Figure 114. <u>Left</u>: Pharmacogenic beta-activity of approximately 20/s of anterior dominance; temporo-posterior a 9/s alpha-activity dominates; uncontrolled self-medication with benzodiazepine because of an anxiety syndrome (K. A., 19 y., m., EEG-nr. 555/93). <u>Right</u>: Over all regions a pharmacogenic beta-activity of approximately 18/s prevails, intermittently with temporo-posterior accentuatuation. Uncontrolled self-medication with clomethiazol in alcoholism (R. S., 54 y., m., EEG-nr. 665/93).

The EEG-effects of all these substances in therapeutic dosages - for inhalation narcotics we are referring to the induction phase of narcosis - are rather similar. We typically find an EEG with an anterior-accentuated 15-30/s beta-activity, which supersedes all other activities, often in connection with *formative tendencies* of the B-stage such as amplitude decrease and rarefication of the alpha-activity (Fig. 114, left). If an alpha-background activity is maintained, it is sometimes marked by an increase in frequency. With regard to the magnitude and the topography of these beta-superpositions, a wide array of graduations is possible. The beta-activity can also dominate over the entire convexity to such a degree that a preexisting alpha-background activity can no longer be defined (Fig. 114, right). We consider calling such EEGs "beta-typical" as unfortunate because it obscures the difference with the rather rare EEGs with constitution-related fast background activity. Preexisting dysrhythmias are, contrary to the effect LSD 25 has on them, not influenced by the substances discussed here. To the contrary, typically latent foci of irregular slow waves associated with some well-defined injury often manifest themselves simply because of the pharmacon effects; neurology put this fact to the diagnosis of circumscribed brain lesions before imaging techniques became available. The reactivity of the pharmacogenic beta-activity to sensorial stimuli is variable, but overall, it is less evident than that of the physiological alpha-activity. There are no regular relationships between the plasma level and the abundance of activity of the beta-superpositions. On the one hand, massive effects can be observed after only minor single doses while on the other hand, we sometimes do not find a significant beta-increase even after documented chronic abuse. Finally, we must remember that because of the lipophilic qualities of such substances, the EEG-effect does not necessarily have to correspond to a specific plasma concentration. For instance, we sometimes find beta-superimposed EEGs without being able to supply the chemical proof by testing the urine. Upon intense interrogation, patients in such cases sometimes remember taking a sleeping pill one or even two weeks ago. As far as we know, the significance of this highly impressive beta-increase on behavior/experience has hardly generated littel interest. In any case, there are no indications of a relationship between the degree of the sedating effect and the amount of beta-superposition. On the other hand, a number of examples exist to prove that a hypno-sedating or narcotic pharmacon effect is also possible without increase in the beta-proportion. Thus, paraldehyde, used as mild hypnotic, never leads to beta-activation. An increase of slow waves can only be observed at higher dosages. A general slowing reaching into the beta-range is found with the short-term narcotic **ketamine**, the neuroleptic-analgesic **dehydrobenzperidol,** and the central analgesic **fentanyl**. With increasing plasma concentrations that exceed the therapeutic range, we observe an increase in irregular slow waves with beta-inducing substances. Heavy barbiturate or benzodiazepine intoxications that frequently result from suicide attempts show a diffuse-dysrhythmic EEG without beta-activity. Their reappearance after the efforts of the intensive care unit indicates a positive prognosis.

The dependence of EEG-effects on the plasma concentrations of the common narcotics was also utilized in the electroencephalographic definition of stages of different depths of narcosis (Schneider & Thomalske, 1956). The induction stage is marked by an anterior 14-30/s beta-activity. During the stage of light narcosis, irregular slow waves are subseding and the beta-frequency decreases. The stage of medium narcosis is dominated by 2 - 3/s delta-waves and a decrease in the superseding beta-activity. Under deep narcosis, all beta-waves disappear.

Because of the potential of dependency and the related neuro-adaptation common to most beta-activity inducing substances, we can assume that the acute effects differ considerably from the effects of the long-term consumption and withdrawal. For barbiturate-addicts, Wikler et al. (1955) described a diffuse dysrhythmia (**DD**) with or without paroxysmal potentials on the second or third day of withdrawal as typical EEG-correlate of the clinical withdrawal symptomatology. Without being able to support this with numbers, some observations during routine diagnostics indicate that such changes also occur under benzodiazepine withdrawal.

5.6 ALCOHOL

A special position with regard to the extent of EEG-literature is reserved for our most popular drug, alcohol. The acute effect investigated in numerous studies with volunteers manifests itself in a dosage-related activation of *formative tendencies* of the A-stage, such as slowing of the background activity under increased synchronization to diffuse dysrhythmia under full drunkenness. On the other hand, totally different characterstcs will show up in the EEG of alcoholics (Arikawa, 1970; Bennet et al., 1956; Davis et al., 1941; Funderburk, 1949; Funkhouser et al., 1953; Jones & Holmes, 1976; Kraus, 1992; Little & Mcavoy, 1952; Müller et al., 1985; Naitoh, 1973; Newman, 1978; Varga & Nagy, 1960;). According to general consensus, at least every other alcoholic shows a discontinuous alpha-rhythm with dominating low-voltage desynchronized activity together with increased beta or in rarer cases also theta-activity. According to these descriptions, which coincide with our own observations, the *formative tendencies* of the B-stage dominate the EEG of an alcoholic following a few days of sobriety. In case of sobriety, the EEG will be "normalized" within 2-3 weeks. The fact that this characteristic is not a rapidly passing effect tied to the immediate effect of the noxa but exhibits a certain time course indicates that we are dealing with a potentially reversible "pathological functional change," which can be coordinated to a dissolution via the B-stage (s.a. Fig.43). As far as we can see, only Propping (1977) considered the possibility that the low voltage desynchronized EEG could be the result rather than the cause of alcoholism. Eventually one will have to bear in mind that one can neither infer nor exclude alcoholism by means of dynamically labile EEG-vigilance (**DL**). If, for instance, a typical alcoholic subject consumes a certain quantity of alcohol immediately before EEG recording – as can be observed with level drunkards before undergoing an EEG recording– he/she will possibly show a physiomorphic Alpha-EEG (**PM**). Therefore, a **PM**-EEG does not necessarily prove non-alcoholism. In such a case, **neuroadaptivity** is responsible for a "false negative" finding.

Because desynchronized low-voltage activity - especially when it occurs in connection with an increase of beta-activity - is still exclusively considered as the manifestation of an increased arousal level (Lindsley, 1961), our interpretation is in diametral contradiction of the common opinion. According to the latter, the EEG may be considered a *trait*- indicator of a supposedly genetically determined increased arousal level that is behaviourally reflected by increased psychological tension and anxiety (Tarter et al., 1984). According to them, alcohol – referring to the acute effect in healthy volunteers - would lead to increased alpha-activity counter-acting constitution-related discomforts. The effects of alcohol perceived as "psycholytic" would make the attraction of thus disposed persons understandable (Docter, 1966; Gabrielli et al., 1982; Jones & Holmes, 1976; Naitoh, 1973). Thus, meditative- as well as biofeedback-techniques emerged as new therapy options.

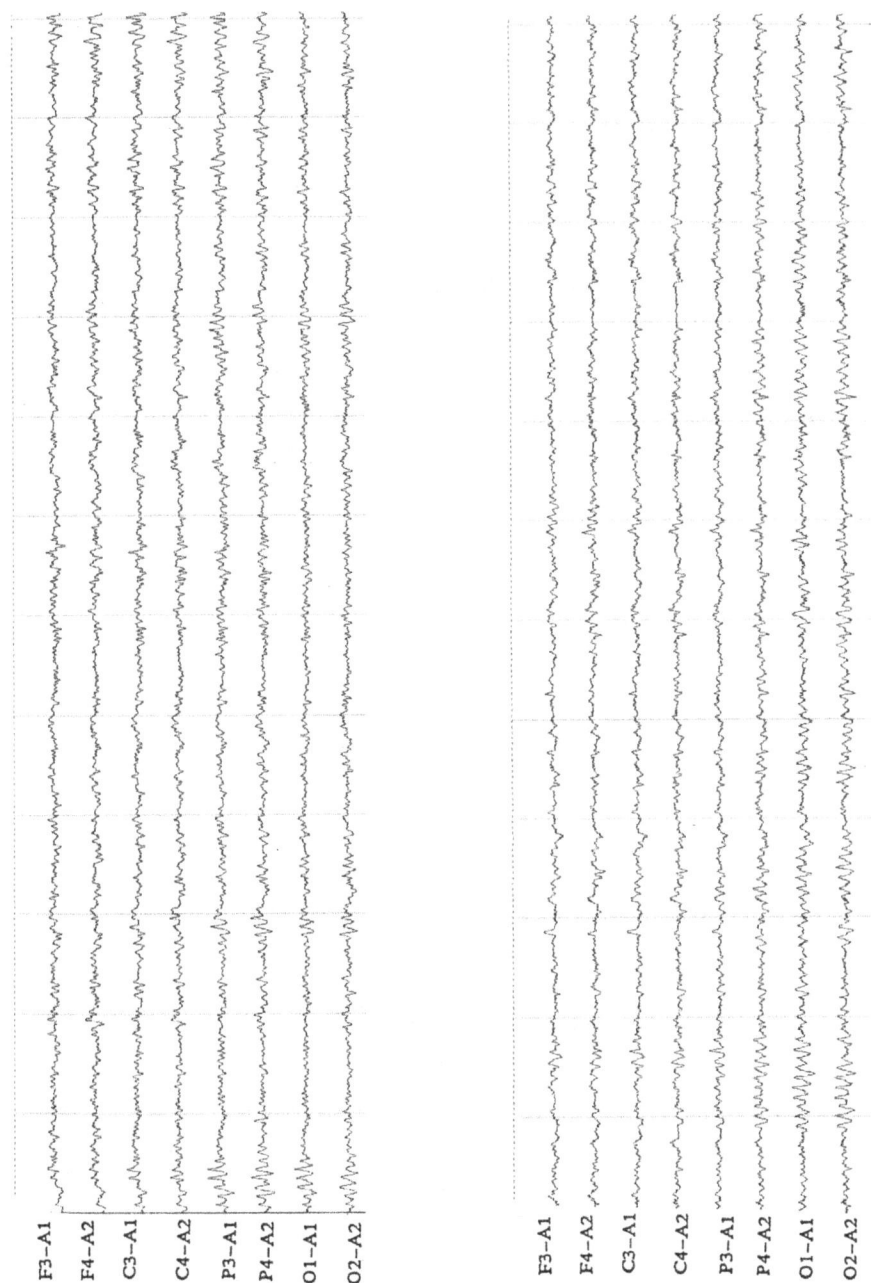

Figure 115. <u>Above</u>: Discontinuous, only sporadically occurring 9-10/s-activity; low-voltage desynchronized phases, partially with fast beta-activity, corresponding to a stage B1 are prevailing; Dynamic lability (**DL**); recorded in medication-free state in an alcoholic, being sober for two weeks; <u>Below</u>: After 3 weeks of withdrawal as inpatient obvious increase in continuity of the now posterior-accentuated 9-10/s-activity in the sense of **PM** (M.N., 44 y., m., EEG-nr. 501/93; EEG-nr. 600/93).

It became evident very quickly that the "training up" of alpha-continuity and -amplitude attempted by such techniques was essentially unattainable in alcoholics (Jones & Holmes, 1976). Instead of re-examining at this point the "arousal"- interpretation that formed the basis of this hypothesis, the negative results were explained by a special inability to cooperate. Moreover, all those well-documented findings, according to which a successful withdrawal is accompanied by a regression of the alpha-discontinuity (**DL**) or the restitution of the physiomorph vigilance dynamics (**PM**) should have been reason to reconsider the "hyperarousal"-theory (Arikawa, 1970; Bennet et al., 1956; Varga & Nagy, 1960;). Especially instructive are the curve examples provided by Arikawa. They document how only three weeks after the beginning of withdrawal, a posteriorly accentuated continuous alpha-rhythm was re-established via an intermediate stage.

The reversibility of the **DL** upon withdrawal of alcohol is a clear indication that we are not dealing with a constitutional variant but with the manifestation of a "pathological gestalt/functional change". This also agrees with more recent neuro-radiological findings. Thus, a number of authors established the reversibility of brain shrinkage under abstinence conditions using CT and NMR (Carlen et al., 1978; Mann et al., 1991; Mann & Bartels, 1992; Ron et al., 1982; Schroth et al., 1988; Zipursky et al., 1989). The potential reversibility of a disturbed brain metabolism can be considered as equally established (Berglund et al., 1987; Schroth et al., 1988; Volkow et al., 1992). Because of the reversibility of the DL in the typical alcoholic-EEG, researchers will have to search for predisposing EEGs *traits* of successfully detoxificated, i. e., long-term sober persons. An interesting alternative are the studies with "high risk" persons, such as the biological sons of alcoholics (e.g., Pollock et al., 1988). However, such efforts can be successful only if attention is paid not only to isolated features, but also to the morphodynamics. It is entirely possible, if not probable, that specific constitutional and possibly also inherited predilection types of the spontaneous dynamics can be defined in such case.

The importance of neuroadaptive mechanisms is reflected with alcohol during the withdrawal delirium. It is not surprising that there are no systematic studies with regard to the EEG-correlates of withdrawal delirium and generally of delirium tremens, if one considers the difficulties interfering with an at least minimally technically acceptable EEG from such patients. A low-voltage EEG with some theta-waves that lacks alpha-activity (Schear, 1985) is viewed as a characteristic of an alcoholic delirium and alcoholic hallucinosis. According to Wikler et al. (1956), generally "mild but definitive dysrhythmias" occur in alcoholics during the withdrawal phase without necessarily being related to a specific psychiatric syndrome. The pertinent recording examples are indicative of a "pathological gestalt/functional change" of the **ILA/IBA** type. In subacute metalcoholic encephalopathies, such as Wernicke's encephalopathy being characterized by an often reversible confusional state and now and then followed by the irreversible findings of Korsakoff's dementia, one usually encounters a diffuse dysrhythmia (**DD**) and sometimes asymmetrically accentuated periodic paroxysmal discharges (Fournet & Langternier, 1956; Niedermeyer et al., 1981).

5.7 Opioids, Psychoanaleptics, Psychodysleptics

The two-phasic nature of the EEG-effects following a single dose that is common to many psychotropic substances has been substantiated in a number of studies on **methadon** (Wikler & Altschul, 1950), **morphine** (Wikler, 1954), **heroine** (Zaks et al., 1969; Volavka et al., 1970) and **cannab**is (Low et al., 1973). Upon the intravenous administration of **opioides**, a clear accentuation of *formative tendencies* of the A-stage occurs initially. Older authors who paid attention mainly to the frequency features considered a slight slowing of the dominant alpha-frequency as a typical acute effect of opiates (Andrews, 1941; 1943; Isbell et al., 1947; 1948; Matejcek et al., 1986).

After a few minutes, *formative tendencies* of the B-stage increasingly dominated the picture. Dependent on the dosage as well as on the constitutional disposition, irregular slow waves and/or paroxysmal potentials may occur. As other centrally dampening substances, such as opioides, can make the EEG-signs of a circumscribed brain lesion more distinct (Schneider & Rémond, 1949). As already mentioned, we must expect, as a matter of principle, that psychotropic substances will induce **neuroadaptive processes**. This is especially true for the potentially addictive substances addressed in this chapter. With long-term consumption of consistently low to medium dosages, a general regression of the initial acute effects can be expected – both of the psychotropic and the electroencephalographic ones - whereas with long-term high dosages the **neuroadaptive capacities** are not sufficient for a complete recovery from the acute effects, leading to the chronic effect. The withdrawal of the substance induces a **readaptation process**. Until the baseline condition is regained, EEG-changes must be expected despite or because of the missing noxa. The studies on the topic of EEG-effects due to addictive substances often do not take into account the various time frames required for adaptation- and readaptation processes (see 5.7). Thus, it is certainly not without significance whether for instance the acute effect of cannabis or cocaine is examined in probands without any drug experience or, as usual, in occasional drug users during a differently defined "drug-free" interval or maybe even in persons who presently are using the drugs. Since usually only the drug addicts with a tendency towards increasing dosages gain medical attention, it is not surprising that relatively little is known about the EEG-effect in socially well-adjusted long-term consumers.

Alper et al. (1990) made a contribution to the topic of **neuroadaption** by means of EEG-quantifying. In habitual **cocaine** users, an anterior-accentuated increase of the alpha-spectral alpha-power was found still two weeks after the last drug consumption, i.e., during the drug-free period. The curve examples, recorded with ear reference show a monomorph, relatively slow and anteriorly spread alpha-activity, i.e., the typical picture of a **DR**. The authors considered this finding a manifestation of a "distinctive syndrome of neuroadaptation" caused by the withdrawal. The performance deficiency induced by the cocaine-withdrawal evidenced itself in the lack of drive, depressive mood, and dysphoria, i.e.,symptoms usually associated with a lack of dopamine (Dackis & Gold, 1985; Gawin & Kleber, 1986). Hardly anything at all is known about the acute effects of cocaine on the EEG. Since there are no medical indications for cocaine, the chances for closing this gap in knowledge are slim. The acute effects observed under dopaminagonists, such as amphetamines probably correspond largely to those of cocaine.

Older observations indicating that the therapeutic effect of amphetamines in hypermotor children did not have an EEG-correlate support the dependence of the effects on the baseline situation that also exists for these substances (Cutts &Jasper, 1939; Lindsley & Henry, 1942), indicating that for hypermotor children, getting addicted to the drug is unlikely. Unfortunately, as far as we know, no recent research about this subject exists.

Neuroadaptation probably also plays a role with **nicotine**. Withdrawal of the noxa led to an evident decrease in the dominating alpha-frequency in nicotine addicts that appeared to be reversible upon resumption of smoking (Ulett & Itil, 1971).

Like Alper et al.'s (1990) study conducted with cocaine users, Struve et al. (1989) found an increased spectral alpha-power in long-term cannabis-users as compared to a control group. The difference was more pronounced in the anterior than in the posterior region. Here, too, the EEG was recorded with ear reference. The assumption that the quantitative findings are an expression of a **DR** is easily supported by the curve examples. The authors do not deem an interpretation of the topographical aspect possible at this time:

"Neurophysiological explanations for the marked hyperfrontality of alpha activity we report with heavy THC users do not readily present themselves nor are they expected to do so soon."

The use of the term "hyperfrontality" expresses an affinity with neuroanatomic/neuropsychological interpretation models that we consider in principle inappropriate for the EEG-phenomena described here. Additionally, regarding the concerns of recording techniques, we do not consider it fitting to talk about "hyperfrontality." In derivations with ear reference (i.e., ear lobe reference may pickup temporal lobe activity from anatomical reasons), the question whether the alpha-focus is frontal or temporal must be left unanswered.

That long-term massive **cannabis** abuse leads to **DR** via an accentuation of the *formative tendencies* of the A-stage, which can be deduced from older research about the topic (Deliyannakis et al., 1970; Fink, 1976; Miras, 1969; Rodin et al., 1970; Volanka et al., 1973b; Wikler & Lloyd, 1945). However, we should not ignore the fact that contradictory findings also exist (f.i., Hollister et al., 1970; Jones & Stone, 1970;). Quite possibly, the dependency of the effects on the baseline condition plays a role as well. Another source of variation might be the two-phasic nature of the EEG-effects that must be assumed for cannabis (Low et al., 1973). Early on, it was noticed that the neuroadaptation with **cannabis** might be particularly pronounced. For instance, previous studies reported that under long-term administration of identical daily doses, the initially evident EEG-effect could no longer be proven after 6 days (Wikler & Lloyd, 1945; Williams et al., 1945). Fink (1976), who was particularly interested in tolerance development, found that long-term users did not present *"abnormal EEG records"* any more frequently than did people in a control group. He stated that in acute tests, long-term users showed a similar EEG-effect as occasional users. The only difference was that for the former, the effect occurred only after comparatively higher dosages.

Our quantitative observations (Winterer et al., 1995) included a 28-year old patient who was admitted for treatment with the diagnosis of "agitated depression" because of a diffuse complaint picture and relationship problems. He informed us about his long-term and regular **cannabis** use. Immediately before being admitted, he had enjoyed another joint. Figs. 116 a, b, and c show representative EEG segments recorded each day at the same time and free of medication on the 2nd, 16th, and 28th day as inpatient. In comparison to the first EEG, the second EEG recorded after a two-week cannabis-free period shows an anteriorization of the alpha voltage maximum corresponding to a stage A2-A3. The third EEG, recorded another 12 days later, is similar to the first one in its morphodynamics. In the average power spectra of track O2-A2 (Fig. 117), but also of any other track, these morphodynamically highly impressive differences are not reflected. As we attempted to substantiate them in another context (Ulrich et al., 1990), the development as well as regression of a **DR** can be objectified by the quotients of anteriorization (AQ), one for the left and one for the right hemisphere (see below, 7.2). For that purpose we first determine, spectral-analytically, the absolute alpha power across the frequency range 8-13 Hz for successive 2s-epochs of an anterior and posterior lead of the left and right hemisphere, respectively.

The quotient is formed for the left side according to:
$$AQ_l = \frac{F3/A1}{F3/A1 + O1/A1}$$
$$AQ_r = \frac{F4/A2}{F4/A2 + O2/A2}$$

The target variable is the average of 300 short-term (2s-) anteriorization quotients as calculated during a 10-minute recording under resting conditions. We express the persistence of the alpha-anteriorization through an amplitude-independent measure of variation of our 2s-anteriorization quotients, i. e., the coefficient of variation (CV).

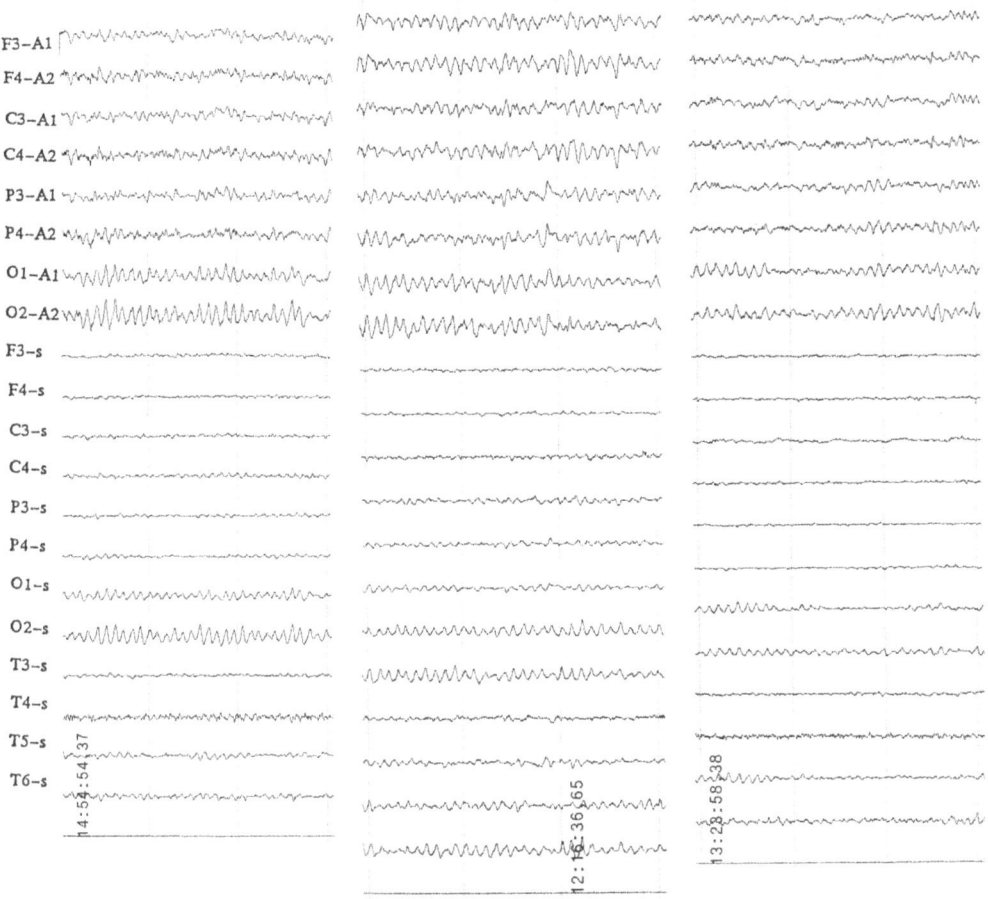

Figure 116. Time course of EEG changes during cannabis withdrawal.
a) Alpha-typically organized EEG with a posterior-accentuated background activity of approximately 9-10/s - recorded medication-free but with assumed residual cannabis influence (F.B., 28 y., m., EEG-nr. 1157/92).

b) 9-10/s alpha-rhythm with an anterior spreading tendency; minor to mid degree **DR** - after two weeks without cannabis (EEG-nr. 1204/92)

c) After another two weeks without cannabis physiomorph EEG; no significant difference from the baseline-EEG (a) (EEG-nr. 1321/92).

The values listed in table 9 confirm and illustrate the impression of an increase in the alpha-anteriorization resulting from a variability decrease in the alpha-topography from day 2 to day 16 and an almost complete return to the baseline EEG on day 28. In relation to day 2, the increase in AQl was 26% and the increase in AQr was 50% on day 16.

Simultaneously, the CV-AQ$_l$ decreased by 34% and the CV-AQ$_r$ by 37%.

Since other possible causes, such as psychoactive drugs, could be ruled out, we can conclude that in our patient, the withdrawal from cannabis led to a passing "pathological gestalt/functional EEG-change" of the type of a dissolution via the A-stage (see Fig. 26). With regard to the "pathological performance change", it is worth mentioning that the patient, approximately one week after admittance, i.e., after a withdrawal period of one week, developed the fluctuating psychopathological picture of a minor-degree organic brain syndrome ("*hypermotorisch-emotioneller Schwächezustand*" sensu Bonhoeffer (1909)). This picture persisted for one week and then faded slowly. The indistinguishability of the EEG recorded while still under cannabis influence and the one after four weeks of withdrawal confirms empirically the principle of **neuroadaptation.**

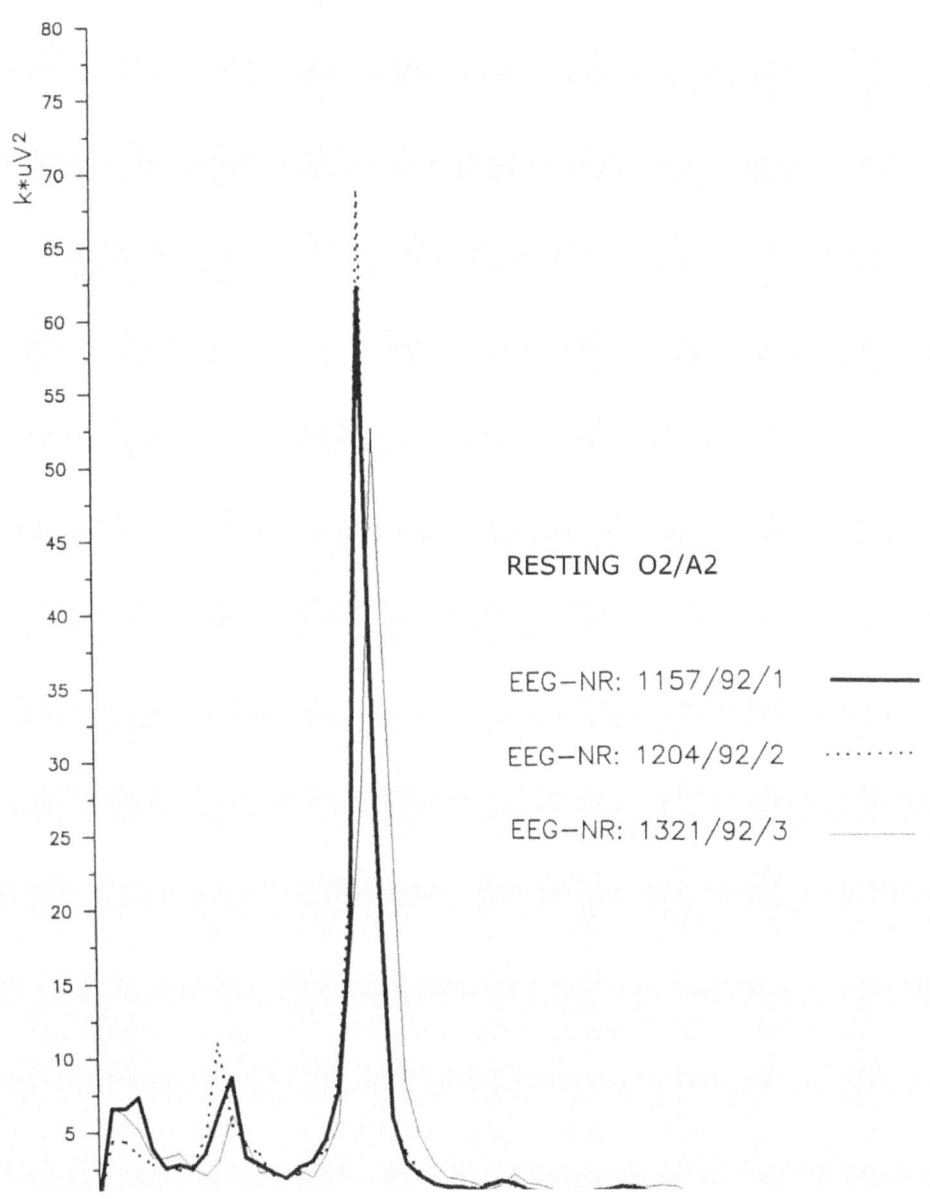

Figure 117. Average power spectra (10-minute resting EEG) corresponding to 300 short-term spectra of 2s each of the track O2-A2 of the 3 EEG-registrations presented in Fig. 116. The obvious morphodynamic difference between the first and the second EEG (Fig. 116a, b) is in in no way reflected in the respective spectra.

	Time of EEG recording		
	Day 2	Day 16	Day 28
AQ_l	0,41	0,52	0,37
$CV\text{-}AQ_l$	0,35	0,23	0,38
AQ_r	0,28	0,42	0,31
$CV\text{-}AQ_r$	0,49	0,31	0,39

Table 10
Mean values from 300 consecutive 2s-epochs of a 10-minute recording under resting conditions, as well as the respective coefficients of variation (CV).

5.8 Psychotomimetics

A pronounced synchronizing initial effect in connection with an acceleration of the background activity followed by a desynchronization corresponding to a stage B is considered typical for hallucinogenics, such as **mescaline** (Borenstein & Cujo, 1969; Denber & Merlis, 1955; Fink, 1969; Wikler, 1954), **psilocybin** (Kolarik et al., 1966), and **LSD 25** (Bente et al., 1958; Borenstein & Cujo, 1969; Brown, 1968; Fink, 1969; Korein & Musacchio, 1968). Several authors agree that the initial synchronization is accompanied by a disappearance of preexisting dysrhythmias or focal changes (f.i., Bente et al., 1958; Borenstein & Cujo, 1969; Itil et al., 1968; Korein & Musacchio, 1968). This is a peculiarity that could not be observed in any other substance with a synchronizing effect. The desynchronization phase (stage B) that follows the synchronization phase (stage A) is considered the correlate of drug-induced hallucinatory experience (ENDO, 1952). Since **hallucinogenics** generally do not lead to addiction, the occasionally discussed question about the chronic effect or the neuroadaptation is of lesser importance (Blackler et al., 1986).

5. 9 Nootropics

We talk about a therapeutically desirable nootropic EEG-effect when a preexisting "pathological functional change" has been counteracted (Bente et al., 1978). This means that the nootropic EEG-effect, as a matter of principle, can only be observed in patients and never in young healthy probands. A methodologically central but generally neglected aspect is that a recovery indicator that is applicable to all patients cannot exist. In the case of dissolution via the A-stage (**DR**), recovery is synonymous with a change in the direction of dynamic labilization (**DL**), i.e., an increase of the alpha-frequency and a retreat of the anteriorized alpha-activity. In the case of dissolution via the B-stage (**DL**), however, a dynamic restriction, i.e., an increase in continuity, amplitude, and synchronization of the alpha-activity indicates therapeutic success. As previously discussed in another context, if we had neglected such premises, we would have missed, for instance, the doubtlessly existing and in the meantime also by other researchers confirmed nootropic effect of the calcium-antagonist nimodipine (Ulrich & Stieglitz, 1988). The same holds true for a study with the partial dopamine antagonist **tergurid** (Ulrich & Suchy, 1987). However, the fact that the therapy goal must be determined individually for each patient based on the baseline condition seems to be beyond the imagination of most EEG-experts as well as gerontopsychiatrists active in the field of nootropics.

CHAPTER 6
The Quantified EEG (QEEG):
Its Present Scientific Status and Eddington's Parable

In order to point out how science may prevent itself from gaining new insights, the famous astrophysicist Sir Eddington (1882-1944) invented the following parable (see „The Philosophy of Natural Sciences", 1939):

After decades of intensive research, an ichthyologist pretended to have found a fundamental law of ichthyology:

Fishes are living beings with a diameter of at least half an inch.

The publication was celebrated as a major breakthrough. None of his peers had any doubts about its truth. Only a close friend who was an ichthyological layman dared to ask (within a face-to-face-talk) about the width of fishing nets' meshes. He learned that every serious ichthyological scientist uses - of course - the scientifically standardized half an inch nets. No prestigious peer reviewed journal would accept an article for publication if an author would violate this profound guideline of the ichthyological society. The friend's proposal to check the truth of the alledgedly new fundamental law was rejected as unscientific metaphysical hairsplitting:

"What I cannot catch with my net lies beyond the bounds of ichthyological knowledge in principle; it does not refer to an object of the kind defined as an object in ichthyology."

Additionally he stressed that even laymen are implicitly convinced based on the newly scientifically proved insight - or had he ever heard from a fish market customer who demanded fishes being thinner than half an inch?

It was totally inconceiveable to our outstanding opinion leader and his peers that the result of any empirical research is essentially determined by the investigator's decision to make use of a particular measurement tool. Using this parable, Eddington argued against the conviction of „naive empirism" that man is principally able to recognize ("see") the nature as it **really** is.

Our "EEG-vigilance"-**framework** can be conceived as analogous to the ichthyologists' fishing nets; however, with a decisive difference. Our framework is much more encompassing compared to any isolated mathematical transformation tool. Any kind of quantification has to be guided by and accomodated with this fundamental conception. Otherwise, the results would lack an interpretative basis.

Originally derived from qualitative visual gestalt-perception, the EEG-vigilance framework delivers a sound basis (the only one that is imaginable to me), at least partially, for the development of mathematical tools to quantitatively reconstruct the originally given highly complex qualitative spatio-temporal information.

No mathematical processing of the EEG signal can be an end in itself. FFT, for instance, does not deliver more clinically relevant information than does the qualitative evaluation by a trained subject. Rather, the contrary is true because FFT totally eliminates the highly important information about **dynamics**! Nevertheless, power spectra are indispensable if they are regarded and used as intermediate steps in order to quantitatively reconstruct the original qualitative signal. The results (given in numbers) of any quantification procedure that are the more precious the better they can be re-translated into the original spatio-temporal signal better. This re-translateability is the lackmus test of the usefulness of quantification tools in principle, notwithstanding the fact that certain parameters (e.g., coherences) or especially differences between succeeding records are hidden to the "naked" eye (even the trained one).

6. 1 Promises, Fictions, Disappointments: A Documentation from the Literature

The present deadlock or even paralysis of clinical electroencephalography in neuropsychiatry accompanies a general disappointment concerning promises and expectations aroused by commercially available quantification techniques. Within the past few decades, serious research has been substituted by commerce.

Experimental physiologists and/or mathematicians with acknowledged merits in basic animal research suggested using EEG-Systems to assist the psychiatrist in making the "correct" diagnosis. The following documentation of selected citations from literature comprises the period between 1987 and 2006.

It may be stated in advance that literature is rather void of arguments justifying correlation, that is, theory-based studies, between the brain-electrical activity on the one hand and behavior (including experiencing as "inner behaviour") on the other. This fundamental problem that has to be deal with before starting empirical investigations has not been discussed up to now. Instead, a trial- and error-strategy seems to be generally accepted as a substitute. We could never obtain insights about the relationship between the domain of **function** (represented by the EEG) and the domain of **performance** (comprising acting and experiencing) through this kind of chance-based research. Thus, stubborn empiricists who are reluctant to deal with the epistemological basis of their work (discredited by them as "metaphysical speculations" or "armchair philosophy") should at least be urged to explicate their arguments in favor of a psychophysiological meaning of mere power spectrum variables.

The Task Force of the "American Psychiatric Association" stated in 1991 that, "*psychiatrists hope that the successful use of q-EEG … may be extended some day to the detection of abnormal features in such illnesses as schizophrenia and affective disorder.*"

However, "hoping" cannot be enough. The "hoping" scientist should also take care of the unsolved problems, methodological shortcomings, and especially the basic errors listed up chronologically in the following.

I. Promises and Fictions:

"*On the other hand, the advantages of this technique are sufficiently clear that in a few years its routine clinical usefulness may well be evident*" (Hughes, 1987).

"*…these results are the first independent validation of clinical nosology*" (John, Prichep, Friedman et al., 1988).

"*.. abnormal profiles distinctive for each disorder….*"
"*Quantitative EEG is far superior to conventional EEG in its detection of true positives and its ability to discriminate among psychiatric disorders*" (John,

1989).

"Extension of the capabilities of the EEG is within easy reach, particularly once techniques are devised for automatic placement of up to 256 electrodes" (Wikswo, Gevins, & Williamson, 1993).

"Q-EEG is clearly of clinical value."
"The raison d'etre of qEEG is to extract, in an objective and quantitative manner, those parameters of clinical EEG that are traditionally obtained by experienced electroencephalographers using unaided visual inspection." *"Issues in application of "Neurometrics" arise primarily from improper application by inexperienced, untrained users"* (Duffy, Hughes, Miranda et al., 1994).

"Relevant biological measurements may become invaluable adjuncts for the selection and evaluation of treatment and may minimize false starts, decrease severity and shorten duration of symptoms, and markedly reduce costs".
"… of all the imaging modalities, the greatest body of replicated evidence regarding pathophysiological concomitants of psychiatric and developmental disorders has been proved by EEG and QEEG studies".
"…QEEG methods offer improved efficacy of patient management and decrease the risk of ineffectual treatment or misdiagnosis" (Hughes & John, 1999).

II. Disappointments

"EEG-based predictions were more accurate when based on DSM-I and DSM-II criteria than when based on Research Diagnostic or Feighner Criteria using the same patients" (Small, Milstein, & Sharpley et al., 1984).

"In fact, evidence to support the clinical use … has not yet proved compelling … have not adequately dealt with the issue of how much new diagnostically relevant information it really provides" (Weiner, 1987).

"Currently, however topographical mapping (TM) findings should not be used as clinical evidence for cerebral dysfunction in the absence of significant changes by

routine testing" (Fish, 1987).

"However, there are no independent studies corroborating the usefulness of Neurometrics in the differential diagnosis of any disorder" (Fish & Pedley, 1989).

"However, the clinical application of EEG brain mapping is still very limited".
"Overall, these techniques have a very limited clinical usefulness" (American Academy of Neurology, AAN, Report, 1989).

"Because qEEG itself contributes only limited information of direct clinical significance, persons otherwise not qualified to perform differential diagnoses of mental disorders, are not qualified to make diagnoses with qEEG".
"The ability of qEEG to help in the diagnosis of (non-organic disorders), such as schizophrenia or depression, is not yet established".
"At this time, the ability of any qEEG procedure to make psychiatric diagnoses or to discriminate between various groups of psychiatric patients and normal subjects is not well established" (APA Report, 1991).

"Although computerized topographical mapping was commercially developed in the 1980s, it did not obviate the need for examination of wave form morphology of the EEG traces and had little impact on clinical practice" (Wikswo, Gevins, & Williamson, 1993).

"CEEG remains highly controversial in the clinical setting, with statements from individual experts and from several medical speciality societies warning against its potential for error, misinterpretation, and abuse. There is a paucity of actual data about the use and validity of CEEG in clinical practice" (Epstein, 1994).

"However no sensitivity, specifity, or other similar accuracy measures were reported, so the applicability of these general results to individual patients is unclear" (Prichep, John, Ferris et al. 1994).

"The practical clinical problem is that even very significant between-group statistical differences on a measure do not necessarily mean that the measure

is capable of classifying individuals into their respective groups with any useful degree of accuracy" (Knott, Bakish, Lusk et al., 1996).

"Although abnormalities have been reported repeatedly in EEG and QEEG studies of patients in the above categories, consistent patterns have not yet been discerned" (Hughes & John, 1999).

"Serious controversy begins when qEEG data recorded from a patient are compared statistically with normative data bases, on the assumption that clinically significant psychiatric disturbances may be accompanied by statistically significant abnormalities in brain activity" (Coburn, Lauterbach, Boutros et al., 2006).

III. Unsolved problems and shortcomings and errors

"Perhaps the most vexing problem in brain mapping is the intersubject and intrasubject reproducibility and variability".
"…the selection of one given epoch to represent the EEG of a given subject offers many potential problems" (Hughes, 1987).

"The portrayal of cortical landmarks … gives the false impression that anatomic resolution to the level of a single cerebral gyrus can be accomplished".
"The mapping of statistical measures has also been questioned, in that the establishment of a difference on statistical grounds does not necessarily imply an abnormality in a pathological sense".
"Furthermore the compressing of many minutes of EEG data into the form of a few maps ignores the time varying nature of the EEG" (Weiner, 1987).

"Up to several thousand variables have been analyzed in patients and control groups often containing fewer than 20 persons".
"Another problem is that many EEG features are correlated. The number of statistical tests is relatively unrestricted. There is no basis for making a priori assumptions about particular quantitative features".
"The validity of the conclusions drawn from the results of John's studies is doubted

because no relationship could be demonstrated to specific brain dysfunctions which could be used for differential diagnosis".

"Manufacturers offer systems containing normative data from control groups and invite the user to determine the statistical significance or likelihood that a given patient belongs to a particular diagnostic group. For this approach to work in practice, however, the user must first have an accurate working diagnosis! Because of the circular reasoning we do not believe that this approach has either scientific or clinical value" (Fish BJ, Pedley TA, 1989).

"…the computer method has the potential drawback that only a brief segment is shown, whereas conventional EEG records display many minutes of activity…"
"Unfortunately, advertisements and promotional material from some manufacturers of qEEG instruments have gone beyond the existing scientific evidence to make claims of diagnostic utility" (APA Report, 1991).

"…results show that changes in EEG power constantly accompany…scale fluctuations…"
"… the exact pattern of correspondence between EEG and behavior differs for different individuals. This relationship, however, appears to remain stable within individuals across sessions …" (Makeig S, Inlow M, 1993).

"But most of the alleged abnormalities lack any definite correlation with … Nonetheless; the interpreters of these CEEGs designated all such findings as consistent with or as almost certainly due to the presenting clinical complaint" (Epstein, 1994).

"In QEEG, multichannel recording of the eyes-closed resting or background EEG … a sample of … usually 1 to 2 minutes is analyzed" (Hughes & John, 1999).

"Since the spectral composition of brain electrical activity changes systematically as a function of normal aging, qEEG systems use either age-stratified normative data bases … or age regression … to enhance sensitivity and specifity while avoiding age-related bias".
(Regarding this specific point, one cannot restrain from referring to the compelling

empirical evidence according to which no essential EEG changes occur along with <u>normal</u> aging. This is one of many reasons why comparisons of an individual EEG with a normative data base might be misleading.)

"However, the acknowledgement of such striking intra-and inter-subjective differences in the correlation between spontaneous alpha rhythm variations and the BOLD signal, mostly overlooked in previous studies, is considered of great interest as the >resting condition< remains the cornerstone of MRI. In this line of reasoning, the question of intersubject variability should be addressed when comparing fMRI results from different subjects"
(Goncalves, De Munck, Pouwels et al., 2006).

"A major problem faced by the psychiatrist wishing to assess the practical usefulness of commercial qEEG systems, is that information about most systems' capabilities is extremely difficult to obtain. The FDA has in the past placed severe restrictions on the information available to potential users, even forbidding a listing of the specific analyses available, and the ludicrous situation has arisen wherein, even after purchasing one major system, the buyer finds no such listing in the user manual.
A partial solution would be to list each discriminant currently available and the specific literature references supporting it, but this has not been done" (Coburn, Lauterbach, & Boutros, 2006).

"The fact that vigilance fluctuations can have strong effects on BOLD signals has considerable consequences for fMRI research on cognition"
(Olbrich, Mulert, Karch et al., 2009).

The general impression from the citations is that EEG has reached its limits and will be replaced by other methods. By the way, the assertion that an increase in electrodes up to 256 will bring the breakthrough (Wikswo et al., 1993) sounds rather ridiculous.

Among the few articles published within the last decade, two revealing reviews need to be mentioned (Hughes, 1996; Hughes & John, 1999). Obviously, they were written to contest the general loss in the importance of and interest in the clinical EEG but had a negatively effect on the selling rate of their products. The arguments delivered in favor of the unchanged usefulness of the EEG in Psychiatry are disappointingly scanty. First, we learn that:

"The major reason for a referral to EEG from Psychiatry is to obtain evidence of an organic etiology for mental disorder" (Hughes, 1996).

This is exactly what the German neurologist Richard Jung stated 60 years ago. In a subsequent article, the authors felt the need to enrich this meagre argument by emphasizing a supposedly more impressive point:

"As many as 64% to 68 % of EEGs in psychiatric patients provide evidence of pathophysiology and these results have additional utility beyond simply ruling out organic brain lesions" (Hughes & John, 1999).

Regrettably, nothing is said wherein this "additional utility" could apply. This informational deficit is easy to explain when one considers the methodological background of the review. The authors restricted themselves to a mere screening of literature, listing up every report about a relationship between a clinical diagnosis and an "EEG abnormality". No attempt was made to weight the respective importance of these (generally not replicated) findings according to their plausibility. Furthermore, the existing literature has not addressed the unsolved or better unsolvable problem of making the "correct" clinical diagnosis in view of competing classification systems and rules nor similarly unsettled problem of defining "EEG-abnormality".

Instead of a theory-based investigation of psycho-physiological correlations, the authors delivered not more than a mere listing of abstracts. Instead of scientific arguments, they preferred formulations like the following: *"There is broad consensus, that ... "* Basically, the authors admitted their failure in dealing with a psychophysiological or psychiatric EEG when they resumed: *"Although abnormalities have been reported in EEG and QEEG studies of patients ... consistent patterns have not yet been discerned."* One can hardly dispute that this clear statement is inconsistent with the assertion of these as well as other authors who have developed the visual EEG towards a highly sophisticated computer based tool that is capable to make psychiatric differential diagnosis more objective or scientific.

To make EEG a neuropsychiatrically useful tool, the new developments would require "going back to the future". Both topography and dynamics would have to be reconsidered. Our unconventional but by no means new view on EEG is clearly inconsistent with the mainstream. Our goal is an EEG based "Psychophysiology" that would be consistent with the project intended by Berger (1929). To Berger "Psychophysiologie" – a term coined by himself – consists of correlating the physiological and the psychological domain of description without reducing the one in favor of the other. Correlating phenomena belonging to different, i.e., mutually irreducible categories, requires an integrative theoretical framework. Performing and experiencing (the psychological domain) may only be coordinated with function (the physiological domain) if both levels of description are being share a common denominator. According to Bente, this common denominator is represented by Head's (1923) theoretical construct of *vigilance*. *Vigilance* is indicated by the morphodynamics of the resting EEG. Therefore, we speak about "EEG-vigilance," which can be assessed objectively.

6. 2 THE REASONS FOR THE PRESENT DEADLOCK OF QEEG

6. 2. 1 THE "NORMALITY"- PROBLEM

In the forgoing (3.3.1), we have already specified general arguments for the renunciation of the value judgement "normal vs abnormal!" Above all, we have stressed that value judgements make sense only if they relate to a given reference. One may add that "normality" is generally understood as a statistical term indicating "normal distribution" of the phenomenon under consideration. Defining "abnormal" as a certain degree of deviation from the "normal distribution" implies that one deals with a social construct that does not contribute to a proper explanation of the phenomenon. Less familiar investigator will be inclined to rely on statistical normality. A stiking example is the uncritical use of the so-called Normalized Data Bases (**NBD**), which are a decisive part of the commercially available QEEG software packages. They nourish the self-misunderstanding of psychiatry as an applied exact natural science comparable to context-independent exact physics.

However, "life sciences" are intrinsically context dependent. It is a valid principle of all measuring sciences that exactness can only be obtained from comparison between successive individual measurements but not from the absolute measurement values themselves. If one is confronted with a reasonable, naturally given between-subjects variability, any quantitative evaluation would be restricted to single case study. This means that each single subject would have to be subjected to lagged measurements within the time course. This exactly is the core of the methodological principle of ipsative difference assessment (**ITA**), as we have previously advocated (see 7.2; 7.3).

Incidentally, many examples from medicine show that diagnosis is critically dependent on trend information resulting from comparisons of measures performed in fixed intervals.

6. 2. 2 The Deliberate Assumption of Stationarity of the SR-EEG and the Central Limit Theorem

The stationarity assumption of the SR-EEG requires a random process. A time function like the EEG can only be regarded as stationary if the mathematized segment represents the signal in its entirety. Thus, for instance, one can tacitly as well as erroneously impute that the first and the sixth recording minute of a SR-EEG are indiscernible. Accordingly, the spectral frequency parameters, as calculated by FFT, are considered to randomly distributed. This coincides with the mathematical definition according to which random variables are the product of a greater number of influencing quantities of which the single contribution to the total sum is negligible small.

In line with the Central Limit Theorem, random variables are normally distributed. They are represented by Gaussian distribution curve with the mean value and spread. The geometric characteristic of this curve reflects a strict unimodality. Only unimodality is compatible with randomness. Bimodal or multimodal distribution of measurement values are evidence for nonrandomness of the underlying act of generation. In such a case, the decisive precondition for parametric transformations and significance tests is omitted. Processing of nonrandom distributed parameters requires nonparametric methods. Instead of performing primary-quantitative analysis that implies the stationarity assumption as usual, the task consists of finding an explanation for the observable and demonstrable nonrandomness of the measures.

6.2.3 The Unrecognized Arterial Pulse Impedance Artifact (APIA)

Literature and diagnostic practice has hitherto ignored this type of a biological artefact. We became aware of this phenomenon by considering the peculiar coincidence of the well known observational facts:

1. Fourier-spectrograms often exhibit typical steep peaks in the 1.0 - 1.5 Hz frequency range (see Fig. 118).
2. This peak typically prefers temporal regions corresponding to the electrode-placements F7, F8, T3, T4, T5 and T6; occasionally, O1 and O2 are involved. There is no hemispheric predilection.
3. By visual inspection, no corresponding focal accentuation can be detected. Therefore, one has to conclude that the "Delta-waves" underlying the spectrographic peaks must be of such low amplitude that they remain below the threshold of visual recognition. In order to explain the steepness of the peaks, it has to be assumed that the underlying low voltage "Delta" waves occur with rather high regularity, i.e., in a systematic manner.
4. Generally, the spectrographic peaks cannot be reproduced.

Viewed in context, the causative nature of superficial scalp arteries, specifically the Aa. temporalis superficialis and Aa. occipitalis superficialis, deserve consideration (s.a., Ulrich, 2001, Chapt. 6, pp. 214-235). **APIA** is distinct from technical artefacts, as for instance those being due to sloppy fixed electrodes, which may be easily recognized by inspection of the raw signal.

It is a well substantiated fact that blood has a far better electric conductivity than water or organic tissues, like bones, muscles, or fat, because of a higher concentration of electrolytes. This means that the impedance between the surface of the brain and the electrodes placed upon the scalp will decrease during the phase of systolic blood filling of the superficial head arteries and increase during the subsequent diastolic phase. Thus, the arterial pulse induces rhythmical changes of the electrical impedance between the cortical generator inside the skull and the recording electrode outside. This will be show up in the EEG if a recording electrode is being fixed over or very close to the artery. Even exact electrode placement according to the 10-20 system will not prevent such a situation due to the biological variability of arterial topography. Accordingly, a heart beat generated rhythmical variation of the electric field will result. Corresponding to a mean heart rate of 60-90/min, the impedance artefact is to be expected exactly within the actually observed range of 1.0-1.5 Hz. The **APIA** phenomenon vanishes upon minimal shifting of respective electrodes. The most susceptible areas are those corresponding to the run of the above mentioned electrodes (Aa. superficialis temporalis and Aa. superficialis occipitalis (s.a. Figs. 118; 119).

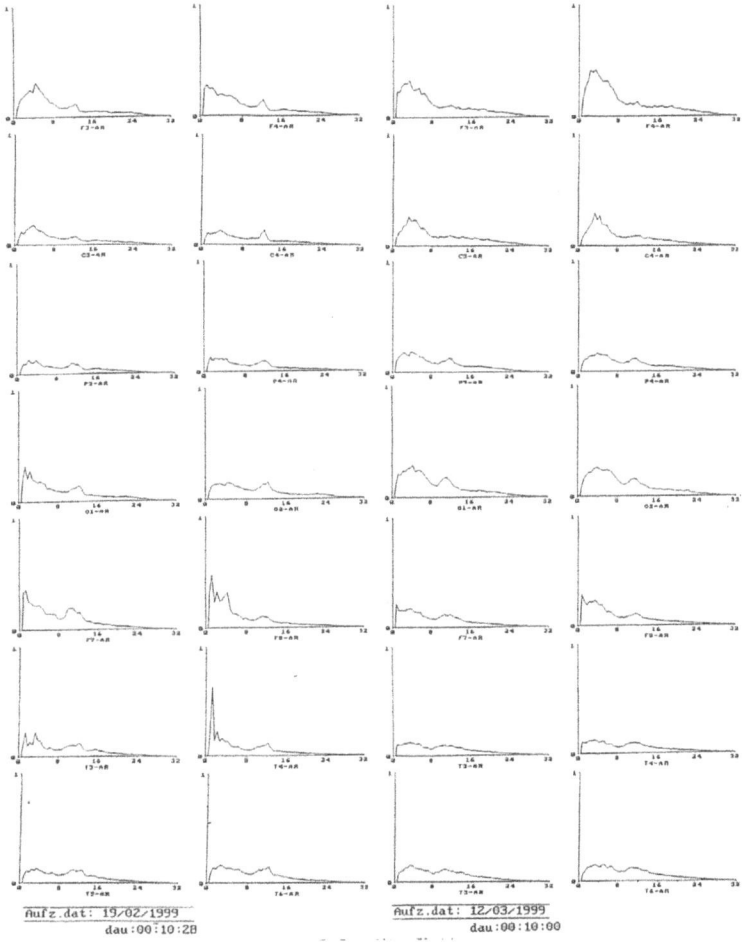

Figure 118. Mean value spectrogramms of two SR-EEGs from a healthy subject, aged 31 y., recorded with an interval of 23 days. First record: The two left-sided vertical columns. Second record: The two right-sided columns; placement of homologous electrodes in vertical direction F3,F4,C3,C4,P3,P4,O1,O2,F7,F8, T3,T4,T5,T6 against Common Average Reference.

With the first EEG, steep peaks around 1.0 -1.5 Hz are distinct over T4 and F8 and less distinct over O1, F3, and T3. With the second EEG, steep peaks are reduced onlyvover F7 and F8. On the whole, a cardial origin, mediated by the superficial head arteries, is suggested (Fig. 119). As can this as well other synopses of FFT spectrograms suggest, the steep peaks around 1.0 – 2.0 Hz occur preferently over the temporal regions F7, F8, T3, T4, T5,T6 and above average over O1 and O2. This localization may be corroborated by the means of Hjorth's (1990) source derivations. The steep peaks appear unilateral and without a hemisperal preference, as a rule. They are generally not reproducible by repeating of the recording. By visual inspection of the underlying raw EEG, no focal lesion-type change can be proven. Thus, one has to conclude that the amplitudes of the generating slow waves must be so low that they remain below the threshold of visual perception. An amplification effect, which occurs from a considerable frequency stability of rather low voltage potentials, can explain the detectability of these waves by FFT. Systematic amplification also explains the steepness, which is uncommon with focal lesions.

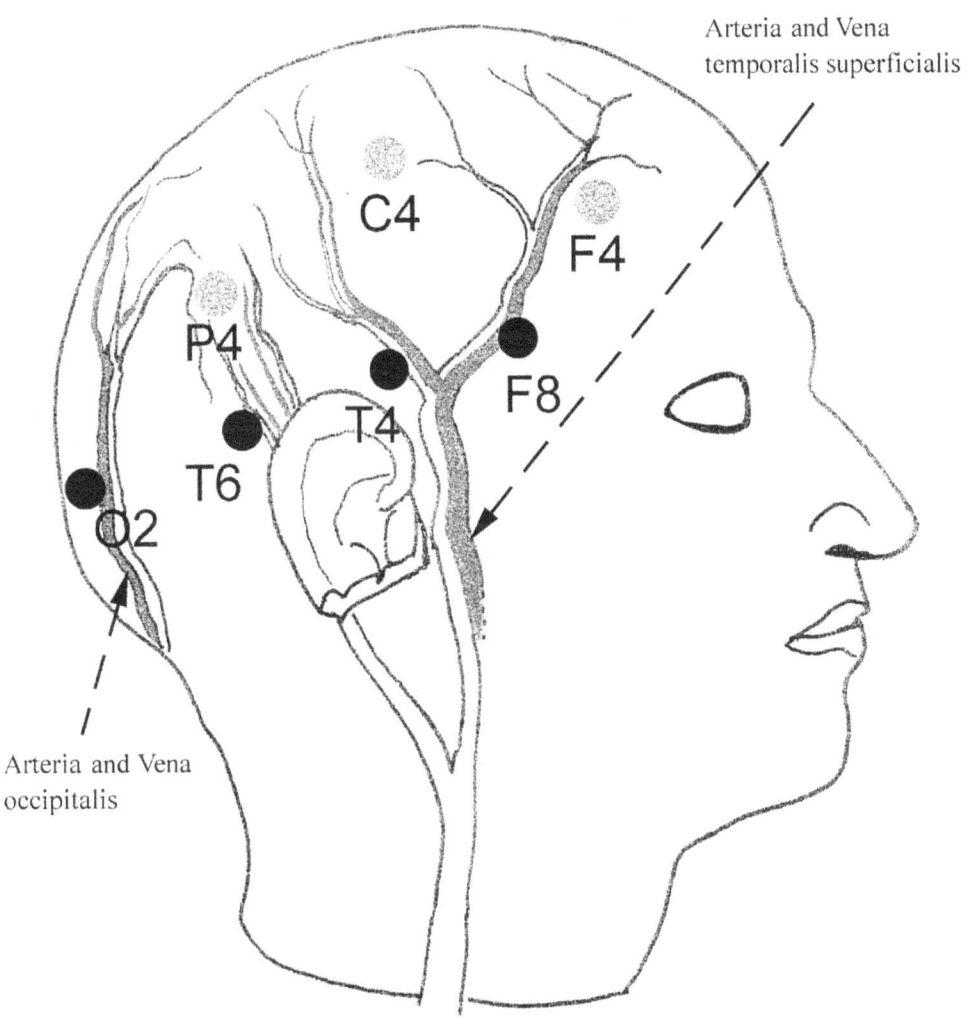

Figure 119. The topographical relationship between certain electrodes as placed according to the international 10-20 scheme and the run of the superficial head arteries.

6.2.4 THE NON-CONSIDERATION OF THE DYNAMICS OF SR-EEG AS MACROINDICATOR OF CEREBRAL GLOBAL FUNCTION (CGF)

It has already been determined that any process of control comprises oscillations about a desired value (3.4.1; 3.4.2; 3.4.4). Characteristically, man-made artificial systems have only one single system status targeted by the design engineer. In living systems, in contrast, a whole range of hierarchically ordered states can be distinguished, which reflect differentiation and goodness of adaptive capability (Bente, 1963).

The SR-EEG can be conceived both as a macroindicator of brain's bioelectric mass activity, i.e., of Cerebral Global Function (CGF), and as a self-organizing process with cyclic order (Bente, 1963; Creutzfeldt, 1975; Freeman, 1975; Storm van Leuwen, 1978). Among the different biorhythms, only the EEG seems to be adequate with respect to the level of systemic integration. Our task consists of the quantitative reconstruction of the different systems' states or levels of brain-electric integration. In doing so, we are guided by the ever changing Gestalt (*Verlaufsgestalt*) of the SR-EEG; thus, explicitly consider the temporal information. The methodological basis of our quantification procedure (see 7.0; 7.1; 7.2) consists of BENTE'S concept of electroencephalographic vigilance dynamics (3.4.3), which has been put forward about half a century ago.

6.2.5 THE MISUNDERSTANDING OF HEAD'S THEORETICAL CONSTRUCT OF VIGILANCE

As already mentioned, *vigilance* is overwhelmingy understood as a certain psychological performance without EEG-connotation, namely "sustained attention", a definition given by Mackworth (1948). As can be deduced from the thematic frame, "Vigilance Regulation in Psychiatric Patients" of an international scientific symposium recently organized by the psychiatric university clinic in Leipzig, there has been a renewed interest in this term in spite of the conceptual confusion. Though being anglophone himself, one of the opinion leaders and author of a rather comprehensive review article, Oken (2006), demanded to abandon *Vigilance* because of continuing semantic inconsistencies.

If under *vigilance* one subsumes different terms, such as *Alertness, Sustained Attention,* and *Selective Attention*, one is in danger of a "categorical fallacy".

Sustained- as well as selective attention refer to certain measurable **performances** of the mind (resulting from an interaction between a living organism and its environment) and therefore to **psychology** (comprising all kinds of behavior, being outward- or inward-directed).

Vigilance (sensu Head, 1923), on the other side, does not refer to functions, the domain of **physiology,** either. Instead, it refers to the disposition enabling a certain performance. The importance of distinguishing between the physiological and the psychological level of description can be demonstrated by an overwhelming amount of empirical findings, excluding the naïve assumption of an unequivocally mutual reduction. An intriguing example concerns the low correlation between experienced (self-assessed) fatigue and certain EEG patterns ($r = 0.20$ or even less!), the so-called sleep inertia following awakening from sleep, or the subgroup of insomnic maniacs who exhibit "paradoxical" drowsiness patterns in their **SR-EEG. Psychological phenomena are neither caused by physiological phenomena nor are they reducible to them.**

Instead, they represent logically and ontologically different categories of description, existing coincidentally (see Jackson's [1884] "Doctrine of Concomitance"). To state that the "power of thoughts" (mind or soul) may steer physiological processes is not more than an unscientific facon de parler. It becomes misleading when it is taken as a scientific statement. A psychological state appears **coincidently** with a defined physiological state, not as an effect of the latter or vice versa. Thus, the notion of "psycho-physic interactions" has no scientific meaning. It is just a way of colloquial speaking (Ulrich: www.journal-fuer-psychology.de/jfp-3-2007-7.98.html). To Head (1923), "*vigilance*" was indispensable in explaining both the clinical fact of spontaneous recovery of the CNS following damage and the characteristical fluctuations with impaired performances. The theoretical influence of Head's concept essentially remained unrecognized in the following decades. As already stated, *vigilance* is neither a function nor a performance. It has the semantic status of an *explanatory principle* (Bateson, 1982).

Explanatory principle is synonymous to *Theoretical Construct* (Carnap, 1956)**,** *Ordering term, or Ordnungsbegriff* (Bente,1975)**,** or Kant's (1784) time-honoured *Regulative Ideen.*

Such terms are needed to explain other phenomena. They cannot be explained by themselves because they represent human creations. One may add that a term, which cannot be explained by itself, cannot be defined operationally.

Whether one prefers to do without *"Vigilance,"* as recommended by Oken (2006) in his review article on vigilance without mentioning Head (1923), or whether one regards *"vigilance"* as an indispensable epistemological term, depends on the position one holds with respect to the theoretical foundation of science as such. To avoid further misunderstandings, it has to be stressed quite unequivocally that Head's *vigilance* makes sense only to a scientist who is primarily interested in the reality behind the overt empirical phenomena. If one, on the other hand assumes the strictly antimetaphysical mainstream position, accepting only objectively measurable facts (to be grasped by our senses and by introspection), Head's *vigilance* must appear nonsensical (Ulrich & Gschwilmg, 1988). Merit has to be given to Bente, who proved the practical usefulness of EEG when already half a century ago, he envisaged a concept of clinical EEG-research based on Head's *vigilance* by recognizing the EEG as an ideal physiological macroindicator thereof. Bente's epistemological position seems somehow inconsistent because he generally committed himself to Logical Positivism (or pure empirism). Notwithstanding, he occupied a clear metaphysical position when he insisted on a categorical separation of physiology and psychology as well as their mutual irreducibility. This might be the deeper reason of his largely unsuccessful endeavour to convince the scientific community of the heuristic value of Head's *vigilance* and his own conception of *EEG-vigilance* that was *based* on the former. Accordingly, it is undisputable to us that a psychophysiological or psychiatric EEG in its proper sense requires Head's *vigilance* (3.4.7). It may be regarded as a sign that EEG-*vigilance* is undergoing revitalization (Hegerl et al., 2008; Olbrich et al., 2009). These authors refered to the work of our Berlin research group that has been conducted during the last decades. Regrettably, they obviously misinterpreted the theoretical term as a psychological one. Such a misunderstanding suffices to discredit the conception as a whole. Thus, we have to read: *"Arousal, activation, vigilance, alertness, sleep wake dimension are overlapping notions and concepts which are broadly used in literature without a commonly accepted definition"* (Hegerl et al., 2008).

Therewith, the authors recapitulated the keynote of the review article by Oken et al. (2006), culminating in the demand to totally abandon *vigilance* because of the seemingly unsolvable confusion concerning its meaning. This is even more disconcerting, as the attentive reading of Head's writings clarifies his intentions in an absolutely unambiguous manner.

Another major difficulty concerns an obstacle to the clinical reception of EEG-*vigilance*. As has already been substantiated, the assessment of *vigilance-* dynamics requires a minimum of 10 minutes of uninterrupted *SR-EEG-* recording (7.2). Before the introduction of the "paperless" digital EEG technique, such a demand was hardly fulfilled. A 30 minutes total recording, for instance, consisted of a sequence of 10 to 20 short-term **SR-EEGs,** each one of about 2-3 minutes length, which was due to the switching between the different electrode montages.

The psychophysiological EEG conception of Bente (1975) is in line with the epistemological foundation of neuropsychiatry initiated by Jackson (1884) and promoted by the most outstanding neuroscientists of the 20th century. In this connection, one should remember to Sittig (1931) when he wrote, more than 80 years ago, that it could be taken for granted that nobody except Jackson (1884) has thought more profoundly about the theoretical foundations of our discipline; thus, it would be wise to follow his traces. According to Sittig, Jackson's teachings were not the teachings of today but the teachings of tomorrow.

(*"Niemand hat vielleicht so tief wie Jackson über die theoretischen Grundlagen unserer Wissenschaft nachgedacht und darin sollten wir ihm folgen."* und weiter: *"Seine Lehren sind nicht die Lehren von heute, sondern die von morgen;"* German original text).

6. 2. 6 THE PRIMARY QUANTIFICATION OF SR-EEG

The quantification of dynamic information, for instance, concerning mimics, gait, or just SR-EEG, focuses on the dimension of time. Time affords a sequential structuring of ever changing dynamic gestalts. Their sequential structure can objectify differences between them. The latter were destroyed by statistical averaging across successively analyzed short-term segments aimed at the calculation of mean values. Since the recognition of a dynamic gestalt depends primarily on visual pattern recognition by a human observer, it represents first and foremost a subjective phenomenon (*quale* in philosophical terms). As such, it is not easily accepted as a real *scientific fact* (Fleck, 1935) within an empiristically funded science. Moreover, the acceptance of such patterns would compromise the tacit assumption of stationarity of the EEG (6.2.2). Nevertheless, subjective phenomena are no fiction. Their real existence can be proved by intersubjectively communicable descriptions and clear cut discriminability. Quantitative reconstructions of dynamic gestalts require simplified models suited for parametrization. Furthermore, they must persist unchanged across a certain timeframe. Otherwise they could not be delimited in a defined pattern.

Literature on this topic is void. The self-critical advisements of Künkel (1980), as published in a German handbook on Psychiatry, deserve more attention:

"One has to ask oneself honestly whether we are treading the right path when we focus on the search of frequency bands ... We will have to face the fact that our model concepts will become much more intricate if we also considered topographical differentiation together with temporal variability. As long as we do not accept this challenge, we may not pretend to have a model at our disposalm which even only roughly describes EEG activity (transl. from German).

Such self-criticism sharply contradicts the practice that has prevailed till now. The influential creators and vendors of q-softwares refer to the so-called z-transformation in defending the stationarity assumption. Z-transformation is a mathematical procedure that brings different frequency distributions to an even standard, known as standard normal distribution. However, if the decisive precondition consisting in unimodal normal distributions of the single EEG parameters is not fulfilled, this is nothing but a baloney. Therefore, this precondition, although it has been ignored, needs to be examined at first. Research founded on a certain unverified assumption will always deliver results that are in line with and conforms to this assumption. Such research has to be dimissed as tautological. Unverified assumptions of normal distribution, linearity, and stationarity/randomness must not be treated as self-evident truths. The existing alternatives of multimodal distribution, non-linearity, non-stationarity/nonrandomness must be given a chance. Otherwise, the editorial remarks, which Freeman formulated to embody the 1992 world congress of the Society of Biological Psychiatry, will be valid also for all forthcoming scientific meetings in this domain:

"The data were expensive to obtain and now are not worth replicating or even retrieving because there was little or no theory to specify what to measure, in what ancillary conditions, and with what expected outcomes. This is not the kind of chaos of which we can be proud" and further: *„When just two parts that are well-known in isolation are interconnected, each to give input to the other, the performance of the coupled unit cannot be predicted,"* moreover: *"...we require the help of concepts taken from dynamics but most psychiatrists do not know what dynamics is,"* and finally: *"Our libraries are filled with volumes of old research results from played out areas, which no one consults or remembers."*

6. 2. 7 THE ABUSE OF EEG FOR NEUROANATOMICAL DEMARCATION OF NEOPHRENOLOGICAL "MODULS"

EEG, as an indicator of brain functions with its unique time resolution, is being increasingly more replaced by various brain imaging techniques with a unique spatial resolution. Functional Magnetic Resonance Imaging (f-MRI) has gained central importance. However, the advantages obtained with respect to the fine differention of **structure** are offset by the disadvantage of time resolution, i.e., of **function**. Whereas neuroimaging has brought an immense progress with respect to neurological diagnostics, its dominance in brain research reflects a doubtful development. It can hardly be disputed that the new imaging methods have revitalized a neuroantomical doctrine, which has been considered obsolete for several decades (e.g., Goldstein, 1934; 1942; Jackson, 1884; Sittig, 1927).

This doctrine, which has to be regarded as a step backwards, is termed "Neophrenology" (Uttal, 2001). It has its roots in the pseudo-scientific, if not fraudulent, assertions of the Viennese anatomist Gall proclaimed about 250 years ago. Gall contented that he was able to infer complex characterologic traits from locally palpable protrusions of the human skull. Whereas today such unsubstantiated assertions will be dismissed as a historical curiosity or charlatanry, one may easily overlook that we are nevertheless in danger to fall back to a comparable primitive and erroneous level of scientific thinking. Modern neuroscience seeks *"rigidly encapsulated moduls"*, as Fodor (1984) put it in his influential book "The Modularity of Mind". This contradicts the painstakingly achieved insight of outstanding clinical scientists – especially Goldstein (1934; 1936) – according to whom the "higher cortical functions" or psychologically defined performances, respectively, do **not reside** in neuroanatomically circumscribed sites of the brain. It seems to be forgotten that clinical anlyses have shown that psychological capabilities are not localized in an anatomical sense but instead are particularly vulnerable to lesions in defined brain sites. Moreover, well-founded consent has been achieved that CNS always works as a functional unity consisting of spatially disparate substrata the integration of which is warranted by a superordinate synchronizing rhythm of about 40 cps (Basar, 1980; Freeman, 1975; Singer, 2002).

Finally, commercial qEEG softwares are being adjusted to reflect the trend towards imaging. Accordingly, EEG is being advertized as a tomographic technique just as powerful as fMRI:

"*Reliance solely of surface EEG patterns ... has resulted in only moderate clinical utility of the qEEG. A new era of tomographic EEG has arisen that ... will affect the convergence of Neurology, Neuropsychology and Neuropsychiatry in the decades to come*" (Thatcher, 2011; see also 6.1).

CHAPTER 7
Limits and Possibilities of QEEG in Clinical Psychiatry

In the early 1980s, q-EEG softwares were propagated with the explicit claim of enabling objective diagnoses of psychiatric diseases. An exact corrrespondance to the then valid classification system DSM III was promised (see 6.1). In the wake of a worldwide initial euphoria celebrated as a major breakthrough, the advertising slogans became increasingly modest. Eventually, program designers stated that their softwares should not be misused as "stand alone" devices. Psychiatric experience was, of course, a prerequisite for making the right use of them..

In the long term, this retreat was compelling since only subjects who are not at all acquainted with psychiatry may assume or believe that psychiatry encompasses naturally given disease entities (see 3.4.8). A far reaching agreement among serious psychiatrists concerns the boundaries between ill and sound that are believed to be essentially determined by social conventions.

According to different perspectives, qEEG does not allow an orientation to a normal reference. What remains are single case analyses consisting of quantitative comparisons between temporally lagged recordings, i.e., ipsative or within-subject measurements of change. We are well aware that such a statement is in stark contradiction with the conventionally practised group-statistical mean value comparisons, including great numbers of subjects.

"As is evident to all clinicians, single case demonstrations, even when data are consistent across repetitions and are nonartifactual, cannot be used to prove the value of a laboratory procedure" (Duffy, 1989).

With our proposal of within-subject measurements of change, we take up again the time-honoured concept of "Functional Electroencephalography" endorsed by Liberson (1944; 1945) more than 70 years ago. From whatever reasons, Liberson's work remained without any resonance. Even those few authors who followed in his footprints seemed to be unaware of his publications.

"Thus, it is only by knowing what is normal for a person that the EEG pattern at a given time can be interpreted as reflecting some pathological brain process."

In the same direction, Makeig & Inlow (1993) stated:

"A healthy individual may display an abnormal EEG while the EEG can be unaffected in a patient with a brain lesion. The presence of a change is more important than the presence of an abnormality as such. In serial examinations, the patient serves as his own control, which is a well-established method of reducing unwanted interindividual variability, e.g., in pharmacological research."

Though serial or ipsative examinations are considered highly desireable when informally discussing with collegues, they have not existed in psychiatry until recently.

7.1 ABOUT THE QUANTIFICATION OF QUALITIES: GENERAL PRINCIPLES

The current mainstream research comprises a methods and data driven strategy. Research-guiding conceptual frameworks have been increasingly superseded by "tacit assumptions" (Polyani, 1966). A striking example of a "tacit assumption" is the deeply rooted mainstream conviction that frequency bands or their power spectral values represent self-explanatory variables, which do not need further psychophysiological interpretation. The undisputable fact, namely that a mathematical transformation from the time- into the frequency domain (for example by means of Fast Fourier Transform) must by no way result in similar spectrograms and vice versa, has not been given the due attention. Furthermore, it has to be stressed that to avoid asking questions about the **meaning** of FFT and other metrics is equivalent to restricting oneself to applied physics or **Brain Physics.** It is erroneous to assume that **meaning** of any metrics with respect to the behaviour and experiences of living beings would automatically result from systematically correlating data obtained by mathematical transformations of the EEG on the one hand and behavioral data provided by physicians/psychologists on the other. **Psychophysiology** is a genuine biological discipline in itself. In contrast to the exact natural sciences, as represented by exact context-independent physics, psychophysiology can be characterized as a context-dependent **biological natural science**. Its questions and problems differ profoundly from those of physics. Physics and math can never supersede a biology discipline, but they can and must be used as very valuable, even indispensable auxiliary tools.

From a methodological point of view, it has to be pointed out critically that ratings of **qualities** require the movie-like integration of changing "pictures" across a temporally extended non-stationary process. This will inevitably lead to inter-rater-reliability problems, which can only be overcome using a quantitative approach. A quantitative assessment of subgroups according to the EEG patterning would require the analysis of longer EEGs than the 2-3 minutes segment ones, which are commonly evaluated by the above mentioned qualitative studies. An objective assessment of both the mean level of EEG-vigilance and its time course profile requires a minimum of 10 minutes of resting EEG uninterrupted by artifact editing (see 6.2.2; 6.2.4; 6.2.5).

According to Bente, the SR-EEG can be understood as a **macroindicator of cerebral global** (highly integrated) **functioning** (**CGF**) (e.g., Bente, 1984; Bente et al., 1964). To him, the lawful sequence of visually easily discernible patterns of ongoing EEG-activity between the poles of feeling alert and drowsy/asleep reflected different levels of global functioning (Bente at al., 1963). This means that the psychophysiologically relevant information consists of the **proportioning and the dynamics** of visually defined recording-time-dependent EEG patterns, which Bente called **higher structural features** ("höhere Strukturmerkmale").

Alterations in the **CGF** or its main determinants, for example, its **dynamics,** are unspecific in a nosological sense. The SR-EEG reflects distinct types of control (Ulrich, 1994; 2001; 2002; 2003). With healthy subjects, the smooth adaptive control prevails (3.4.1). It corresponds to our **physiomorphic** EEG (**PM**). Another type consists of overshooting control and corresponds to the **dynamically labile** EEG (**DL**). The third type consists of delayed control and corresponds to the dynamically rigid EEG (**DR**). This tripartition of control types does not imply discrete categories. As long as there are no empirical data available, a continuous Gaussian distribution of healthy sampling populations has to be assumed. Both overshooting and delayed control may be regarded as dysfunctional but nosologically non-specific. Nosological non-specificity is not equivalent to clinical irrelevance. Half a century ago, this has been convincingly demonstrated by Selye (1952) who coined the scientific terms "Stress" and "General Adaptation syndrome" (GAS) and described the neuroendocrine HPA-Axis.

PM, DL, and **DR** may be distinguished visuo-morphologically if a long-enough record of undisturbed resting EEG is available. Additionally, it has to be reminded that an algorithm, which reliably discriminates the EEG-vigilance dynamics at a single case level quantitatively, has been developed long ago (Ulrich & Frick, 1986). This algorithm is based upon a spectral analysis of 300 consecutive 2-second epochs of an uninterrupted artifact-free 10-minute resting EEG restricted to the 4 derivations, F3-A1; F4-A2; O1-A1; O2-A2 (Ulrich & Frick, 1986). As a new as well as fertile tool in neuropsychiatric research, this approach to quantitative reconstruction of EEG dynamics has repeatedly proved useful (e.g., Bschor et al., 2001; Bräu & Ulrich, 1990; Ulrich et al., 1988; Ulrich et al., 1990; Ulrich et al., 1993; Ulrich, 1994; Ulrich & Fürstenberg, 1999; Ulrich, 2001; Ulrich, 2002; Ulrich, 2003). Our seemingly ignored or forgotten quantification method was rediscovered only recently (Hegerl et al., 2008). Regrettably, the indispensable role of the time course profiles in the characterization of EEG-vigilance dynamics was overlooked.

To apply our algorithm, the following preconditions must be fulfilled:

- an EEG-resting record of at least **10 minute** duration,
- undistorted by visual artifact editing,
- 4 ear-referenced derivations, 2 from the anterior quadrants (**F3-A1** and **F4-A2**) and 2 from the posterior quadrants (**O1-A1** and **O2-A2** or P3-A1 and P4-A2) and
- a Fast Fourier Transform (FFT) of 300 successive 2-second epochs with assessment of the **absolute Alpha-Power** (in the 7.5-13/s range).

Each of the successive 2s epochs has to be determined by our algorithm to represent an A - or non-A stage. This procedure has been proved to be optimal with respect to the cost-benefit relation. As a rule, a two-partitioned time course profile can be expected with healthy subjects (Fig. 120). By counting the rate of non-A epochs within successive minutes (maximally 30 epochs per minute), one gets the time course profile. Up to the fifth minute, a rather continuous Alpha activity prevails, followed by a more or less steady increase of non-A epochs. It is not uncommon to observe, from one minute to the next, shortlasting, counter-regulatory response shiftings.against the general trend .

The possibility to objectively measure EEG-vigilance dynamics and to reliably localize an individual EEG on a continuum between the extreme poles of dynamic lability (**DL**) and rigidity (**DR**) with ideal smooth control as the "golden middle course" (**PM**) has opened new and potentially productive prospects for psychiatric research. To pursue this line of thought, one has to consider that a reversible unequivocal matching between **function** (systems' physiology) and **performance/experiencing** (psychology) cannot be assumed.

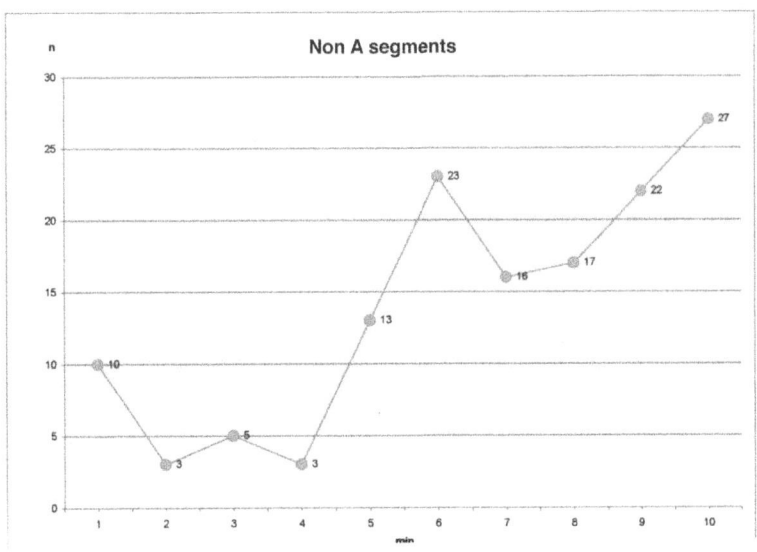

Figure 120. Two-partitioned time course profile characterizing physiomorphic vigilance dynamics (PM).

In order to consider the individual subject, additional information out of the scope of EEG-vigilance dynamics is needed. Information from heterogeneous sources and by profoundly different methods has to be weighted and integrated and will probably become the guiding principle. This demands a structural-mathematical combination of different, already available tools, e.g., Bayes-nets, Petri-nets, Fuzzy logic etc., as well as the support from experts of information technology.

Decades ago, the outstanding US American psychiatrist, Zubin (1950), demanded a methodical completion of group analyses by single case studies:

"In the study of a single individual, especially of a so-called abnormal individual, we must treat each case as an independent universe. Later, when the characteristics of each of these universes become known, we may be able to classify them into groups or like structured or similar universes. Until such knowledge becomes available, it is unwarranted to classify individuals as equivalent even if they have made identical scores on a series of tests."(p. 1 - 6).

7.2 Longitudinal, Serial, Dynamical, or Ipsative Trend Assessment (ITA)

About one decade ago, we had begun to conceptualize a quantification procedure for practical psychiatric purposes. We aimed at reconciling user-friendliness with fault tolerance and sensitivity as much as possible. The underlying main idea was to objectify quantitatively changes in the organizational level of Cerebral Global Function (**CGF**) ascertainable from the Spontaneous Resting EEG (**SR-EEG**) along with the clinical course. Such an endeavour complies with a quantitative reconstruction of the time course of the visuo-morphological quality of the **SR-EEG**. Thus, variables had to be selected with both a sensitivity towards changes in the **CGF** and a mutual independence from each other. Assuming that the complex spatio-temporal organization of the EEG cannot be fully expressed within a single parameter, the assessment of functional impairment will become more reliable when more relevant information is extracted from EEG.

In this respect, it has to be considered that psychophysiological relevance of quantitative parameters as well as their independence from each other rather than their number is decisive. In the first step towards quantitative reconstruction, these variables had to be parametrized by **FFT**. In order to achieve a sufficient exhaustion of the dynamical information, two constraints are indispensable:

- An uninterrupted SR-EEG with a minimal length of 10 minutes;
- No manipulation of the SR-EEG in advance of the mathematical transformation (FFT), in particular no visual artefact editing.

To obtain a time resolution of 0.5 Hz, successive 2 second epochs need to be submitted to FFT (according to the NYQUIST-theorem). The solid proof of the characteristic pattern along with the time course, i.e., the inherent non-stationarity of the SR-EEG, requires using a uniform time-window with respect to the target variables. A width of 2 seconds has turned out as the optimum in preliminary investigations. Both closer and wider time windows tend to conceal the naturally given non-stationarity. We remind that the same is affected by the conventionally performed averaging across short-term epochs in order to obtain spectral mean values. We hold that visual artefact editing can be avoided if one excludes artefact-prone spectral components below 2 Hz and above 15 Hz from further processing (see 6.2.3). This corresponds to a digital filtering in the sense of "cut off." As a source of abundant artefacts, one may in addition exclude the frontopolar leads FP1 and FP2. The skull and the earlobe electrodes are to be placed according to the 10-20 system.

Subsequently, a stringent description of the selected variables is given:

Variable 1: **Absolute Alpha-power** (squared amplitudes) for O1-A1 and O2-A2.
With earlobe- or mastoid-reference, a rhythmic activity of 8-13 Hz accentuated over the posterior regions (parietal, occipital or temporo-posterior) is conventionally expected in healthy subjects. This applies especially for the first 5 minutes of the SR-EEG. This rhythm is also denoted as background activity or basic rhythm. It is considered as a substantial sign of more or less undisturbed cerebral global brain function (CGF).

Variable 2: **Barycentric Frequency (BF)** is defined as the frequency median across the spectral power range. It is therefore also denoted as the "weighted mean frequency" and considered as a "geometrical descriptor of the frequency power spectrum" (Tolonen & Sulg, 1981; Tolonen et al., 1981). Though **BF** reflects the relation between the slow and the fast spectral components, it differs from the quotients, which result from simply relating the power-values of the slow and fast frequencies. **BF** is of high clinical importance since it has been shown to correlate especially well with cortical oxygen intake (Ingvar et al., 1976). Moreover, it has been shown to be the most valid indicator of the restitution of brain infarctions (Tolonen et al., 1981), remarkably not only over the lesioned, but also the unaffected contralateral hemisphere. According to our restriction of the resticted frequency range for parameter calculation, **BF** is assessed for the artifact-free range of 2.0-15.0 Hz.

Variable 3: **Anterior spreading of the Alpha-activity** indicates a slight to medium decrease in the level of EEG-vigilance (3.4.3), which can be quantitatively expressed by a quotient of anteriorization, both for the left and the right hemisphere -**AQl** and **AQr**. The AQ is calculated from absolute Alpha-power values (8-13 Hz) for successive 2 second epochs according to the anterior/ anterior+posterior relationship.

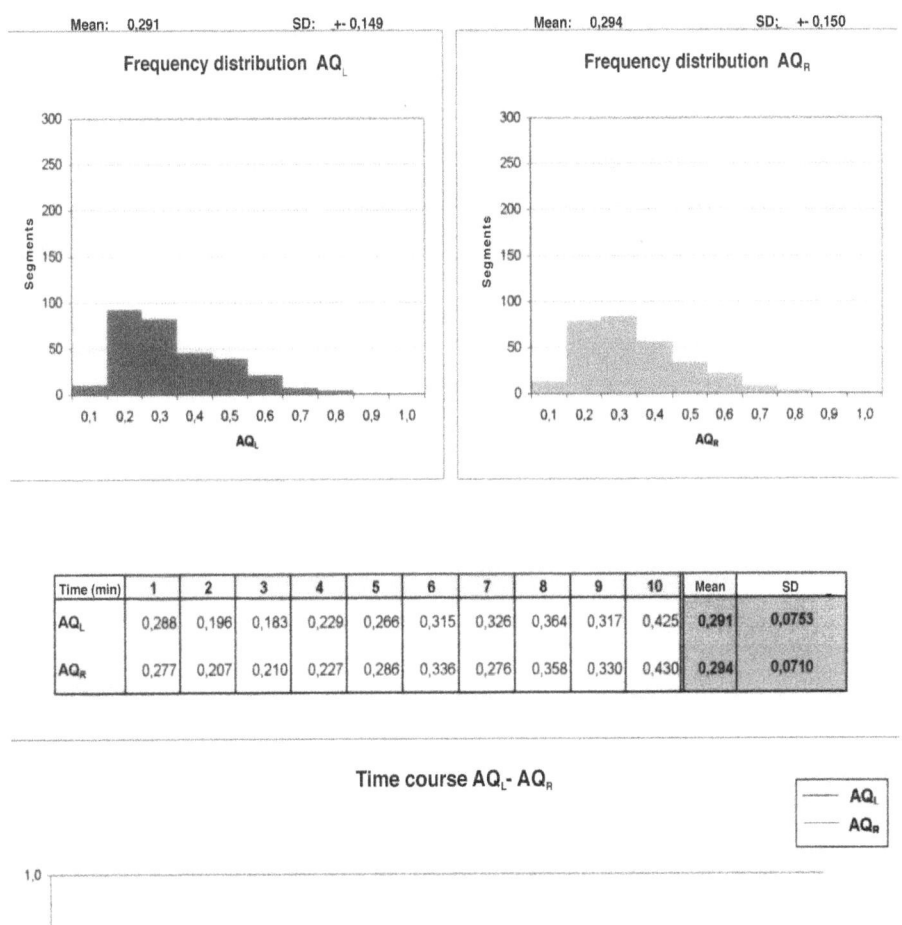

Figure 121. Frequency profiles of the AQ value (AQl and AQr) as calculated for 10 consecutive recording minutes. Each value represents the average across 30 2-second epoch, same EEG as Fig. 120.

***Variable 4*: Alpha continuity** (number and frequency profile of the non-A-segments)

As already mentioned, ideally, Alpha-background activity should show a certain degree of continuity. This feature may be expressed by the number of non-A segments within successive recording minutes (Ulrich & Frick, 1986; Ulrich, 1994). A non-segment is referred to when the absolute Alpha-power (8-13 Hz) does not exceed more than 50 % of the artifact-free total power (2.0 - 15.0 Hz) in any one of the 4 leads F3-A1; F4-A2, O1-A1 and O2-A2. Calculation is performed with successive 2-second epochs. Within a standardized recording time of 10 minutes, maximally 300 non-A epochs may be obtained.

Non A segments

Patient-ID: 037-131201
Patient: 0
recorded: 13.12.2001 time: 15:35:42

Untersuchungs-ID: 01
born: 05.11.1989

time (min)	1	2	3	4	5	6	7	8	9	10	total
2s segments	30	30	30	30	30	30	30	30	30	30	**300**
Non A segments	0	1	7	14	17	17	13	20	22	26	**137**

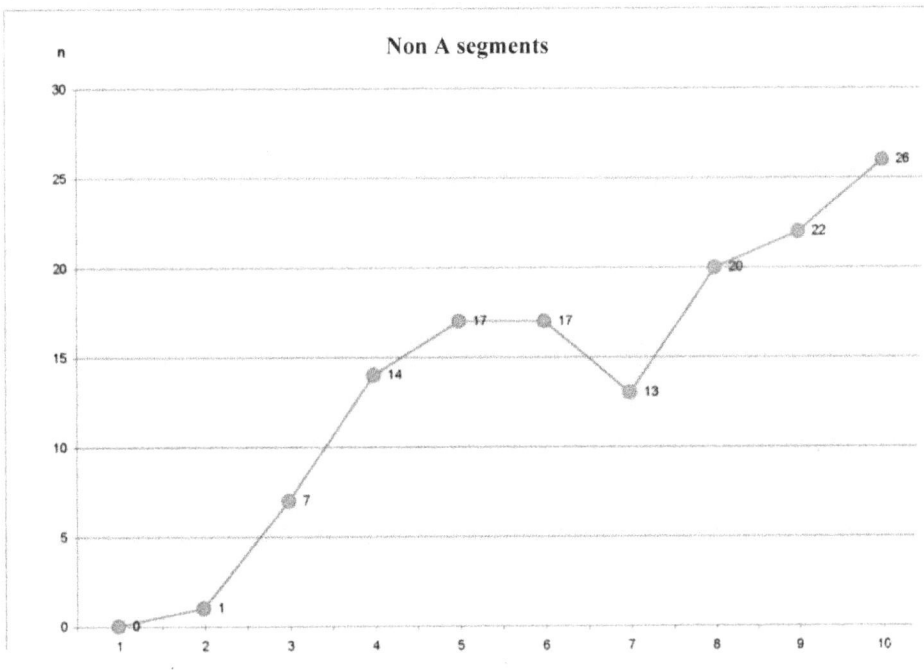

Figure 122. Frequencies of non-A segments calculated for consecutive minutes with an analysis time window of 2 seconds. Maximally 30 non-A epochs may be obtained per minute.

The number of the non-A segments delivers information about the mean level of EEG-vigilance but not about the dynamics of the time function (Fig.122, numbers). The latter can be learned from the time course profile (Fig. 122, graph). A greater number of non-A epochs correspond to more Alpha discontinuity or an Alpha rarefication, respectively.

As can be inferred from a comparison between Fig. 120 and 121, the time course profiles of the **AQl** and **AQr** on the one hand and of the number of non-A segments on the other are nearly congruent. The distinctness of such a mutual validation of these two indicators of the EEG vigilance level could not be expected since Alpha-topography and Alpha-continuity can be viewed as quite disparate aspects of the EEG time function.

Variable 5: **Absolute power of the slow frequency range (2.0-7.5 Hz)** calculated for the 4 quadrants, i.e. F3-A1, F4-A2, O1-A1 and O2-A2.

The visual impression of Diffuse Dysrhythmia (**DD**) essentially results from the predominance of irregular slow waves belonging to the Theta and Delta band.

DD is conventionally regarded as an indicator of a pronounced disturbance of cerebral global function (**CGF**).

	Ableitedatum	Ableitedatum	Score Δ Sens. I	Score Δ Sens. II
1. Alpha -Leistung (8 - 13 Hz, µV², Ln-Wert)				
O1 - A1				
O2 - A2				
2. Baryzentrische Frequenz (0.5 - 32 Hz)				
O1 - A2				
O2 - A2				
3. Anteriorisierungsquotient AQ (100x, Ln-Wert) (als Mittelwert aus 300 konsekutiven 2s-Segmenten)				
AQ_l				
AQ_r				
4. Anzahl der non-A-Segmente (Ln-Wert) (Kriterien 70%, 60%, 50%, 40%, 30%, 20% rel. Alpha-Leistung)				
5. Delta- / Theta-Leistung (0.5 - 7,5 Hz , µV², Ln-Wert)				
F3 - A1				
F4 - A2				
O1 - A1				
O2 - A2				
Δ - Totalscore:				

Figure 123. Ipsative Trend Assessment (ITA) –
Variables and Score-differences between two successive records

The measurement differences between the 5 main parameters were transformed into difference scores using a glossary (Ulrich, 2001). Within the pilot stage, it turned out that re-test reliability could be improved by logarithmical transformation of the originally measured values. Furthermore, the usage of different sensitivity steps has proved successful (sens I and sens II). With lower sensitivity (sens I), differences are treated more conservatively than with higher sensitivity (sens II). The total difference score, resulting from adding up of the single difference-scores indicates the degree of clinical improvement or deterioration. In view of the alleged mutual independence of the 5 selected variables, one has to take into account that changes may not always take place in the same direction. According to the Law of Initial Value (Wilder, 1932), the possibility of seemingly paradoxical effects has to be considered. In particular, one has to take into account that with an initial pathomorphic degree of the DR, a decrease in Alpha-continuity (variable 4) indicates an improvement of GCF while with an initial pathomorphic degree of DL, an increase in Alpha-continuity will indicate an improvement of the GCF. Thus, all 5 variables can be added to form a Total Difference Score only with PM in the initial EEG. Notice that in the table in Fig. 123, the conventionally assessed frequency spectrum 0.5-32.0 Hz is still taken as a basis. As explained in detail, there are sound reasons to exclude the slow and the fast frequencies from parametrization (6.2.3). In order to prevent any misunderstanding, it shall be pointed out again that ITA has no meaning at all with regard to cross sectional diagnosis.

7. 3 Validity and Reliability of ITA as well as examples of use

It goes without saying that the procedure must show a satisfactory test-retest-reliability. Therefore, special attention has to be paid to the transition resistancies of the electrodes F3, F4, O1, O2 as well as A1 and A2, which play a decisive role with regard to the parametrization of the selected variable. The proof of clinical usefulness of **ITA** comes from the external validation using, for instance, rating scales and even the global judgement of the experienced physician.

7.3.1 Senile Dementia (SD) or Dementia of Alzheimer Type (DAT or AD)

Today, there is a far-reaching agreement that the great expectations in quantitative EEG analysis of **DAT** have been disappointing. Nearly all studies on Alzheimer's pathophysiology are based on the *let's - try- it - and - see* strategy. No arguments are given why these but no other quantitative parameters are assessed. Literally, not a single study relied upon hypotheses about the **meaning** of visually or quantitatively distinguished EEG-features. Thus, it is all but amazing that EEG was discredited in the lump over the last two decades. As a rule, the authors restricted themselves to an estimation of frequency power values by means of Fast Fourier Transformation (FFT), dispensing with any kind of information about recording-time dependent changes, be it across time course of one single EEG under resting conditions or between EEG recordings repeated at weekly or monthly intervals (e.g., Brenner et al., 1987; Coben et al., 1983; Duffy et al., 1989; Johanneson et.al., 1979; Penttilä et al., 1985; Soininen et al., 1989; Stigsby et al., 1981).

A rule-confirming exception is the approach of Soininen et al. (1989) who longitudinally evaluated patients with slight to moderate dementia. Only one in two patients who deteriorated within a 12 months observation period also showed the expected general slowing down of frequencies. The authors inquired about how it can be that patients with distinct dementia may present with normal EEGs and concluded that simple spectral analysis probably does not deliver the kind of information that is needed to obtain differences across repeated measurements. We entirely concur with this opinion, which led us to a more profound exploitation of relevant EEG-information. The hitherto disappointing results with quantitative EEG have contributed to a shift in interest to brain imaging. Nowadays, it becomes increasingly evident that even the most elaborate neuroimaging techniques can only be the second choice when dealing with the central challenge of early recognition of the disease within the clinically silent stage (see Hyman et al., 2004).

Since the EEG, by its nature, reflects the self-organized neuronal mass activity of the cortex, no other investigative or diagnostic tool should be more appropriate.

Notwithstanding a wealth of visual EEG findings that have been accumulated over the years (see 4.5; Ulrich, 1994, 2001), the significance of EEG in involutive-degenerative brain syndromes has remained rather low. Moreover, one has to state a general decline of expertise in clinically oriented EEG. As such, we refer to the erroneous assumption of age-dependence of certain EEG features (in adults) and especially of the frequency of the background activity (Tharcher, 2011; Ulrich, 1994; 2012;). This kind of ignorance is being fostered by the so-called Normative Data Bases (**NBD**), which are the core of the well-known qEEG software-packages.

When developing and scrutinizing **ITA,** we relied primarily on gerontopsychiatric patients with a probable diagnosis of **AD**. On theone hand, we were interested whether it is possible to objectify the inherent tendency towards deterioration across a longer time course and how. On the other hand, we wondered how AChE Inhibitors would act upon this trend. A number of individual longitudinal case studies, performed up to two years in a prospective manner, were published in a monography (in German) together with further examples of a clinically useful application of **ITA** (Ulrich, 2001).

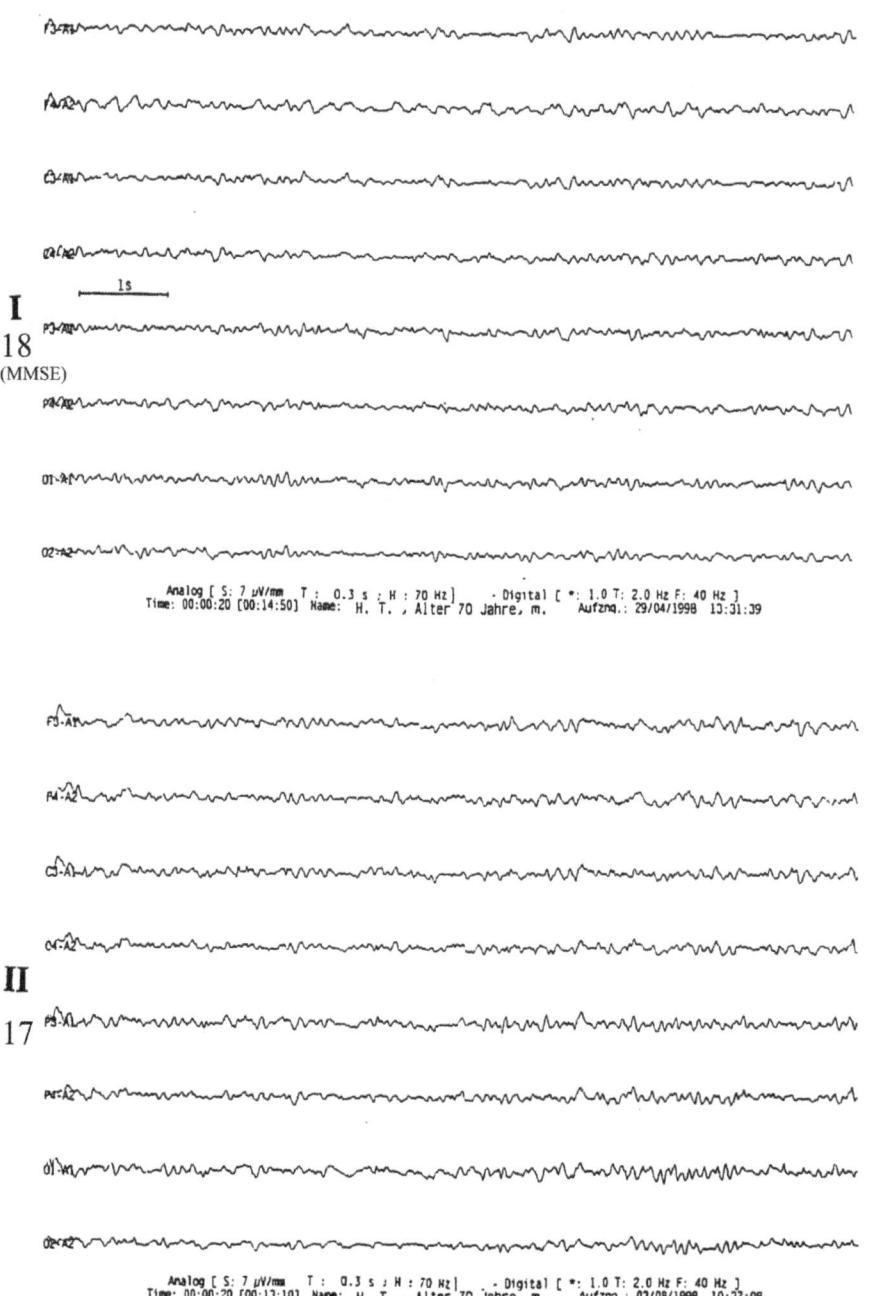

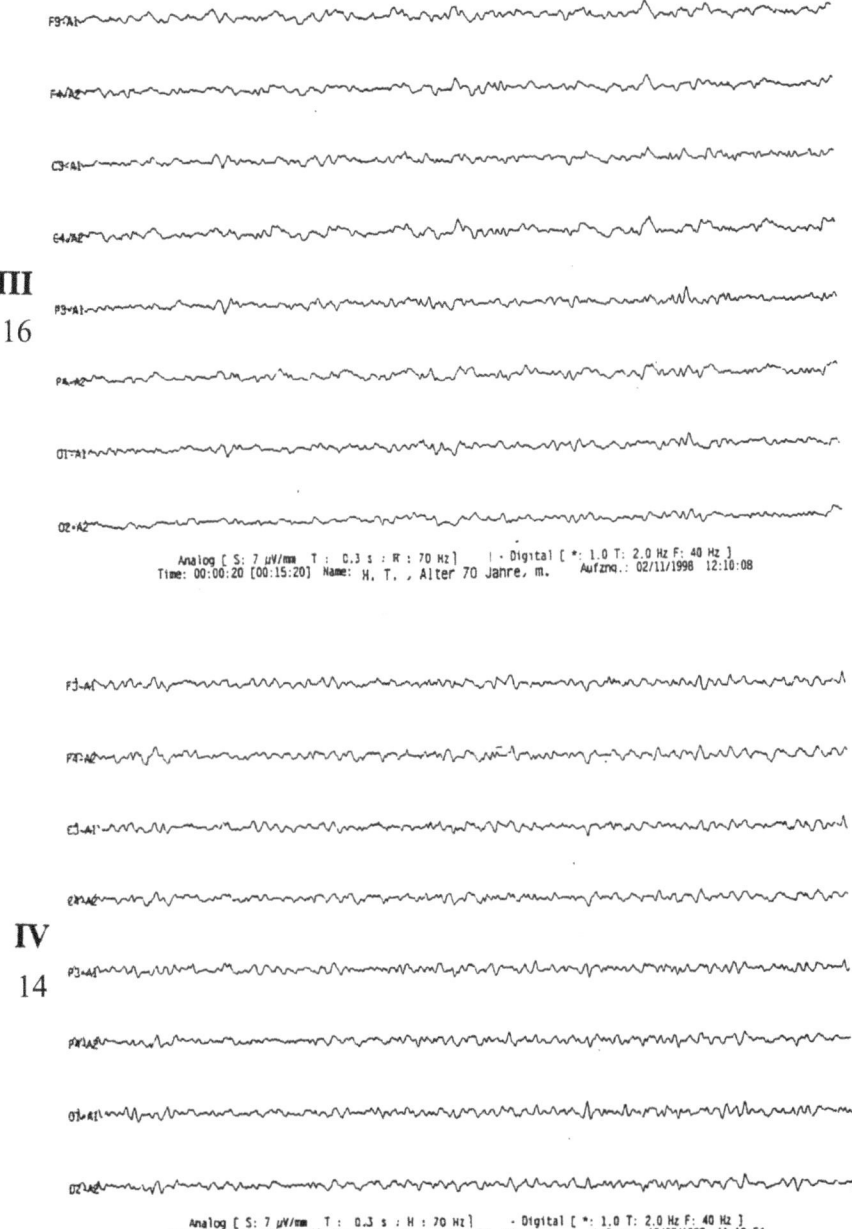

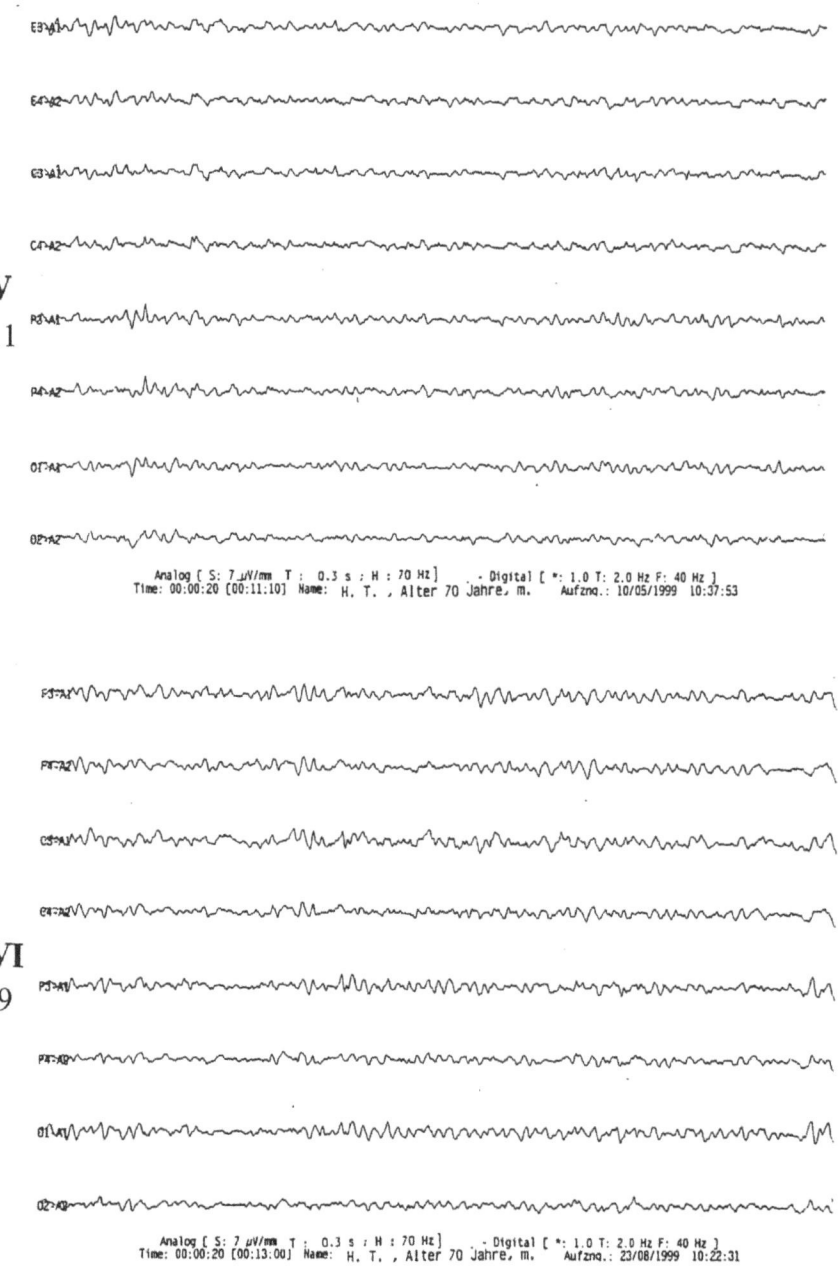

Figure 124 (Pages 314-316). Exemplary documentation of the changing SR-EEG with a male patient (W.G.), 68 years of age, suffering from DAT – 6 recordings with fixed 3-months intervals together with the MMSE-Scores.

Differences between **I** (MMSE:18), **II** (MMSE:17), and **III** (MMSE : 16) are hardly visually recognizable. From **IV** (MMSE: 14) to **V** (MMSE : 11) and to **VI** (MMSE : 9); a progressive increase in Delta waves becomes obvious (MMSE = Mini Mental State Examination according to Folstein et al., 1975).

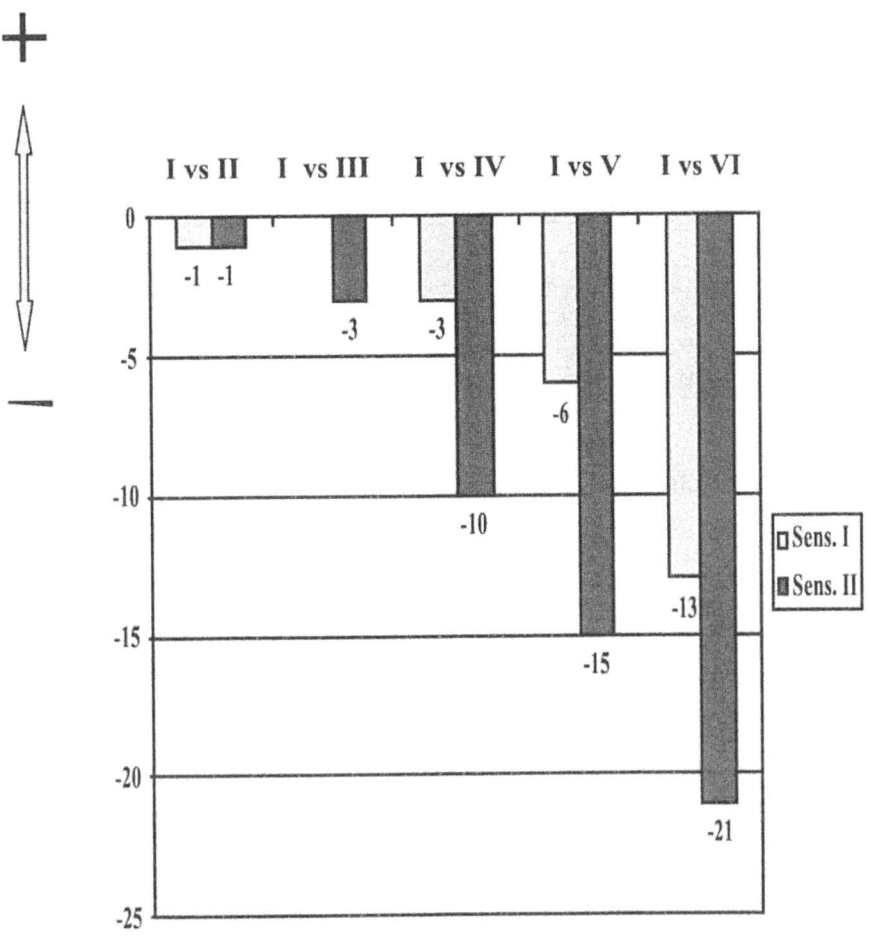

Figure 125. Diagrammatic representation of the ITA Total-Difference Scores related to the initial SR-EEG recording (I, Fig. 124)

Figures 124 & 125. Epicrisis Pat. W.G. 6 SR-EEG recordings with a fixed 3 months interval show a trend towards clinical deterioration, as objectified by ITA and validated by MMSE –Scores.

Our hitherto obtained results differ from the prevailing conviction concerning the fruitlessness of the SR-EEG in gerontopsychiatry (see Ulrich, 2001). We could demonstrate that the EEG is an eminent sensitive tool for objectifying a pathological change of function (pathological *Funktionswandel*). This sensitivity sufficiently objectifies a spontaneously occurring functional deterioration as well as passing effects of antidementive drugs. Till now, spurious effects could have been inferred from psychological testing (Corey-Bloom et al., 1998; Cummings et al., 1998; Rogers et al., 1998; Rogers & Friedhoff, 1998). Therefore, the possibility of objective measurement reflects an important enrichment of our diagnostical equipment. This also concerns a frequently unanswered question on psychpathological grounds, namely whether an irreversible DAT or a principally reversible, long-lasting involutional pseudo-dementia exists in a particular patient (Alexopoulos et al., 1993; Jordan et al., 1989; Lazarus et al., 1987; Sachdev et al., 1990;). The most important achievement of the ITA-EEG might involves the **true** early-detection of the DAT disease, i.e., the intravital diagnosis of the neuropathological disease process, which precedes the clinical manifestation by several years (4.6). Early diagnosis of DAT in the proper sense is increasingly becoming the central challenge of gerontopsychiatric research.

"Detecting ALZHEIMER'S disease in its early stages challenges researchers and clinicians alike. Early detection and treatment of the preclinical AD syndrome might offer far better outcomes than treatment of symptomatic mild-to moderate AD" (Knopman, 1998).

This is fully in line with a more recent statement:

"The optimal subjects in whom to intervene therapeutically are those who are destined but not yet manifest" (Jack, 2004).

In spite of intensive research, there is no objective measuring tool for diagnosing the asymptomatic phase of the disease equivalent to progressive neuronal rarefication. In view of the extensive literature on Alzheimer disease in general, one may ask why such an important topic as true early recognition has not been investigated with a greater rigor. It has been proposed (Finger, 1988) that systemic thinking, as signified by terms like *Neuroadaptation* or *Neuroplasticity,* is inconsistent with the prevailing paradigm of the *brain as a mosaic of rigidly encapsulated moduls* (Fodor, 1984).

Neuropathologists are guessing that within a random sample of 100 subjects belonging to the age group of 50-70 years, 20 subjects belong to the preclinical phase (Beyereuther et al., 1993). Whether ITA-EEG will be the ideal tool for making up an early diagnosis of DAT can only be proven by a comprehensive, time-consuming prospective epidemiological study. We hold that for ethical reasons, it is imperative not to wait but to act. A strong argument supports the rather solid findings according to which the progression of the disease can be assessed rather reliably (see Ulrich, 2001). We propose to start a preventive- or screening program immediately whereby the present state of knowledge is taken as a basis. The proram should include healthy persons between 50 and 65 years of age. A trend towards deterioration across 3 measuring points with intervals of 3 months would be a sound rationale to assume a pathological process in progress. Consequently, certain recommended unspecific long-term measures concerning conduct of life as well as certain drug therapies could be tested in a systematical manner, aiming at an delay or even inhibition of the process.

To sum up, we found:
- Measurement intervals of 12 weeks confirmed the deterioration to be expected in AD-patients.
- The parameters elected by means of our conceptual framework changed more or less uniformly with respect to clinical deterioration or improvement.
- A deterioration assessed by ITA (corresponding to a lowering of the organizational level of the brain electric activity) was always found to be in agreement with the clinical deterioration of the MMSE-Score.
- Slight to moderate changes of the total difference score towards deterioration or improvement could not be foreshadowed visually ("eye ball evaluation").
- A therapeutic effect of AChE inhibitors (as indicated by an improvement of the MMSE score) could be made probable – if at all - by a transitory delay of the EEG deterioration.

7. 3. 2 Acute Alcohol Withdrawal (detoxification)

As already addressed (5.6), the SR-EEG of an alcoholic is typically characterized by a more or less distinct **DL**, with preponderance of low voltage desynchronized activity corresponding to the subvigil stage B1 associated with frequent transitions into short-lasting stage A segments. On condition of sobriety, this characteristic shows up as reversible. Within 2-3 weeks, it generally changes into physiomorphic dynamics (**PM**). **DL** had been demonstrated only with every other alcoholic (5.6), which argues against an interpretation of a rapidly passing effect being tied to the immediate effect of the noxa. Instead, it indicates that we are dealing here with a potentially reversible pathological change of the cerebral global function (**CGF**), which can be interpreted as an acute withdrawal effect. It is realistic to assume that the typical alcoholic, when sent to the EEG laboratory, would be inclined to consume a certain quantity of alcohol that would stabilize his/her mood and anxious tension. In such a case, a "normalization" of his/her pre-existent **DL** towards PM may be expected. This is in line with the well founded assumption that the DL-EEG in alcoholics is the result but not the cause of alcoholism (5.6). A strong argument against the prevailing assumption of a predisposing factor corresponding to a genetically determined hyperarousal is the failure of the therapeutic strategies aiming at a stabilization of th latter by means of, e.g., "training up" Alpha-continuity with biofeedback.

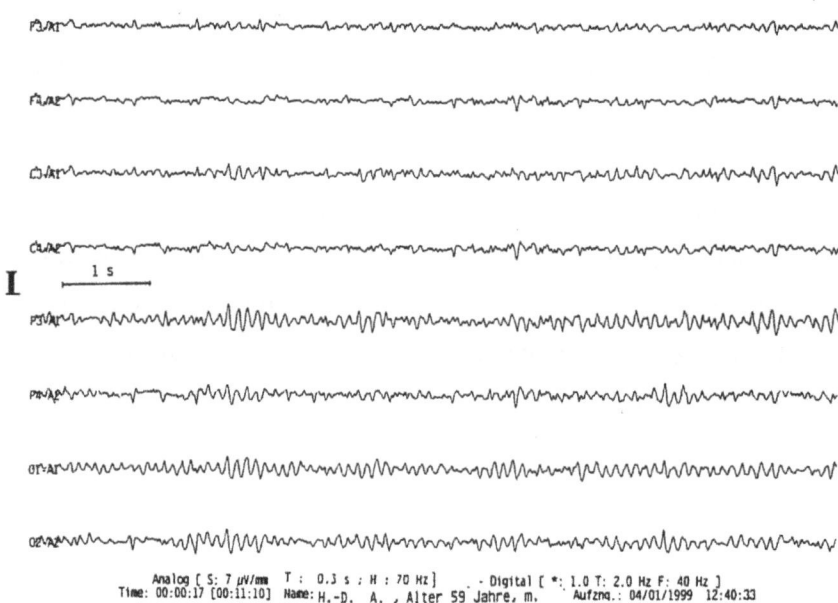

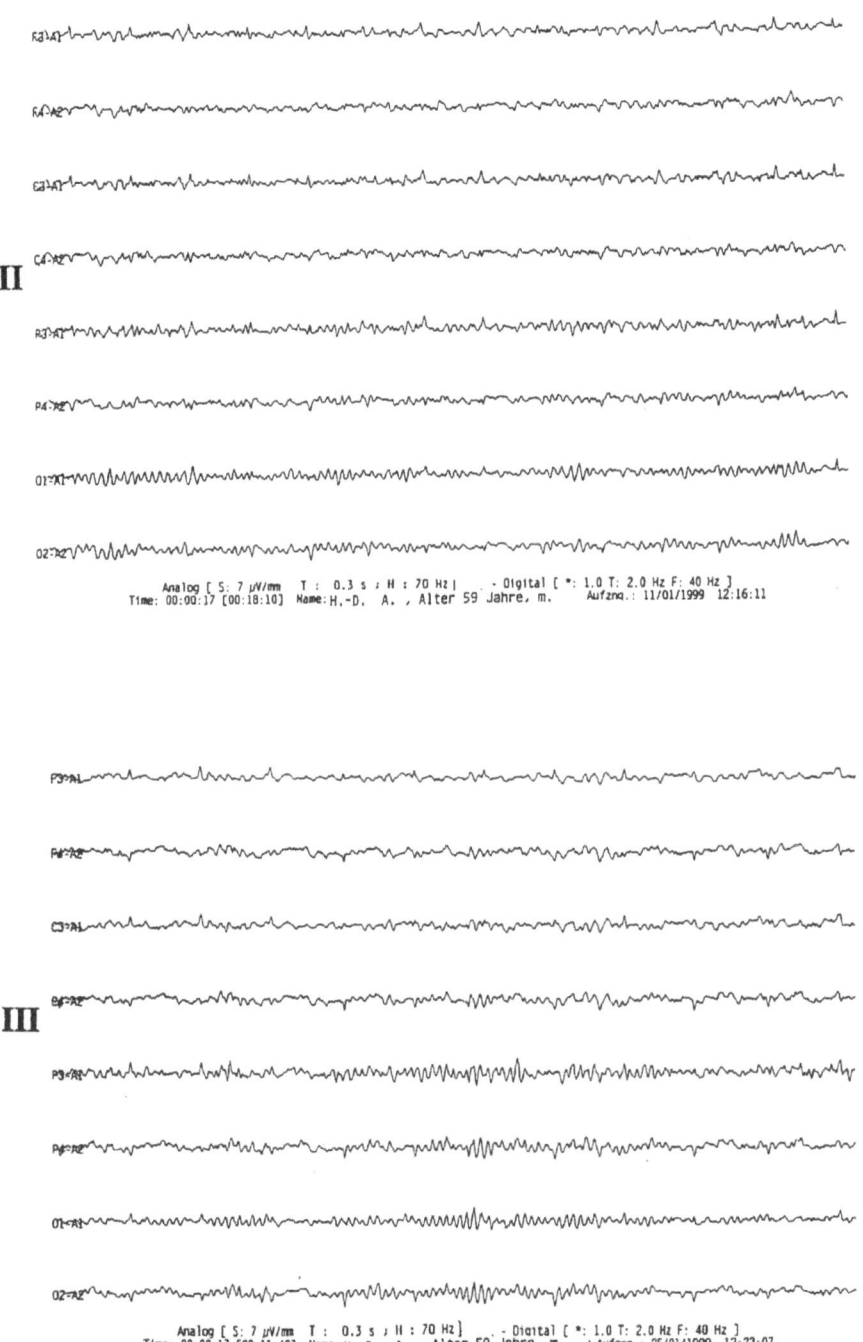

Figure 126. Inpatient alcohol-withdrawal therapy across 30 days; SR-EEG recorded on day 9 (**I**), day 16 (**II**), and day 30 (**III**) from F3-A1, F4-A2, C3-A1, C4-A2, P3-A1, P4-A2, O1-O2, O2-A2; for the sake of comparability, the seconds 10-19 from the first recording minute are shown. From **I** (day 9) to **II** (day 16), a distinct increase of Alpha-continuity may be observed; no further change from **II** (day 16) to **III** (day30).

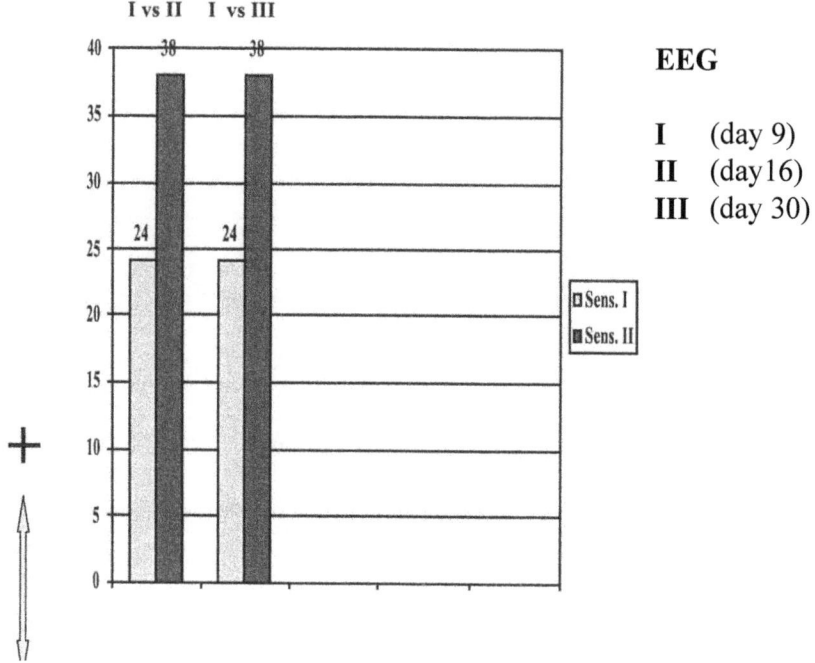

Figure 127. Changes of the ITA Total-Difference score in relation to the initial EEG (Fig. 125, **I**)

Figures 126 and 127. Distinct increase in the EEG vigilance level from day 9 (**I**) to day 16 (**II**) : **+ 24/+38**, going along with remission of a predelirant syndrome; additionally with (day 30, **III**) no change. (Compare with Figure 125)

7. 3. 3 Depressive Syndromes

An essentially untreated topic of psychiatric **qEEG** is that of affective psychoses. As opposed to this, older literature comprises numerous articles dealing with visuo-morphological characterizations of the **SR-EEG** addressing a coordination with different psychopathological types (4.7). Much has been been written about the EEG with melancholias, especially those of the involutional age, which are clinically hallmarked by an organic note. The description of the SR-EEG given by different authors essentially corresponds to our description of Dynamic Rigidity (**DR**). Compared with this, the SR-EEG descriptions of the patients which were formely denoted as "neurotic" or "reactive" may be summarized under our Dynamic Lability (DL). Regrettably, literature is totally void with concerning changes of the EEG-dynamics dependent on the changes of the clinical state. It is amazing that literallly noone spent time to compare EEG accompanying the full-blown syndrome on the one side and the remitted state with dismissal. Therefore, we regard our few quantitative correlational studies as preliminary attempts to remedy shortcomings, which will have to be reconsidered by other investigators. Though we performed only 10 single case studies, the results seem to be encouraging (Ulrich, 2001). With all 10 patients, clinical improvement or deterioration coincided with a theoretically expected increase or decrease in the mean EEG-vigilance level, as assessed by ITA. The following graph of such a single case study may bee regarded as exemplarily.

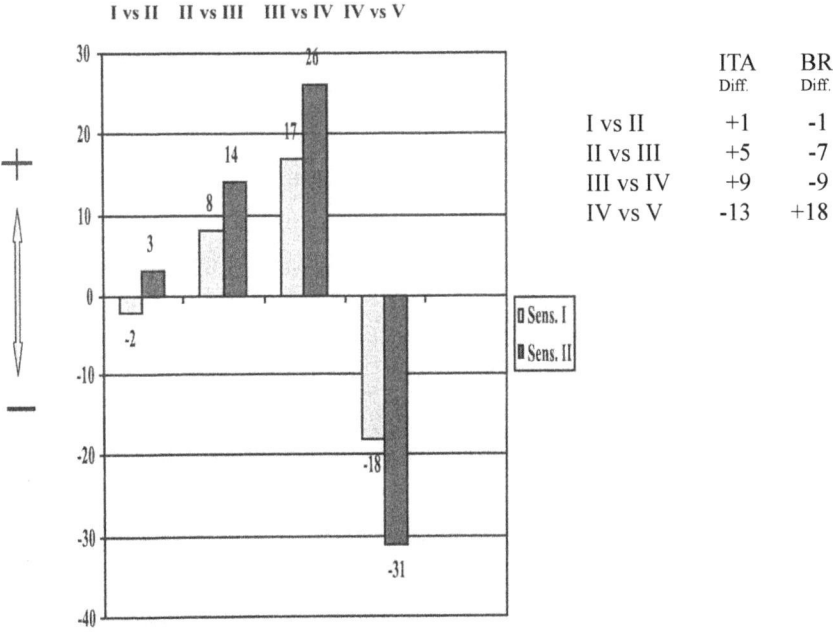

Figure 128. ITA Total-Difference-Scores as dependent on the clinically assessed Depression Scores (Bech-Rafaelsen Depression Scale, **BR**); Comparisons between days 3 (**I**), 6(**II**), 21(**III**), day 28(**IV**, dismissal) of inpatient treatment and a further assessment on the day of readmission because of suddenly occurring relapse day 63 after dismissal (**V**). The recordings depended on clinically distinct imposing changes in the syndrome; Qualitatively (visually) no change from **I** to **V** between consecutive comparisons. Quantitatively, a consistent concordance between decrease and increase in the mean EEG-Vigilance level on the one hand and decrease and increase of the severity of the Depressive syndrome (BR) on the other shows up.

7. 3. 4 Manic Syndromes

It is well-known from the era of visuo-morphological EEG-analysis that a certain percentage – about one third or more – of patients with acute mania are presenting a typical drowsiness-EEG, i.e., they show subvigil drowsiness patterns from the very beginning of the record. This feature is essentially independent of medication. A further peculiarity is that a feeling of tiredness does not accompany this patterning. Furthermore, maniacs with and without this EEG-characteristic do not differ with respect to symptomatology and prognosis (see 4.7). This issue did not receive appropriate attention up to now. The open question to be answered is whether the maniacs with a decrease of EEG-vigilance would respond favourably to psychostimulants, e.g., to methylphenidate. We, therefore compared two acutely manic in-patients who were similar in every respect with the exception of the EEG. Pat. A exhibited a classical drowsiness-EEG, Pat. B an ordinary physiomorphic Alpha-Type-EEG. For Pat.A, but not Pat. B, a sedative antimanic effect was expected following a single test-dose of 20 mg methylphenidate per os and an increase of the mean level of SR-EEG-vigilance.

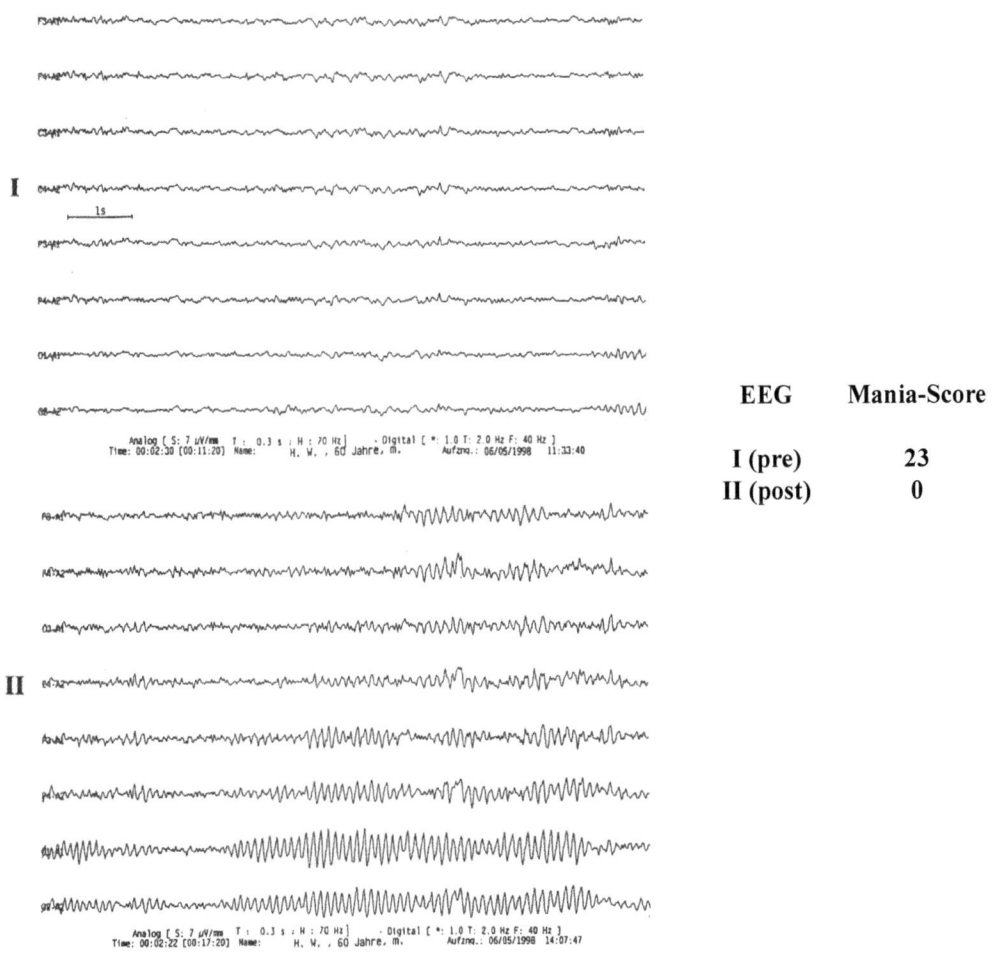

Figure 129. Pat. **A** male, 60 y. acute mania (BECH-RAFAELSON- Mania Score: pre: 23; post: 0; triple long-term prophylaxis with Lithium, Carbamazepin and Valproat; pre-/post comparison of the SR-EEGs before (I) and after (II) oral intake of a test dose of 20 mg methylphenidate; electrodes F3, F4, C3, C4, P3, P4, O1, O2 with reference to the ipsilateral ear;
<u>Above</u> (I): Before test-dose intake prevalence of irregular desynchronized activity, corresponding to the subvigil stages B1-B2;
<u>Below</u> (II): 2 hours after test-dose intake posteriorly accentuated 9/s Alpha basic rhythm, corresponding to stage A1.

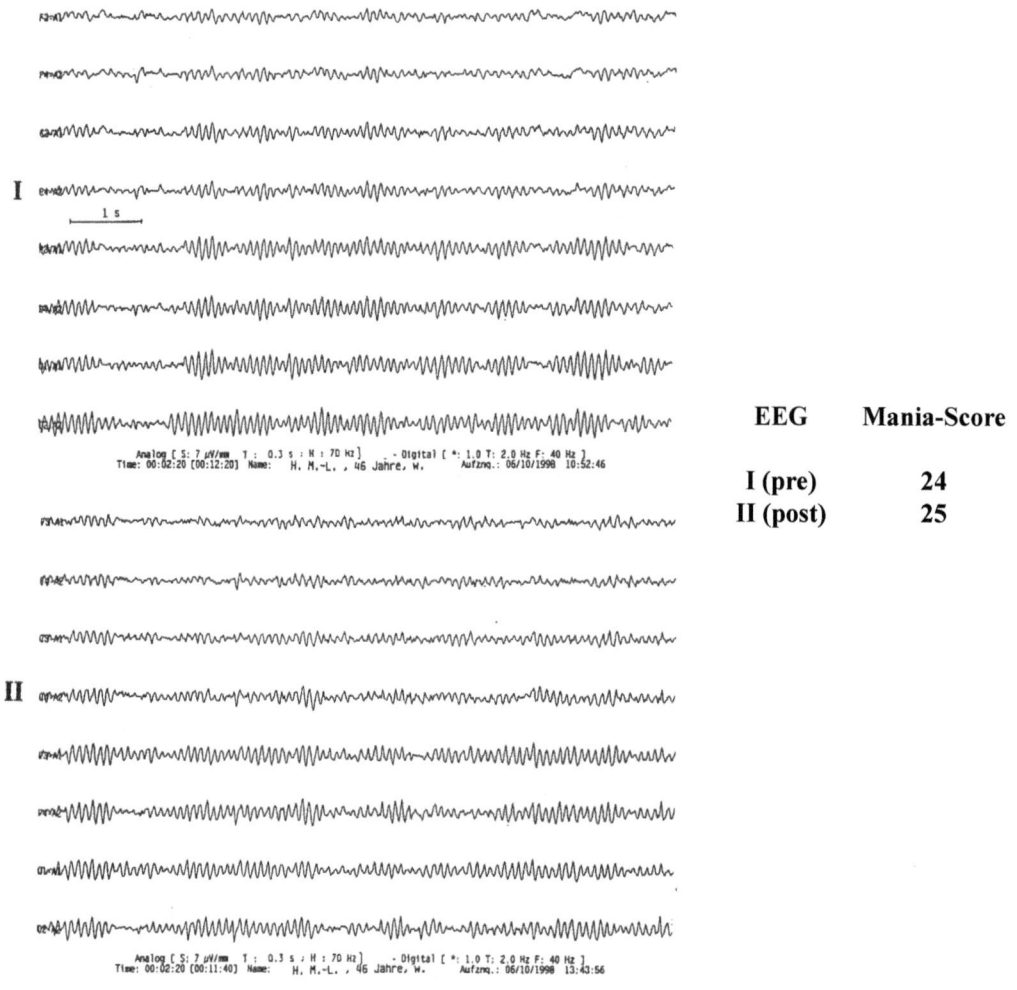

Fig. 130 Pat. **B** female, 47 y. acute mania (Bech-Rafaelson- Mania Score: pre: 24; post: 25; double long-term prophylaxis with Lithium and Carbamazepin; pre-/post comparison of the SR-EEGs before (I) and after (II) oral intake of a test dose of 20 mg methylphenidate; psychopathologic status similar to Pat. **A**; electrode montages as with Fig. 129.
<u>Above</u>: Before test dose intake ordinary Alpha-typical EEG,
<u>Below</u>: 2 hours after test dose intake no essential change.

In contrast to Pat. **A**, Pat. **B** showed, along with previous manic phases, a rather "normal" Alpha-EEG instead of a "Drowsiness-EEG". The reactions to the test dose medication were likewise different. Pat. **B** showed no drug effect at all, both with respect to psychopathology and the EEG-vigilance (ITA -Totaldifference-Scores: (-4/0). Therefore, we immediately commenced with a conventional "dampening" neuroleptic acute therapy. The ITA-EEG supported the observation that pathophysiological homogeneity can not be inferred from psychopathological homogeneity, e.g., between Pat. **A** and **B**. We had to learn that the "right" therapy must not always follow from the "right" diagnosis. If a statistician objected that these studies may not be regarded as representative of the general population of patients, one may argue that in principle, even very copious samples can never be regarded as representative. Moreover, one should consider that the large numbers of subjects as demanded by parametric statistics rather impede the discovery of certain lawfulnesses. (e.g., Significant differences may be obtained due to the greater number of subjects within groups, but these significances are without meaning. For example, a correlation coefficient of rs = 0.20 is very low but it may be highly significant if the number of subjects compared is high [p = 0.0000001]). It can be expected that with an increase of cases, group inhomogeneity inevitably increases. Thus, a finding, regardless of the attained level of statistical significance, would become more and more difficult to interpret.

7.3 5 SCHIZOPHRENIC PSYCHOSES

As already mentioned (4.9), electroencephalographic research in the domain of schizophrenic psychoses is particularly deplorable example of data driven and method-guided empiristic research without guiding theoretical ideas. This applies both to the older qualitative visuo-morphological and the newer quantitative efforts. No attempt was made to distinguish subgroups based on different SR-EEG pictures or their dynamics. As a result, we are facing a plentitude of useless and uninterpretable data. So-called *choppy activity* (Fig. 40), a low voltage desynchronized activity with interspersed fast waves, might be the only notion that could be used to tackle the problem. Davis (1939, 1942) described *choppy activity* as typical for a certain proportion of schizophrenic in-patients. In the pre-neuroleptic era, it was viewed as a prognostically unfavourable sign. Later on, this characteristic was considered as comparable to the norm-variant of the *Low voltage EEG*, which was perceived as nosologically unspecific and therefore meaningless in clinical respect. From the physiological point of view (4.0), *choppy activity* indicates the predilection type of the dynamic labile control (**DL**, Fig. 47). Comparably less attention was given to the counterpart of *Choppy activity*, the dynamic rigid type of control to be coordinated to our Dynamic Rigidity (**DR**, Fig. 46). This characteristic of *hypovariability* was inferred from a decreased variability of the voltage values determined for successive time intervals integrated over the total frequency spectrum (4.8).

In Chapter 4.8, we have outlined three main domains for further research. The most obvious question concerns the mutual changes in psychopathology and EEG over the course of the disease. The question with the highest practical interest is that of the predictability of the therapy response. The third question centres around the possibilities to delay or even prevent the clinical manifestation by making an early or pre-clinical diagnosis. In the following section, we will consider own investigations concerning the second question. The reason is that the principle of the generally avoided longitudinal single case stude is indispensable for this kind of research.

Several years ago, we found, by means of the Test-dose-model, a distinctly worse response to neuroleptics among acute schizophrenic in-patients with a **DR** characteristic of their SR-EEG compared to patients with a **DL** characteristic (Ulrich et al.,1988). We recapitulate (3.4.1) that from a systemic point of view, **DR** is distinguished by a *low systems' tension* or by a *diminished number* of *degrees of freedom concerning the adaptive control of function*. In contrast, **DL** is distinguished by a *high systems' tension* and *increased number of degrees of freedom with respect to the adaptive control of function*.

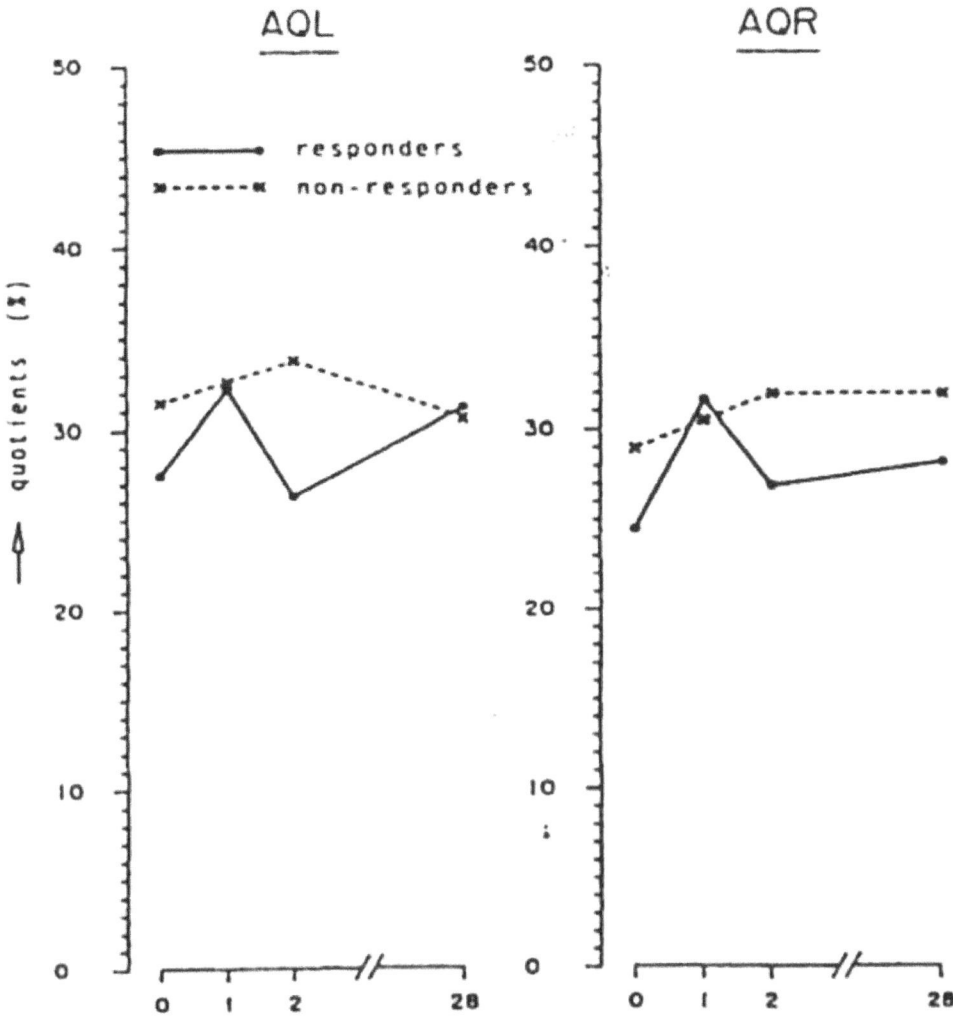

Figure 131. Prediction of the Response to Neuroleptics in Schizophrenics by means of the Test-dose model. Mean values of the Anteriorization- Quotients AQl and AQr as calculated for the group with clinically defined Response (n = 20) and Nonresponse (n = 14).
0 : medication-free initial value; **1**: two hours after oral intake of a test dose of 150 mg perazine; **2** : 28 days later after a medication-free period with variable dosage.

Inpatients who reacted positively to a 4-week treatment with neuroleptics (responder) showed, in the medication-free recorded EEG at the beginning of the treatment more non-A-epochs corresponding to a predominance of low-voltage desynchronized activity phases compared to patients with rather unfavorable treatment results (non-responder). The group of responders, but not the group of non-responders, showed increase in non-A-epoch rates with increasing recording time. A lesser therapeutic response to neuroleptics therefore indicates a deficiency of the spontaneous vigilance dynamics of the type of a dynamic rigidity (**DR**).

That non-response is related to deficient vigilance dynamics could also be deduced from the reaction of the anterior-posterior alpha-quotient as assessed by means of spectral analysis to a single dose of neuroleptics. While in responders, a prompt and extensive increase occurred in the quotient corresponding to an anteriorization of the alpha-activity followed by a counter-reactive restitution of the same kind, the non-responders showed no significant changes at all.

7.3.6 Attention-Deficit-Hyperactivity-Disorder (ADHD)

ADHD is an ambiguously defined behavioural impairment of childhood and early adulthood. To a certain degree, ADHD overlaps with the outdated diagnoses of MCD and MBD. In recent years, it has been referred to as a disturbance of the "execution functions", a somewhat ambiguous definition. The numerous attempts to assess an underlying dysfunction of neuroanatomically delimited modules by means of neuroimaging have been largely unsuccessful. For a number of reasons, it seems plausible that the pathophysiology of ADHD consists of a disturbance of the Global Cerebral Function (**GCF**) as being reflected by the dynamics of the SR-EEG. Such a working hypothesis is supported by observations, which assume a bimodal frequency distribution of the two contrary dynamic predilection types **DL** and **DR** (Fig. 46, 47) in clinically homogenous groups. On the contrary, the in-between type of physiomorphic dynamics (**PM**, Fig. 45) seems to be clearly underrepresented.

Clinical ADHD research still consists in correlating psychopathology with EEG features assessed by expert rating. Arns et al. (2008) recently distinguished 8 *EEG phenotypes* in a sample of clinically homogeneous ADHD diagnosed subjects. The authors emphasized the large variability of EEG- pictures in a diagnostically homogenous population of children with ADHD. This is consistent with nearly all other findings (e.g., Barry et al., 2003; Chabot & Serfontain, 1996; Clarke et al., 1998; 2002; 2003). Regrettably, no study has provided an exemplary documentation of the pretended differences. An additional flaw is the lack of studies that would test test-retest reliability. Therefore, it remains unsettled whether the *phenotypes* represent invariant/outlasting state-independent *Traits* (being of relevance to ADHD or not) or transitory *States* being dependent on the actually given context. Despite the methodological shortcomings, the descriptions given are to be reconciled with our three predilective types of dynamic control, i.e., **DR**, **DL,** and **PM** (Fig. 45, 46, 47).

According to Arns et al. (2008), the *Frontal Slow* and *Slow Alpha Peak Frequency (phenotypes 2 and 3)* and the *Low Voltage EEG (phenotype 5)* discriminate best between ADHD subjects and controls . *Phenotypes 2 and 3* correspond to Bente's (1964a, b) description of the subvigil stage A2. If this pattern persisted for a couple of minutes, one may speak about Dynamic Rigidity (DR). In a similar vein, a persisting *Low Voltage EEG (phenotype 5)* - corresponding to a subvigil stage B1 - indicates Dynamic Lability (DL). Our tripartition into DR and DL through PM does not imply discrete categories. As long as not challenged by research data, a continuous Gaussian frequency distribution has to be assumed in samples of healthy subjects. Both overshooting and delayed control has to be regarded as dysfunctional or maladaptive but non-specific in a nosological sense. However, nosological non-specifity does not mean clinical irrelevance. With healthy subjects, the smooth adaptive control (Physiomorphic Dynamics, PM) is observed.

Generalizing, one may state that subjects with a neuropsychiatric disorder differ from healthy control groups with respect to the frequency distribution of the predilective types of dynamic control of CGF.

With regard to the behavioral importance of the constitutionally bound character of systems' control, an older study of Rémond & Lesèvre (1957) is enlightening. A sample of 60 healthy adult subjects was subdivided into 3 even subgroups (n= 20). The criterion of subdivision was the visually assessed degree of the Alpha rhythm continuity. Therefore, it may be rather safe to infer that this tripartition corresponded to our tripartition of systems' control dynamics **DR, DL,** and **PM**. The assumed **DR**-subgroup showed a low psychomotor speed, slowed sensorial reactivity, and general passivity. For each of the mentioned behaviours, the assumed **DL**-subgroup showed the contrary results as well as increased impulsivity and emotional instability.

These findings support the idea that the behavioral domain reflects the individual characteristics of systems' control. One may conclude that exceeding a certain medium range, be it upwards into the direction of *overshooting* (**DL**) or downwards into the direction of *delayed control* (**DR**), will turn out to be **maladaptive.** This will become especially apparent with attentional behavior because of its particular sensitivity to impaired dynamics. The possibility to objectively measure vigilance dynamics and to localize a subject with its individual EEG on continuum between the extreme poles of **DR** and **DL** with ideal smooth- control in-between has opened new and fecund prospects for research. Thereby, one has to take into account that a reversible unequivocal matching between the description levels of **function** (physiology) and **performance** (psychology) does not exist. Hence, one has to reckon that even extreme deviations of EEG-vigilance need not be accompanied by disturbed behaviour and vice versa. At a first glance, it seems paradoxical that the same attentional impairment may occur both with overshooting and delayed control of systems' dynamics. This paradox subsides if we bring to mind that **DL** – in systemic terms – may be conceived as a maladaptive increase of degrees of freedom. The subject becomes a a plaything of his environment since attention cannot be concentrated to a certain focus due to overshooting activity. **DR**, on the other hand, may be conceived as a maladaptive decrease in degrees of freedom associated with a general psychomotor slowing or a delayed (re)activity. The accompanying behavior has been termed *Umstellerschwerung* (Goldstein, 1934, disablement of adjustment, transl. from German), *erhöhte Umweltkohärenz* (Uexküll, 1920, increased coherence to the environment, transl. from German) or *Reizgebundenheit* (Weizsäcker, 1948, functional fixedness, transl. from German). From a systemic viewpoint, one may summarize that both a maladptive increase and decrease in the degrees of freedom may bring about the same attentional disturbance. Assessing the characteristics of the systems' control quantitatively by means of the test dose model provides an answer to the question of response prediction in the individual subject. An easily testable working hypothesis may be formulated as:

> --- A drug effected improvement of attentional deficits in ADHD-patients (e.g., by the central analeptic methylphenidate) with discontinuous SR-EEG (**DL**) follows an increased Alpha-continuity, which can be objectified by a decrease in the number of non-A-epochs. This decrease is equivalent to a "normalization" of a pre-existent maladaptive DL towards **PM**.

> --- A drug effected improvement of attentional deficits in ADHD-patients (e.g., by the central analeptic methylphenidate) with exaggerated or "hyperstable" SR-EEG (**DR**) follows an increase in the number of non-A-epochs. This increase is equivalent to a "normalization" of the pre-existent maladaptive **DR** towards **PM**.

--- If the central analeptic methylphenidate given as a test-dose has marginal or no effect on the preexistent dynamic system characteristics, a therapeutic effect upon the attentional deficits cannot be expected. In such case, other test-dose drugs may be tried, for instance, serotonin agonists, the Noradrenalin-Reuptake-Inhibitor Atomexetin , cyclic antidepressants, or others.

If we wanted to adopt the idea of the newly proposed *Individualized Medicine* in its literal sense, we would have to concern ourselves with the individually given systems control. Thereby, we dispose with only one single indicator of the highest level of central nervous integration, i.e., the SR-EEG. It gives us hope in the future development that this insight seems to forge ahead:

" .. *The EEG is the privileged method because it reflects the temporo-spatial pattern of synchronized cortical neuronal mass activity and is the only non-invasive method to measure directly and with sufficient time resolution neuronal activity"* (Hegerl et al., 2008).

7. 3. 7 OTHER PSYCHIATRIC DISORDERS: OBSESSIVE COMPULSIVE DIOSORDER (OCD) AND BORDERLINE PERSONALIY DISORDER (BPD)

Hegerl et al. (2008) recently compared a sample of patients diagnosed with Obsessive Compulsive Disorder (n = 20) with a sample of patients diagnosed with Borderline Personality Disorder (n = 20) in terms of EEG vigilance-dynamics. All patients were unmedicated. The control-group consisted of 20 healthy, gender- and age-matched persons. We learn that the vigilance classification was performed with a computer algorithm ("vigilance macro" that has been developed with the assistance of Dr. Gutberlet, BlindSight Consulting TM). Regrettable, the "re-discoverers" of our algorithm, which has been published a quarter century before (Ulrich & Frick, 1986) missed a fundamental aspect of the concept, which is the time-course of the EEG-vigilance level (Fig. 119; 120). The graph offers a visual representation of the dynamic information. We repeat that such representation requires a minimal recording time of 10 minutes. The authors self-critically admitted in the discussion part that this condition was not fulfilled. A second shortcoming concerns artefact editing, which by all means should have been omitted, particularly as the patient samples proved to be significantly different with respect to their artefact load. Despite such weighty methodological flaws, statistical differences between the patient groups could be obtained, supporting the underlying concept of assessing spontaneous vigilance dynamics.

Compared to the OCD sample, the BPS sample exhibited distinctly more subvigil non-A-epochs, which corresponds to a greater discontinuity of the Alpha-rhythm. In other words, BPS accompanies a lower mean level of EEG-vigilance than OCD. If BPS and OCD also represent the antithetical predilection types of overshooting control (DL) and of delayed control (DR) cannot be answered on the account of the missing assessment of the time course of non-A epochs. The finding indicating that the control group of healthy subjects did not differ significantly from the BPS- or the OCG-group might be due to the mentioned methodological flaws.

7.4 Non-linear Complexity Analysis: An important supplement and extension to traditional linear Q-EEG analysis

As already pointed out, the EEG may only be described and analyzed by stochastic or linear concepts with respect to short segments in the range of few seconds (e.g., 6.2.2). Longer time-segments could be regarded as a extremely nonlinear as well as nonstationary (Brodsky et al., 1999; Kaplan et al., 2001; Nunez, 1995; Steriade et al., 1990, etc.).

It has been demonstrated that nonlinear EEG measures convey behaviorally relevant information beyond the information to be extracted by spectral analysis. With this kind of quantitative analysis, the phase information suppressed by FFT spectral analysis plays an important role (Debus & Kuenkel, 1991). Visually indistinguishable EEGs or power spectra may correspond to completely different nonlinear complexity measure values. By means of the so-called surrogate method, the basic nonlinearity of the SR-EEG could be substantiated (Ehlers et al., 1998; Jelles et al., 1999; Jeong et al., 2004; Pijn et al., 1991; Soong & Stuart, 1989; Stam et al., 2003). "Surrogate data" are construed by phase randomization of the original EEG data. Thereby, the original nonlinear structure of the naturally given time function is destroyed. The linear properties, such as power spectra, coherences etc., remain unchanged.

The quantitative analysis of nonlinear systems is performed in a so-called **phase space**. Each state of the system is represented by a point within such a n-dimensional space. The time-sequence of the single states defines a **trajectory**. The trajectories converge to a subset of the **phase space,** which is denoted as **attractor**. All nonlinear methods of time series analysis are based on the so-called Takens theorem (1981). The most important metric property of an attractor or of a transient trajectory under study is the so-called **correlation dimension D2,** a measure of the complexity of a dynamical system (Grassberger et al., 1991). **D2** is the lower boundary of the degrees of freedom of signal possesses. It determines the number of independent variables that are necessary to describe the dynamics of the the original system, and it characterizes the distribution of the points within the phase space. Larger D2 value of the attractor indicates more complicated behavior of the nonlinear system. In the case of a steady state behaviour, the D2 of the attractor is zero, in the case of a periodic attractor, D2 is 1. In chaotic states, D2 takes on noninteger values.

Regarding other measures of complexity, Lyapunov's exponents estimate the mean exponential divergence or convergence of nearby trajectories of the attractor in the phase space. They reflect the sensitive dependence on the initial conditions. The reconstruction of the attractor in phase space is carried out through the technique of delay coordinates. **Tau** is the **time delay** between the time series considered and **d** is the embedding dimension (Eckmann & Ruelle, 1985). The choice of an appropriate time delay Tau and embedding dimension d determines the result. Therefore, an absolute measurement of D2 is not considered with empirical series of finite lengths. What exclusively matters are changes (Babloyantz & Destexhed, 1986; Elbert et al., 1994; Lutzenberger et al., 1992; Pritchard & Duke, 1992).

A number of studies convincingly demonstrated that D2 is related to a diversity of human behaviors. Most studies concerned sleep stage differentiation (Babloyantz, 1986; Babloyantz & Salzar, 1985;Ehlers et al. 1991; Roeschke & Aldenhoff, 1992; Roeschke & Aldenhoff, 1992; Roeschke & Basar, 1988; 1989).

Further topics concern information processing in healthy subjects under defined cognitive load (Gregson et al., 1990; Lutzenberger et al., 1992; Schupp et al., 1994) as well as deficient information processing in patients with Alzheimer's disease (Besthorn et al., 1995; Jelles et al., 1999; Jeong et al., 2004; Stam et al., 1996) and in patients diagnosed as schizophrenics (Elbert et al., 1994; Koukkou et al., 1993). Eventually, D2 was found to be related to psychotropic agents (Ulrich et al., 1993; Wackermann et al., 1993).

From a theoretical viewpoint, it deserves attention that D2 monotonously increases along with years of age. Anokhin et al. (1996) speculated that the "wisdom of age" may find its neurophysiological basis in an increase in the complexity of brain dynamics compared to young ages. The authors found that after a rapid increase in the brain dynamics complexity during puberty, a linear increase with age showed up during maturation (7-25 years). According to Anokhin et al., it was obvious that the life span adds to the long-term assemblies by the sheer increase of incoming information. This gain in complexity of brain dynamics would be reflected in the EEG.

Overall, convincing evidence suggests that the EEG's finite noninteger correlation dimension indicates *deterministic chaos* (Schuster, 1984). This means that any quantitative characterization of the *EEG- vigilance* control mechanisms will have to consider this very basic nonlinearity. The traditional linearity-based q-EEG analysis of two manic-depressive patients representing visuo-morphologically opposing predilection types of EEG-vigilance, who were both excellent responders to long-term Lithium prophylaxis, gave no hint concerning drug prediction (Ulrich et al., 1993). As opposed to this, the nonlinearity-based complexity analysis for both patients showed a distinct decrease of D2 under Lithium, which was not expected, neither from inspection of the raw signal nor from any linearity-related parameters. As pointed out in detail, there are convincing reasons to assume that Lithium may unfold its prophylactic efficiency by a decrease in the of brain dynamics complexity. Because of that, it might be worthwhile to make use of nonlinear complexity analysis to answer the practically extremely important question of individual drug response.

It is quite reasonable that the vendors of the commercial q-EEG software packages are very critical with nonlinear complexity analysis, particularly since it is almost impossible to realign it with the conventional linearity based tools. Moreover, nonlinear analyses are hardly suited for group-statistical purposes if one takes into account the inherently free choice of the **time delay Tau** and the number of embedding dimensions **d**. It goes without saying that such specialties are incompatible with the seemingly sacrosanct but nevertheless unsound principle of **Normative Data Base** (see 6.2.1) comparisons.

CHAPTER 8
Outlook

If we draw a preliminary résumé, we cannot help but notice that the psychophysiological electroencephalography, as targeted by Berger, has been suppressed from its beginnings. One may speculate whether the endeavour would have run another course if biocyberneticists would have discovered the SR-EEG as a central vehicle of systemic thinking. As pointed out, SR-EEG may be conceived as a macroindicator of Cerebral Global Function (**CGF**), reflecting the interaction of the brains with its environment. The SR-EEG has also been denoted as an **integrated wholeness** or as a **network of cooperative neuronal elements that are coherent across the entire derivation area** (3.4.4; 3.4.7). If we are pondering on the nature of the SR-EEG, its presently utilised practical and theoretical possibilities, as well its possible future perspectives, we cannot forger an ingenious clinician and scientist Hans Selye (1907-1982), who realized, without conducting EEG research, that all acute diseases, although etiopathogenetically different, have a non-specific symptom complex of very similar in appearance in common. Selye referred to the **General Adaptation Syndrome** (**GAS**), commonly referred to as **stress**. If a person feels exhausted, listless, tired, or irritable, if appetite is missing as well as relaxing sleep, than he/she will probably state to be **ill**. This conviction is not induced by "specific" phenomena but by phenomena assigned to the GAS-symptom- complex. By means of animal experiments, Selye was able to demonstrate that GAS corresponded to disturbances of functional axis: hypothalamus –pituitary gland – adrenocortex (**HPA**), which he postulated. By detecting this anatomical and endocrine connexion, the indivisible body–mind unity of the living organism no longer has to be considered a metaphor. It has become empirical reality. The SR-EEG reflects functional relations within the HPA-axis. Both descriptive domains, that of the "body" (material, physiological) on the one hand and of the "soul" (immaterial psychological) on the other, are indivisibly entangled.

Each illness finds its expression with **both** level of description. Different modes of illness behaviour can be localized on a dimension between the extreme poles of the somatological and psychological continuum. Even with the illnesses generally regarded as pure examples of somatogenic or psychogenic origin, a dual domains description has to be given as a matter of principle. Thus, SR-EEG overcomes the apparent contradistinction between the somatic and the mental aspects. Consequently, the EEG is not only defined as an indicator of the neurophysiological or the material aspect of the brain (according to a hidden assumption). It is not easy to grasp that it is can also be conceived as an indicator of the immaterial aspect of an organism interacting with its environment. In other words, the SR-EEG is also an indicator of the mental or the psychophysiological states. This kind of biperspectivism ensures the special status of the SR-EG within a medicine based upon the epistemic position of aspect-dualistic monism. Accordingly, the patient is neither pure body nor pure mind but a indivisible organismic unity which will be seen more in terms of the one or the other aspect, depending on the changing of the interactional processes. Viewing the SR-EEG as a diagnostical tool, it has to be inferred that the scope of application must not be restricted to material changes along the lines of physics. It is, for the most part, responsible for the EEG to be considered primarily as a means for neurological exclusion diagnostics. However, if we considered the EEG as an expression of the interaction between the brain and its environment, we would perceive it as a diagnostical means to objectify intangibles, for instance, differentiate the quality as well as the adaptability of the currently viable level of interaction. Therewith, the SR-EEG gains go beyond the conventional neurophysiologic or neurologic exclusion diagnostics. It becomes more important for psychology and hence psychiatry. We must not forget that all kinds of ipsative change measurements belong to this non-conventional kind of objectifying intangibles. Each change measurement refers to a past interaction between an organism and its environment. If one desists from the topographical neuroanatomical diagnostics of lesions and considers that the brain works as an integrating and controlling organ within an hierarchical order of functional layers, then it immediately becomes clear that the SR-EEG primarily serves in finding of intangible facts.

In contrast to the specifity paradigm, the premise of indivisible mind-body units demands that no disease is being restricted to a "target organ" but that other organ systems are always involved in an intricate fashion. The fashionable method of structural diagnosis by means of brain imaging, which aims at *an mosaic of rigidly encapsulated moduls* (Fodor, 1984), encourages a mechanistic and materialistic image of humanity. According to this, illness is nothig but the disturbance of certain spots of brain tissue and/or the strictly determined connections with other spots. As it seems, the EEG provides the only possibility for diagnosing complex interactions, be it between the structures of an organism or between an organism and its environment. There is no other way to diagnose changes in the unspecific components of any disease than by means of objectively assessing the differences between the organizational levels of the EEG within the time course. Moreover, one does not get around the insight that it is only by means of the nosologically unspecific information provided by the SR-EEG to numerically objectify the spontaneous restitution of an illness.

The same holds true for the effectiveness of therapeutic interventions, as for instance with:
- Traumatic brain injuries;
- Inflammatory, toxic and degenerative encephalopathies;
- Cerebral lesions of vascular or neoplastic origin;
- Persistent Vegetative State (Coma Vigile);
- Psychosomatic Disorders:
- The so-called Burn-out syndrome.

Therefore, it seems warranted to give the method of Ipsative Trend Assessment (**ITA**) a chance.

Transitory Ischemic Attacks (**TIA**) requires a special annotation. Though, by nature, the EEG will never reach the spatial resolution of our marvellous brain-imaging techniques, it may nevertheless be an indispensable adjunct with this special vascular problem. It is common that a **TIA** syndrome evades the verification by MRI. This is epecially true with the early acute phase of a vascular infarction, where the initial perifocal edema or penumbra impedes a sufficient structural differentiation.

A major reason for the negligence of the EEG method should be a lack of intimate knowledge about the intricate dynamic patterning of the SR-EEG. An adequate state of knowledge, which goes far beyond excluding of neurological disorders, which has been usually taught, can only be acquired by a longstanding employment of an EEG consultant within a psychiatric institution. Thereby, a special kind of visual pattern recognition can be acquired, which may serve as a scientifically legitimate tool to advance of new insights (Lorenz, 1959).

On these grounds, it has to be stated that despite multifarious assertions of the contrary, a genuine psychiatric EEG does not yet exist. Notwithstanding, few authors who aimed to conceptualize and practically elaborate on Berger's original idea deserve attention. The authors rely upon the SR-EEG as an indicator of the theoretical construct of *vigilance* proposed by Head (see 6.2.5). As already pointed out, it was essentially Bente who half a century ago adapted Head's conception for a psychophysiologically oriented EEG. This conception has been systematically elaborated by our Berlin research group over the years. It is sad to say that basic misunderstandings still hamper propagation and general appreciation of our EEG-vigilance concept. Thus, for instance, one may read:

"Arousal, activation, vigilance, alertness, sleep wake dimension are overlapping notions and concepts which are broadly used in literature without a commonly accepted definition" (Hegerl et al., 2008).

This misunderstanding of the theoretical term *vigilance* (sensu Head) as a psychological one is suited for discrediting the whole approach. Moreover, it puts the project of a *Psychophysiological* or *Psychiatric EEG* or of *Functional Electroencephalography* (Liberson, 1944; 1945) at risk. The other major difficulty, which is still counteracting clinical utilazation, is of technical nature and should therefore be overcome much easier than theoretical pondering. As we have already pointed out, a valid characterization of the SR-EEG dynamics is bound to 10 minutes of undisturbed and uninterrupted EEG as the lower limit of recording time. Generally, 10 minutes can be regarded both as the minimum but also as the optimum (3.4.2; 3.4.3; 7.1; 7.2). Such a condition would have been absolutely unrealistic up to the introduction of the "paperless" digital recording and processing technique in the beginning 1990s. Because of the multitude of prescribed electrode montages, the final record consisted of a stringing together of a number of rather short SR-EEGs, each one lasting maximally 1-2 minutes.

If we bring to mind that the subvigil patterns, particularly those corresponding to the later B-stages will generally not appear within short records, then it would not be surprising at all if the lawful changes of patterning were unnoticed. Today, there is no longer a need to record with different montages. Every montage can be displayed by conversion of the digitally stored raw EEG. Nevertheless, our proposals to make use of this technical advance and to record undisturbed and uninterrupted across longer periods – e.g., 10 minutes at least – meet with reluctance, resistance, or even refusal. Longer recordings than 2 to 3 minutes were purported as unpractical, especially with artefact prone psychiatric patients.

Since the future of the EEG hinges on the question of test-retest reliability, a radical methodological realignment seems to be worth pondering.

The heart of the reliability problem is the artefact problem. No artefact editing will be able to guarantee an artefact-free EEG. The most vicious kind of an artefact is the essentially unknown **APIA** (see 6.2.3). Because of the naturally given variability of both the topography of the superficial head arteries and of the shape of the skull, it is impossible to circumvent this artefact by conventional means. **APIA**, as well other artefacts, may be excluded if the frequency spectrum to be used for parametrization is restricted to **2.0 - 15.0 Hz.** Visual artefact editing would become pointless because thereby the complete spectral power due to artefacts would be practically excluded. With regard to the slow spectral components, this concerns the loco-motor effects due to ocular and facial muscle activity as well as the the DC voltage generated by sweating, the QRS-complexes from ECG, the cardioballistic effects, and last but not least the Arterial Pulse Impedance Artefact (APIA, see 6.2.3). With regard to the fast components, muscle activity of any kind and pharmacogenic beta waves are excluded.

To prevent a misunderstanding, it shall be stressed that our procedure has nothing to do with conventional filtering, be it in the analog or the digital mode. What we propose is simply a cut off of frequencies. The test-retest reliability may be further improved if we spared electrodes, which are especially prone to the conventional artefacts, e.g., Fp1 and Fp2. With digital recording and processing technique, one may safely restrict to the electrodes F3,F4,C3,C4,P3,P4,O1,O2 and to both earlobe- or mastoid electrodes. There is no reason to assume that reliability can improve on the account of losing validity of information. We firmly hold that such a radical methodological realignment represents both the absolute minimum of technical expenditure as well as the optimum with regard to the attainable reliability and validity. The limitation of electrodes and therewith of spatial resolution is just the contrary to the demanded increase of up to 256 electrodes (Wikswo et al., 1993). In the era of brain-imaging, no weighty argument suggests using the time function EEG for structural diagnosis. This especially holds for the Loreta-algorithm (Pascual-Marqui et al., 1994; Pascual- Marqui, 2002).

ITA, in contrast, offers many possibilities towards enhancing user-friendliness and applied flexibility. Thus, it has been criticized, for instance, that ITA is strictly commited to the assessment of differences/changes between consecutive recordings. Some minor changes of the algorithm will provide the possibility to assess the absolute values and thus characterise the cross sectional state by determining the frequency distributions of the single ITA variables within defined pathological or healthy control samples. Such a modification of **ITA** could be denoted as *R*esting *D*ynamics *A*ssessment (**RDA**).

As a further modification of **ITA**, one could envisage the dynamic information to be obtained at the single wave level, i.e., the level of the *lower structural elements*. Whereas **ITA** focuses on the dynamic information resulting from the quantitative reconstruction of the subvigil patterns occuring in the range of several seconds, it would interesting to learn additional information that can be found, by default of time windows, in the range of Alpha basic frequency, i.e., of about 1/10 seconds. That the morphology of a single graphoelement contains bahaviorally relevant information can be followed from the spindle-like modulation of Alpha activity being characteristic of subvigil stage A1 and from the progressive decomposition of spindles with the beginning subvigil stage A2. We may also refer to own experimental investigations showing that a defined senso-motor load exactly coincides with a certain change of the Alpha amplitude (Ulrich & Kriebitzsch, 1990). Overall, it may be concluded that there exist lawful relationships between the microdynamics of graphoelements constituting the basic rhythm on the one side and of the macrodynamics generated by the higher structural characteristics or patterns of EEG-vigilance on the other. Dealing with such relationships could possibly open a hitherto untreated and possibly industrious field of future research. Without going into more details, I will only mention some methodological challenges being posed by this approach. If one would analyze the microdynamics by means of FFT, this would require a high sampling rate that the commercial softwares do not provide. A solution consists of making use of a "sliding window" of a certain width (e.g., 0.2 seconds) being moved in steps of 0.1 seconds across the EEG. The computation is performed by the Root-Mean-Squared (RMS) algorithm for short segments (Ulrich & Kriebitzsch, 1990). Each single value is to be compared in a following step with the mean value of the first recording minute. A decrease in the amplitude within a 0.2 segment by more than a default criterion value (e.g., standard criterion: 65%; optional: 40 %) is defined as an **AAD-event** (Abrupt Amplitude Decrease).

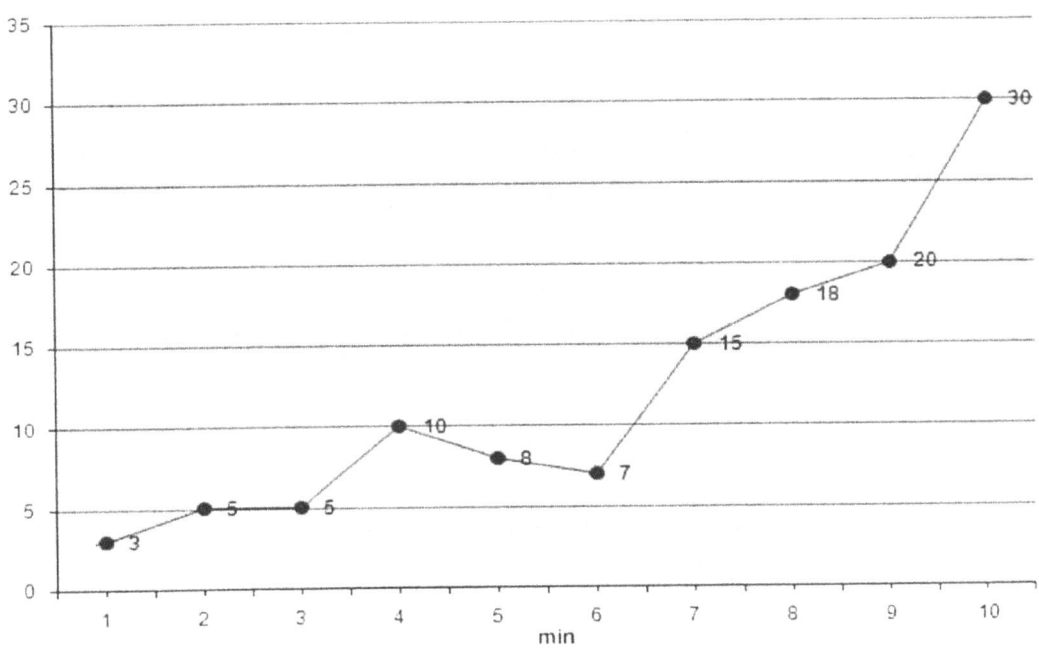

Figure 132. Fictional graph of the frequency course of AAD events within successive 1 minute-segments (out of 10 minutes SR-EEG); lead F3-A1.

AAD-analysis-windows: **0.2s**　　　　Step width of the sliding window : **0.1s**

Time (minutes)	1	2	3	4	5	6	7	8	9	10	Total
AAD segments (max)	600	600	600	600	600	600	600	600	600	600	6000
AAD events	3	5	5	10	8	7	15	18	20	30	121

Both **RDA** and **AAD** have not been realized as commercial software up to now. Nevertheless, if the concept along with methodological details were disclosed, we would deliberately abandon the possibility of applying patent protection. The intention behind this idea is that it could encourage other research groups to further develop the basic concept.

References

AIRD, R. B., GASTAUT, Y. (1959). Occipital and posterior electroencephalographic rhythms. EEG Clin. Neurophysiol. **11**, 637-656.

AIZENSTEIN, R.C., COCHRAN, J.,SAXTON, J. et al. (2005). Functional neuroimaging indicators of successful executive control in the oldest old. Neuroimage **289** 881-889

AJMONE-MARSAN, C., RALSTON, B. R. (1957). The Epileptic Seizure. Its Functional Morphology and Diagnostic Significance. Thomas, Springfield, Ill.

ALBERT, E. (1950). Die Diagnose der symptomatischen Psychosen nach ihrem Zustandsbild. Psychiat. Neurol. med. Psychol. (Lpz.) **2**, 97-104.

ALEXOPOULOS, G.,S., MEYERS, B. S., YOUNG, R.C. et al. (1993). The course of geriatric depression with 'reversible dementia': a controlled study. Am. J. Psychiat. **150**,1693-1699.

ALPER, K. R., CHABOT, R. J., KIM, A. H., et al. (1990) Quantitative EEG correlates of crack cocaine dependence. Psychiatry Res.: Neuroimaging **35**, 95-105. AMDP (1982). Arbeitsgemeinschaft für Methodik und Dokumentation in der Psychiatrie - Manual for the assessment and documentation of psychopathology. Guy, W., Ban T. A. (eds.) Springer, Berlin - Heidelberg-New York.

AMERICAN ACADEMY OF NEUROLOGY (1989). Report of the Therapeutics and Technology Assessment Subcommittee: Assessment brain mapping. Neurology **39** 1100-1101.

AMERICAN REPORT OF THE TASK FORCE ON QUANTITATIVE ELECTROPHYSIOLOGICAL ASSESSMENT (APA) (1991). Report of the Task Force on Quantitative Electrophysiological Assessment: Quantitative electroencephalography. A report on the present state of computerized EEG techniques. Am J Psychiatry 148 961-964.

ANAND, B. K., CHHINA, G., SINGH, B. (1961). Some aspects of electroencephalographic studies in Yogis. EEG Clin. Neurophysiol. **13**, 452 – 456.

ANDERMANN, F., ROBB, J. P. (1972). Absence status. A re-appraisal following a review of 38 patients. Epilepsia **13**, 77-187.

ANDREANI, G., CASELLI, A., MARTELLI, G. (1958). Clinical and electrographic findings in the treatment of mania with lithium salts. Psychiat. Neuropat. **83**, 273-328.

ANDREOLI, V. (1992). The complexity of psychiatric nosography and the "simplicity" of molecular genetics.J. psychiat. Res. **26**, 279-284.

ANOKHIN, A. P., Birbaumer, N., Lutzenberger,W. et al. (1996). Age increases brain complexity. EEG Clin. Neurophysiol. **99**, 63-68.

ANTONOVSKY, A. (1997). Salutogenese. Zur Entmystifizierung der Gesundheit ; dgvt-Verlag, Tübingen.

ANTONOVSKY, A. (1979) Health, Stress and Coping: New Perspectives on Mental and Physical Wellbeing Jossey-Braas, San Francisco.

ARENAS, A. M., BRENNER, R. P., REYNOLDS, Ch. F. (1986). Temporal slowing in the elderly revisted. Am. J. EEG Technol. **26**, 105- 114

ARIAS BAL, M. A., VAZQUEZ-BARQUERO, J. L., PENA, C., et al.: Psychiatric aspects of multiple sclerosis. Acta Psychiatr. Scand. **83**, 292-296 (1991)

ARIKAWA, D.: An electrophysiological study on the alcohol withdrawal in chronic alcoholics.Psychiat. Neurol. Jap. **72**, 596 - 617 (1970)

ARNS, M., GUNKELMAN J, BRETELER, M.et al. EEG phenotypes predict treatment outcome to stimulants in children with ADHD.J. Integ. Neurosci. **7**, 421-438 (2009)

ASHBY, W.,R. Principles of the self-organizing system (pp 122-142) In von Foerster H, Zopf GW (eds.) Principles of Technology of Self-Organizing Systems Pergamon Press, London, 1962

AU, W. J., GABOR, A. J., VIJAYAN, N., et al.: Periodic lateralized epileptiform complexes (PLEDs) in Creutzfeld-Jakob disease. Neurology **30**, 611-617 (1980)

BABLOYANTZ, A. Chaotic dynamics in brain activity (pp. 196-202) In: Basar, F.(ed) Dynamics of Sensory and Cognitive Processing by the Brain. Springer,Berlin, 1988

BABLOYANTZ, A., SALAZAR, J. M., NICOLIS, C.: Evidence of chaotic dynamics of brain activity during the sleep cycle. Physics Letters **111A**, 152 - 156 (1985)

BABLOYANTZ, A., DESTEXHE, A. Low-dimensional chaos in a case of epilepsy. Proc. Natl. Acad. Sci. USA **83**, 3513-3517 (1986)

BAEYER, W. v.: Die moderne Schockbehandlung. G.Thieme, Stuttgart 1951

BAGCHI, B. K., LISS, L., MOORE, K., et al.: The significance of disagreement between EEG, clinical and pathological findings. Presented at the tenth annual meeting of the American Electroencephalographic Society, 1956

BANCAUD, J.: Correlation of neuro-psycho-pathological and EEG findings in cases with cerebral tumours. EEG Clin. Neurophysiol. Suppl. **19**, 204-248 (1961)

BANCAUD, J., HECAEN, H., LAIRY, G. C.: Modifications de la reactivite electroencephalographique, troubles des fonctions symboliques et troubles confusionnels dans les Iesions hemispheriques localisees. EEG Clin. Neurophysiol. **7**, 179 (1955)

BANQUET, J. P.: EEG and meditation. EEG Clin. Neurophysiol. **33**, 454 (1972)

BANQUET, J. P.Spectral analysis of the EEG in meditation. EEG Clin. Neurophysiol. **35**, 143-151 (1973)

BARAHONA-FERNANDEZ, J.: Über die Syndrome bei symptomatischen Psychosen. Zbl. ges. Neurol. Psychiat. **137**, 132-133 (1956)

BARNES, R. H., BUSSE, E. W., FRIEDMAN, E. L.: The psychological functioning of aged individuals with normal and abnormal encephalograms. II. A Study of hospitalized individuals. J. Nerv. Ment. Dis. **124**, 585-593 (1956)

BARRY, R.J., CLARKE, A.R., JOHNSTONE, S.J. A review of lectroencephalography in attention-deficit/hyperactivity disorder: I. Qualitative and quantitative electroencephalography.*Clin Neurophysiol.* **114** 171-183 (2003)

BASAR, E. EEG - Brain Dynamics. Elsevier, Amsterdam - New York—Oxford 1980

BASH, K. W. Epilepsia sine ictu. Schweiz. Arch. Neurol. Neurochir. Psychiat. **103**, 351-353 (1969)

BATESON, G., Geist und Natur; Suhrkamp, Frankfurt a.M. 1982

BAUER, J., DRUSCHKY, K. F., ERBGUTH, F.: Status epilepticus: Ursachen, Verlauf und Therapie bei 100 Patienten. Akt. Neurol. **19,** 165 - 170 (1992)

BECKMANN, H., HEINEMANN, H.D. Amphetamin beim manischen Syndrom. Arzneim. Forsch./Drug Res. **26** 1185-1186 (1976)

BELLAK, L.: Schizophrenic syndrome related to minimal brain dysfunction: a possible neurologic subgroup. Schizophr. Bull. **5**, 480-489 (1979)

BENNET, A. E., DOI, L. T., MOWREY, G. L.: The value of electroencephalography in alcoholism. J. Nerv. Ment. Dis. **124**, 27-32 (1956)

BENTE, D.: Elektroencephalographische Gesichtspunkte zur Klassifikation neuro- und thymoleptischer Pharmaka. Med. exp. **5**, 337-346 (1961)

BENTE, D.: Elektroencephalographische und psychiatrische Pharmakotherapie, S.75-99. In: Anthropologische und naturwissenschaftlich-klinische Grundprobleme der Pharmakopsychiatrie. Achelis J. D., v. Ditfurth H. (Hrsg.). Thieme, Stuttgart 1963

BENTE, D.: Vigilanz, dissoziative Vigilanzverschiebung und Insuffizienz des Vigilitätstonus, S,13-28. In: Begleitwirkungen und Mißerfolge der psychiatrischen Pharmakotherapie. Kranz H., Heinrich K. (Hrsg.). Thieme, Stuttgart 1964a

BENTE, D.: Die Insuffizienz des Vigilitätstonus. Habilitationsschrift, Universität Erlangen 1964b

BENTE, D.: The effects of psychotropic drugs on the EEG in man, S. 162-168. In: Second Advanced Course in Electroencephalography of the International Federation Societies for Electroencephalography and Clinical Neurophysiology (Salzburg). Verl. Wiener Med. Akad., 1965a

BENTE, D.: Das Elektroenzephalogramm bei Psychosen: Befunde und Probleme. Hippokrates **36**, 817-823 (1965b)

BENTE, D.: Episodische Psychosen im Rahmen der Epilepsie, klinische und elektroencephalographische Aspekte. Das ärztliche Gespräch (Tropon, Köln) **11**, 33 - 49 (1969a)

BENTE, D.: Veränderungen der Vigilanzregulierung bei Schlafentzug, S. 185-189. In: Der Schlaf - Neurophysiologische Aspekte. Jovanovic, V. J. (Hrsg.). Barth, München 1969b

BENTE, D.: Vorwort zu: Die Quantifizierung des Elektroenzephalogramms. Schenk, G. K. (Hrsg.). Symposium der Arbeitsgemeinschaft für Methodik in der Elektroencephalographie, Jongny sur Vevey 1973. AEG-Telefunken, Konstanz 1973a.

BENTE, D.: Differentielle und generelle Wirkungen psychotroper Pharmaka auf das menschliche EEG, S.149-156. In: Psychopharmacology, Sexual Disorders and Drug Abuse. Ban, T. et al. (eds..).North-Holland Publ. Co., Amsterdam 1973b

BENTE, D.: Psychophysiologische Hypothesen zur Genese depressiver Erkrankungen. Ärztl. Praxis **27**, 3641-3643 (1975)

BENTE, D.: Elektroenzephalographische Gesichtspunkte zum Wach-Schlaf-Verhalten und zur Chronophysiologie endogener Depressionen. Arzneimittelforsch./Drug Res. **26**, 1058-1061 (1976)

BENTE, D.:Vigilanz: psychophysiologische Aspekte, S. 945-952. In: Verh. dtsch. Ges. f. inn. Med. Schlegel, B. (Hrsg.). Bergmann, München 1977

BENTE, D.: Vigilance and evaluation of psychotropic drug effect on EEG. Pharmacopsychiat. **12**, 137-147 (1979)

BENTE, D.: Möglichkeiten und Grenzen der Elektroenzephalographie in der geriatrisch-pharmakotherapeutischen Forschung, S. 137-144. In: Funktionsstörungen des Gehirns im Alter. Platt, D. (Hrsg.). Schattauer, Stuttgart - New York 1981

BENTE, D.: Vigilanzregulation hirnorganischer Psychosyndrome und Alterserkrankungen: ein psychophysiologisches Modell, S. 63-73. In: Hirnorganische Psychosyndrome im Alter. Bente, D., Coper, H., Kanowski, S. (Hrsg.). Springer, Berlin - Heidelberg - New York 1982

BENTE, D.:Elektroenzephalographische Vigilanzbestimmungen: Methoden und Beispiele. Z. EEG. EMG **15**, 173 - 179 (1984)

BENTE, D., ITIL, T.: Zur Wirkung des Phenothiazinkörpers Megaphen auf das menschliche Hirnstrombild. Arzneimittelforsch./Drug Res. **4**, 418-423 (1954)

BENTE, D., ITIL, T., SCHMID, E. E.: Elektroencephalographische Studien zur Wirkungsweise des LSD 25. Psychiat. Neurol., Basel **135**, 273-284 (1958)

BENTE, D., ITIL, T.: A comparison of the action of various phenothiazine compounds on the human EEG, pp. 496-498.In: Neuro-Psychopharmacology. Bradley, P. B., Deniker, P., Radouco-Thomas, C. (eds.). Elsevier, Amsterdam 1959

BENTE, D., ITIL, T.: EEG-Veränderungen unter chronischer Medikation mit Piperazinyl-Phenothiazinderivaten. Med. exp. **2**, 132-137 (1960)

BENTE, D., MÜLLER, M. L.: Intermittierende Störungen des Vigilitätstonus, S.439 - 441. In: Proc. Ill. World Congress of Psychiatry, Montreal. Univ. of Toronto Press, Toronto 1961

BENTE, D., ENGELMEIER, M.-P, HEINRICH, K. et al.: Psychische Grundaktivität und cerebrale Gesamtfunktion („vigilance"-HEAD). Nervenarzt **34**, 426-430 (1963)

BENTE, D., HARTUNG, H., HARTUNG, M.-L. et al.: Zur Pathophysiologie und Psychopathologie des durch zentrale Anticholinergica erzeugten amentiell-deliranten Syndroms. Arzneimittelforsch./Drug Res. **14,** 513-518 (1964)

BENTE, D., HOFFMEISTER, F., KREISKOTT, H. et al.: Zur Frage pharmakologisch-klinischer Wirkungskorrelate bei zentral dämpfenden psychotropen Pharmaka, S.392-395. In: Neuro-Psychopharmacology. Bente, D., Bradley, P. D. (eds.), Bd. 4. Elsevier, Amsterdam 1965

BENTE, D., FRICK, K., LEWINSKY, M. et al.: Signalanalytische Untersuchungen zur Wirkung des Antidepressivums Nomifensin auf das EEG gesunder Probanden, Arzneimittelforsch./Drug Res. **26**, 1110-1115 (1976)

BENTE, D., GLATTHAAR, G., ULRICH, G. et al.: Piracetam und Vigilanz. Arzneimittelforsch./Drug Res. **28**, 1529-1530 (1978)

BENTE, D., SCHEULER, W., ULRICH, G. et al. Effects of lithium on the EEG of healthy subjects in psychiatric patients: methods, results and hypotheses, pp.369 - 385. In: EEG in Drug Research. Herrmann, W. M. (ed.) G. Fischer, Stuttgart - New York 1982

BERGER, H.: Psychophysiologie in 12 Vorlesungen, G. Fischer, Jena 1921

BERGER, H.: Über das Elektrenkephalogramm des Menschen. I.Mitteilung. Arch. Psychiat. Nervenkr. **87**, 527-570 (1929)

BERGER, H.: Uber das Elektrenkephalogramm des Menschen; Vl. Mitteilung. Arch. Psychiat. Nervenkr. **99**, 555-574 (1933)

BERGES, J. A., HARRISON, A., LAIRY, G. C.: L'asynchronie des rhythmes posterieurs chez l'enfant d'age scolaire non encephalopathe. Rev. neurol. **115**, 162-174 (1966)

BERGLUND, M., HAGSTADIUS S. , RISBERGJ. et al. Normalization of regional cerebral blood flow in alcoholics during the first 7 weeks of abstinence. Acta Psychiatrica Scand. **75**. 202-208 (1987)

BÈRNARD, C. (1878) Lectures on the phenomena common to animals and plants (transl. Hoff, H.E. et al.) Ch. Thomas, Springfield Ill, 1974

v. BERTALANFFY, L. Gesetz oder Zufall: Systemtheorie und Selektion (p 71-95) In A. Koestler J.R. Smythies (eds) Das Neue Menschenbild F. Molden, Wien etc. 1970

v. BERTALANFFY, L., BEIER,.W.,LAUE., R. Biophysik des Fließgleichgewichts (2. Aufl.) Vieweg, Braunschweig, 1977

BERTOLUCCI, P., SILVA, A.: Alternating periodic lateralized epileptiform discharges (cerebral bigeminy). Clin. EEG **23**, 177 - 179 (1992)

BESSER, R., HORNUNG, K., THEISOHN, M. et al.: EEG changes in patients during the introduction of carbamazepine. EEG Clin. Neurophysiol. **83**, 19-23 (1992)

BEST, K., KÖHLER, G.-K.: Psychopathologische und hirnelektrische Befunde bei chronischem Trijodthyroninabusus, S. 253-264. In: Pharmakopsychiatrie / Neuropsychopharmakologie, Bd.4. Coper, H. et al. (Hrsg.). Thieme, Stuttgart 1971

BESTHORN, C, SATTEL, H., GEIGER-KABISCH, C. et al. Parameters of EEG dimensional complexity in Alzheimer's disease. EEG Clin. Neurophysiol. **95**, 84-89 (1995)

BEYREUTHER, K., MULTHAUPT,. G. MASTERS, C.L.: Molecular biology and pathology of Alzheimer's disease (p. 61-73). In: Neuronal Cell Death and Repair. Cuello AC (ed), Elsevier, Amsterdam 1993

BHROLCHAIN, M. N.: Psychotic and neurotic depression: I. some points of method. Brit. J. Psychiat. **134**, 87-92 (1979)

BICKFORD, R. G., BUTT, H. R.: Hepatic coma: The electroencephalographic pattern. J. Clin. Invest. **34**, 790-799 (1955)

BIELSKI, R. J., FRIEDL, R. O.: Predicition of tricyclic antidepressant response: a critical review. Arch. Gen. Psychiat. **33**, 1479 - 1489 (1976)

BINGLEY, T.: Mental symptoms in temporal epilepsy and temporal lobe gliomas. Acta psychiat. scand. suppl. No. 120, Vol. **33**, (1958)

BLACKLER, K. H., JONES, R. T., STONE, G. C. et al.: Chronic users of LSD: the "acidheads". Am. J. Psychiat. **125**, 97-107 (1968)

BLANC, CL.: Les foyers temporaux gauches dans les etats nevrotiques et depressifs. Rev. Neurol. **106**, 141-147 (1962)

BLANC, CL., LAIRY, G. C.: Modifications de l'EEG au cours des syndromes depressifs. Rev. Neurol. **102**, 371-374 (1960)

BLANC, CL., LAIRY, G. C.: Note sur les foyers temporaux gauches en psychiatrie. Rev. Neurol. **104**, 241 (1961)

BLEULER,. E. Dementia praecox oder die Gruppe der Schizophrenien; Deuticke Leipzig-Wien, 1911

BONHOEFFER, K.: Zur Frage der exogenen Psychosen. Zbl. Nervenheilk. Psychiat. **32**, 409 - 505 (1909)

BONHOEFFER, K.: Die Psychosen im Gefolge von akuten Infektionen, Allgemeinerkrankungen und inneren Erkrankungen, S. 1-118. In: Handbuch der Psychiatrie, Spez. Teil, 3. Abt. Aschaffenburg, G. (Hrsg,), Deuticke, Leipzig - Wien 1912

BONNET, H., BONNET, H.: L'endormissement spontane dans les etats d'excitation maniaque - etude electroclinique. Encephale **49**, 305-318 (1960)

BORENSTEIN, P., CUJO, P.: Electroencephalographie clinique et substances psychotropes. Sem. Hop. Paris **45**, 1315 - 1330 (1969)

BORENSTEIN, P., CUJO, P., KRAMARZ, P. et al.: A propos de certains aspects electroencephalographiques de l'action des psychotropes. Sem, Hop. Paris **45**, 1331-1336 (1969)

BOUTROS, N., MIROLO, H.A.,STRUVE, F. : Normative data for the unquantified EEG: examination of adequacy for neuropsychiatric research. Neuropsychiatry Clin Neurosci **17** 84-90 (2003)

BRAAK, H., BRAAK, E.: Neuropathological staging of Alzheimer-related changes. Acta Neuropath **82,** 239-259 (1991)

BRAAK, H., BRAAK, E.: Staging of Alzheimer disease-related neurofibrillary tangles Neurobiol of Aging **16,** 271-284 (1995)

BRAEU, H., ULRICH, G.: Electroencephalographic vigilance dynamics in multiple sclerosis during an acute episode and after remission. Eur. Arch. Psychiatr. Neurol. Sci. **239**, 320-324 (1990)

BRENNER, R. P., SCHWARTZMAN, R. J., RICHEY, E. T.: Prognostic significance of episodic low amplitude or relatively isoelectric EEG patterns. Dis. Nerv. Syst. **36**, 582 - 587 (1975)

BRENNER, R,P., REYNOLDS, C.F., ULRICH, R.F.: EEG findings in depressive pseudodementia and dementia with secondary depression. EEG Clin. Neurophysiol. **72** 298-304 (1989)

BRESLAU, J, STARR, A., SICOTTE, N. et al.: Topographic EEG changes with normal aging and SDAT. EEG Clin. Neurophysiol. **72**, 281-289 (1989)

BRIDGERS, S. L.: Epileptiform abnormalities discovered on electroencephalographic screening of psychiatric inpatients. Arch. Neurol. **44**, 312-316 (1987)

BRODSKY, B.E., DARKOVSKY, B.S., KAPLAN A.Y. A nonparametric method for the segmentation of the EEG. Comp. Meth. Prog. Biomed. **60**, 93-106 (1999)

BRON, B., LEHMANN, K.: The issue of the core syndrome of endogenous depression. Psychopathology **23**, 1-8 (1990)

BROWN, B.B.: Subjective and EEG response to LSD in visualizers and non-visualizer subjects. EEG Clin. Neurophysiol. **25**, 372-379 (1968)

BROWN, W.A.; MUELLER, B. Alleviation of manic symptoms with catecholamine agonists. Am. J. Psychiat. **136,** 230-231 (1979)

BSCHOR T., MUELLER-OERLINGHAUSEN, B.. ULRICH, G. Decreased level of EEG-vigilance in acute mania as a possible predictor for a rapid effect of methylphenidate: a case study. Clin. EEG 32 (2001) 1-4

BUCHSBAUM, M.S., KESSLER, R., KING, A. et al.: Simultaneons cerebral glucography with positron emission tomography and topographic electroencephalography (pp 263-269). In: Pfurtscheller G, Jonkman EJ , Lopes da Silva FH (eds). Brain Ischemia: Quantitative EEG and Imaging Techniques, Progress in Brain Res., Vol. 62, Amsterdam, Elsevier, 1984

v. BÜLOW, I, DIENER, H. C., ROCKSTROH, B. et al.: Zentralnervöse Effekte von Carbamazepin bei Gesunden, S. 264 - 268. In: Epilepsie 86. Speckmann, E. (Hrsg.). Einhorn, Reinbek, 1987

BUENNING, E.: "Ganzheit" in der Biologie. Studium Generale **5** 515-520 (1952)

BUESSOW, H.: Zur Frage der Perniciosa-Psychosen. Z. ges. Neurol. Psychiat. **165,** 314-318 (1939)

BÜSSOW, H.: Uber Psychosen nach Malaria. Allg. Z. Psychiat. **123,** 235-278 (1944)

BURGER, L. J., ROWAN, A. J., GOLDENSOHN, E. S.: Creutzfeld-Jakob-disease. An electroencephalographic study. Arch. Neurol. **26,** 428-433 (1972)

BUSSE, E.W.: Round-table discussion: EEG in Gerontology. Clin. EEG **4,** 153-163 (1973)

BUSSE, E.W.: Electroencephalography, pp. 231 - 236. In: Alzheimer's Disease. Reisberg, B. (ed.). The Free Press, New York 1983

BUSSE, E. W., BARNES, R. H., SILVERMAN, A. J. et al.:Studies of the process of aging: factors that influence the psyche of elderly persons.Am. J. Psychiat. **110,** 897-903 (1954)

BUSSE, E. W., OBRIST, W. D.: Significance of focal electroencephalographic changes in the elderly. Postgraduate Medicine **34,** 179-182 (1963)

BUSSE, E. W., WANG, H. S.: The value of electroencephalography in geriatrics. Geriatrics **20,** 906-924 (1965)

BUTENUTH, J., KUBICKI, S.: Klinisch-elektroenzephalographische Schlafbeobachtungen im apallischen Syndrom. Z. EEG-EMG **6,** 185-188 (1975)

BUTT, M. D., JOHNSON, I. D. A.:Computed tomography and EEG in herpes simpler encephalitis: their value in diagnosis and prognosis. Arch. Neurol. **39,** 99 - 102 (1982)

CAINE, E. D., BAMFORD, K. A., SCHIFFER, R. B. et al.:A controlled neuropsychological comparison of Huntington's disease and multiple sclerosis. Arch. Neurol. **43,** 249-254 (1986)

CANNON, W.B.: Organization for physiological homeostasis. Physiol. Rev. **8** (1929) 399-431
CANU, E.D.G., MAGNANO, I. PAULUS, K.S. et al.:Neuropsychophysiological findings in a case of long-standing overt ventriculo-megaly (LOVA). Neurosci Let 385 (2005) 24-29

CARNAP, R.: The methodological character of theoretical concepts, pp. 34-76.
In: The Foundation of Science and the Concepts of Psychology and Psychoanalysis. Feigl, H., Scriven, M. (eds.). Univ. of Minneapolis Press, Minneapolis 1956

CARPENTER, W. T., BARTKO, J. J., STRAUSS, J. S. et al.: Signs and symptoms as predictors of outcome: a report from the International Pilot Study of Schizophrenia. Am. J. Psychiatry **135**, 940-945 (1978)

CELSIS, P., AGNIEL, A., PUEL, M. et al.: Lateral asymmetries in primary degenerative dementia of the Alzheimer type. A correlative study of cognitive, haemodynamic and EEG data in relation with severity, age of onset and sex. Cortex **26**, 585-596 (1990)

CENTORRINO, F., PRICE BH, TUTTLE M et al.: EEG abnormalities during treatment with typical and atypical antipsychotics. Am J Psychiatry **159** 109-115 (2002)

CHABOT, B., SERFONTEIN, G.: Quantitative electroencephalographic profiles of children with attention deficit disorder. Biol Psychiatry **40** 951-963 (1996)

CHATRIAN, G. E.: The low voltage EEG, 6A-77 - 6A-88. In: Handbook of Electroencephalography and Clinical. Neurophysiology, vol. 6 -The Normal EEG Throughout Life, Part A. Remond, A. (ed.). Elsevier, Amsterdam 1976

CHATRIAN, G. E., SHAW, C. M., LEFFMAN, H.:The significance of periodic lateralized epileptiform discharges in EEG: an electrographic, clinical and neurological study. EEG Clin. Neurophysiol. **17**, 177-193 (1964)

CHRISTIAN, W.: Klinische Elektroenzephalographie, 2. Aufl. G.Thieme, Stuttgart 1975

CHIARAMONTI, R., MUSCAS, G.C., PAGANINI, M. et al.: Correlation of topographical EEG features with clinical severity in mild and moderate dementia of Alzheimer type. Neuropsychobiology 36 (1997) 153–58

CIGANEK, L.: Theta discharges in the middle-line - EEG symptom of temporal lobe epilepsy. EEG Clin. Neurophysiol. **13**, 669 - 673 (1961)

CLARKE, A.R., BARRY.R.J., McCARTHY, R. et al.: EEG analysis in attention-deficit/hyperactivity-disorder. A comparison study of two subtypes. Psychiatry Res **81,** 19-29 (1998)

Clarke, A.R., Barry, R.J., Mc Carthy, R. et al.: Excessive beta activity in children with attention-deficit/hyperactivity disorder: an atypical electrophysiological subgroup. Psychiatry Res **103** 205-218 (2001)

CLARKE, A.R., BARRY,R.J., McCARTHY, R. et al.: EEG differences between good and poor responders to methylphenidate and dexamphetamine in children with attention-deficit/hyperactivity disorder. Clin. Neurophysiol. **113** 194-205 (2002)

CLARKE, A.R., BARRY,R.J., McCARTHY, R. et al.:Effects of stimulant medications on children with attention-deficit/hyperactivity disorder and excessive beta activity in their EEG. Clin Neurophysiol **114** 1729-1737 (2003)

CIOMPI, L, LOMBRINUS, A., MÜLLER, C.: Basisdokumentation in der Gerontopsychiatrie: Das „AGP"-System, S. 130-140. Jansen Symposion Bd. 13. Jansen, Düsseldorf, 1973

CLARENBACH, P., WACHNER, R., LUCIUS, G. et al.: EEG-Befunde, neuroendekrinologische und psychometrische Untersuchungen zur Carbamazepin-Wirkung. Arch. Psychiatr. Nervenkr. **230**, 197 - 207 (1981)

CLARENBACH, P., RIEDEL, R.-R., TACKMANN, W.: AIDS und Nervensystem. Akt. Neurol. **14**, 113-116 (1987)

CLARK, C. M., FLEMING, J. A., Ll, D. et al.: Sleep disturbance, depression, and lesion site in patients with multiple sclerosis. Arch. Neurol. **49**, 641 - 643 (1992)

COBB, W. A.: Rhythmic slow discharges in the electroencephalogram. J. Neurol. Neurosurg. Psychiat.**8**, 65-78 (1945)

COBB, W. A.:Changes in background activity, 11B-12 - 12B-31. In: Handbook of Electroencephalography and Clinical Neurophysiology, vol. 11 Clinical EEG, 1, Part B. Remond, A. (ed.). Elsevier, Amsterdam 1978

COBEN, L. A., DANZIGER, W., BERG, L.:Frequency analysis of the resting awake EEG in mild senile dementia of Alzheimer type.EEG Clin. Neurophysiol. **55**, 372-380 (1983)

COBEN, L. A., DANZIGER, W., STORANDT, M.: A longitudinal EEG study of mild senile dementia of Alzheimer type: changes at 1 year and at 2.5 years. EEG Clin. Neurophysiol. **61**, 101-112 (1985)

COBURN, K.L, LAUTERBACH, E.C, BOUTROS, N.N. et.al. The value of quantitative electroencephalography in clinical psychiatry: A report by the Committee on Research of the American Neuropsychiatric Association.J Neuropsychiatry Clin Neurosci **18**, 460-500 (2006)

COHEN, B.A., BRAVO-FERNANDEZ, E.J., SANCES, A.: Quantification of computer analyzed serial EEGs from stroke patients, EEG Clin. Neurophysiol; **41** 379-386 (1976)

COHN, R.: On the significance of biooccipital slow wave activity in the electroencephalogram of children. EEG Clin. Neurophysiol. **10**, 766-768 (1958)

COHN, R.: Delayed acquisition of reading and writing abilities in children. Arch. Neurol. (Chic.) **4**, 153-164 (1961)

COHN, R., NARDINI, J.:The correlation of bilateral occipital slow activity in the human EEG with certain disorders of behavior. Amer. J. Psychiat. **115**, 44-54 (1958)

COHN, R., TANNHAUSER, M., BENTZEN, F.: On the significance of biooccipital slow wave activity in the electroencephalogram of children. EEG Clin. Neurophysiol. **10**, 766-768 (1958)
COLON, E., HOMMES, O. R., DE WEERD, J. P. C.: Relation between EEG and disability scores in multiple sclerosis. Clin. Neurol. Neurosurg. **83**, 163-168 (1981)

CONRAD, K.: Strukturanalysen hirnpathologischer Fälle: über Struktur- und Gestaltwandel. Deutsch. Z. Nhlk. **158**, 344 - 371 (1947)

CONRAD, K.: Die beginnende Schizophrenie. 1. Aufl. G. Thieme, Stuttgart 1958

CONRAD, K.: Das Problem der „nosologischen Einheit" in der Psychiatrie. Der Nervenarzt **30**, 488 - 494 (1959)

COPPOLA, R., HERRMANN, W. M.: Psychotropic drug profiles: comparison by topographic maps of absolute power. Neuropsychobiology **18**, 97-104 (1987)

COREY-BLOOM, J., GRUNDMAN, M., THAL, L.J. : A randomized trial evaluating the efficacy and safety of ENA-713, a new acetylcholinesterase inhibitor in patients with mild to moderately severe Alzheimer's disease. Int J Geriatr Psychopharmacol. **1** (1998) 55-56

CORNELL, D. G., SUAREZ, R., BERENT, S.: Psychomotor retardation in melancholic and nonmelancholic depression: cognitive and motor components. J. abnorm. Psychol. **93**, 150-157 (1984)

COURJON, J.: A longitudinal electro-clinical study of 80 cases of post-traumatic epilepsy observed from the time of the original trauma. Epilepsia **11**, 29—36 (1970)

CREUTZFELDT, O.: Some problems of cortical organization in the light of ideas of the classical "Hirnpathologie" and the modern neurophysiology. An essay, pp. 217 – 226. In: Cerebral Localization. An Otfrid Foerster Symposium. Zülch, K.J., Creutzfeldt, O., Galbraith, G. C. (eds.). Springer, Berlin - Heidelberg - New York 1975

CUMMINGS, J.L., CYRUS, P.A., BIEBER, F. et al.: Metrifonate treatment of the cognitive deficits of Alzheimer's disease. Neurology **50** 1214-1221 (1998)

CUTTS, K. K., JASPER, H. H.: Effect of benzedrine sulfate and phenobarbital on behavior problem children with abnormal electroencephalograms. Arch. Neurol. Psychiat. **41**, 1138-1145 (1939)

CZERNIK, A.: EEG-Veränderungen unter langjähriger Lithiumbehandlung. Psychiat. clin. **11**, 189-197 (1978)

DACKIS, C., GOLD, M.: New concepts in cocaine addiction: the dopamin depletion hypothesis. Neurosciences Biobeh. Rev. **9**, 469-477 (1985)

DALBY, M. A.: Epilepsy and 3 per second spike and wave rhythms. Acta neurol. scand. **40**, (suppl.) 6-180 (1969)

DALY, D. D., WHELAN, J. L., BICKFORD, R. G. et al.: The electroencephalogram in cases of tumors of the posterior fossa and third ventricle. EEG Clin. Neurophysiol. **5**, 203-216 (1953)

DALY, D. D.: Das EEG in der Diagnose und Beurteilung von epileptischen und nichtepileptischen Anfällen, S. 200 - 244. In: Klinische Elektroenzephalographie. Klass, D. W., Daly, D. D. (Hrsg.). G. Fischer, Stuttgart - New York 1984

DALY, D., WHELAN, J. L., BICKFORD, R. G. et al.: The electroencephalogram in cases of tumors of the posterior fossa and third ventricle. EEG Clin. Neurophysiol. **5**, 203 - 216 (1953)

DANIEL, R. S.: Electroencephalographic pattern quantification and the arousal continuum. Psychophysiology **2**, 146-160 (1966)

DARROW, Ch. W.: Psychological and psychophysiological significance of the electroencephalogram. Psychol. Rev. **54**, 157-168 (1947)

DASBERG, H., ROBINSON, S.: Electroencephalographic variations following anti-psychotic drug treatment. Dis. Nerv. Syst. **32**, 472-478 (1971)

DAUMEZON, G., LAIRY, G. C.: Dynamique du rhythme alpha en psychopathologie. Ann. Med.-Psychol. **115**, 35-51 (1957)

DAVIES, R. K., NEIL, J. F., HIMMELHOCH, J. M.: Cerebral dysrhythmias in schizophrenics receiving phenothiazines: clinical correlates.Clin. Electroenc. **6**, 103-115 (1975)

DAVIS, P. A.: Evaluation of the electroencephalograms of schizophrenic patients. Am. J. Psychiat. **96**, 852-860 (1940)

DAVIS, P. A.: The electroencephalogram in old age. Dis. Nerv. Syst. **2**, 77 (1941a)

DAVIS, P. A.: Electroencephalograms of manic-depressive patients. Am. J. Psychiat. **98**, 430 - 433 (1941b)

DAVIS, P.A.: Comparative study of the EEGs of schizophrenic and manic-depressive patients. Am. J. Psychiat. **99**, 210-217 (1942)

DAVIS, H., DAVIS, P.A.: Action potentials of the brain. Arch. Neurol. Psychiat. (Chic.) **36**, 1214-1224 (1936)

DAVIS, H., DAVIS, P. A., LOOMIS, A. L. et al.: Human brain potentials during the onset of sleep. J. Neurophysiol. **1**, 24-38 (1938)

DAVIS, P., DAVIS, H.: The electroencephalograms of psychotic patients. Am. J. Psychiat. **95**, 1007-1025 (1939)

DAVIS, P., GIBBS, F., DAVIS, H. et al.: The effects of alcohol upon the electroencephalogram (brain waves). Quart. J. Stud. Alcoholism **1**, 626-637 (1941)

Davis RK, Neil JK, Himmelhoch JM. Cerebral dysrhythmias in schizophrenics receiving phenothiazines. Clin EEG 6 103-115 (1975)

DEBUS, S., KÜNKEL, H.: Zur Interpretation der chaotischen Dynamik im EEG. Z. EEG-EMG **89**, 89 (1991)

D'ELIA G, PERRIS C.: Cerebral functional dominance and depression. Acta psychiat scand. **49** 191-197 (1973)

DELIYANNAKIS, E., PANAGOPOULOS, CH., HUOTT, A. D.: The influence of hashish on human. EEG. Clin. EEG **1**, 128 - 140 (1970)

DELL, P.: Some basic mechanisms of the translation of bodily needs into behaviour, pp. 187-200. In: Ciba Foundation Symposium on the Neurological Basis of Behaviour. Churchill, London 1958

DEMENT, W., KLEITMAN, N.: Cyclic variations in EEG during sleep and their relation to eye movements, body motility, and dreaming. EEG Clin. Neurophysiol. **9**, 673-690 (1957)

DENBER, H. C. B., MERLIS, S.: Studies on Mescaline action in schizophrenic patients. Psychiat. Quart. **29**, 421-429 (1955)

DESAI, B., WHITMAN, S., BOUFFARD, D. A.: The role of the EEG in epilepsy of long duration. Epilepsia **29**, 601 - 606 (1988)

DESMURGET, M., BONNETBLANC, F., DUFFAU, H. Contrasting acute and slow growing lesions: a new door to brain plasticity. Brain **130** 898-914 (2007)

DEVINSKY, O., HONIGFELD, G., PATIN, J.: Clozapin-related seizures. Neurology **41**, 369-371 (1991)

DIEHL, D. J., GERSHON, S.: The role of dopamine in mood disorders. Comp. Psychiatry **33**, 115-119 (1992)

DIERKS, T., PERISIC, I., FRÖLICH, L. et al.: Topography of the quantitative electroencephalogram in dementia of the Alzheimer type: relation to soverity of dementia. Psychiatry Res.: Neuroimaging **40**, 181-194 (1991)

DIERKS, T., IHL, R., FRÖLICH, L. et al.: Dementia of Alzheimer type: effect on the spontaneous EEG described by dipole sources Psychiat Res 50 (1993) 151-162

DIMASCIO, A., MEYER, R. E., STIFLER, L.: Effects of imipramine on individuals varying in level of depression. Amer. J. Psychiat. **124**, 55 - 58 (1968)

van DIS H., CORNER, M., DAPPER, R. et al.: Individual differences in the human electroencephalogram during quiet wakefulness EEG Clin Neurophysiol **47**, 87-94 (1979)

DOCTER, R. F., NAITOH, P., SMITH, J. C.: Electroencephalographic changes and vigilance behavior during experimentally induced intoxication with alcoholic subjects. Psychosom. Med. **28**, 605 - 615 (1966)

DONDEY, M., GACHES, J.: Semiology in clinical E EG, 11-A3 - 11-A-39. In: Handbook of Electroencephalography and Clinical Neurophysiology, vol. 11 - Clinical EEG, III, Part A. Remond, A. (ed.). Elsevier, Amsterdam 1977

DONGIER, S.: Statistical study of clinical and electroencephalographic manifestations of 536 psychotic episodes occurring in 516 epileptics between clinical seizures. Epilepsia **1**, 117-142 (1959)

DONGIER, S.:A apropos des etats de mal generalises a expression confusionelle. Etude psychologique de la destructuration de la conscience au cours de l'etat de petit mal.pp. 110-118. In: Les etats de mal epileptiques. Gastaut, H., Roger, J., Lob, H. (eds.). Masson, Paris, 1967

DONGIER, M.: Mental diseases, 13B-3 - 13B-65. In: Handbook of Electroencephalography and Clinical Neurophysiology, vol. 13 - Clinical EEG, III, Part B. Remond, A. (ed.). Elsevier, Amsterdam 1977

DONGIER,S.,DE TOURNADRE, N., NAQUET, R.: A psychological study of 34 subjects presenting a posterior 4c/sec rhythm. EEG Clin. Neurophysiol. **18**, 722P (1965)

DONSELAAR C. A. VAN,SCHIMSHEIMER, R.-J., GEERTS, A. T. et al.: Value of the electroencephalogram in adult patients with untreated idiopathic first seizures. Arch. Neurol. **49**, 231-237 (1992)

DRACHMAN, D. A., HUGHES, J. R.: Memory and hippocampal complexes. III: aging and temporal EEG abnormalities. Neurology **21**, 1 - 14 (1971)

DREYER, R.: Zur Frage des Status epilepticus mit psychomotorischen Anfällen. Der Nervenarzt **36**, 221-223 (1965)

DRISCHEL, H. Einführung in die Biokybernetik Akad. Verlag Berlin, 1973

DUENSING, F.: Das Elektroencephalogramm bei Störungen der Bewußtseinslage. Arch. Psychiat. Z. Neurol. **183**, 71-115 (1949)

DUFFY, F.H. : Brain electrical activity mapping: clinical applications Psychiat Res 29 (1989) 379-384

DUFFY, F. H., ALBERT, M. S., McANULTY, G. et al.: Age-related differences in brain electrical activity of healthy subjects. Ann. Neurol. **16**, 430-438 (1984)

DUFFY F.H., HUGHES, J.R., MIRANDA, F. et al.: Status of quantitative EEG (QEEG) in clinical practice; Report of an "Ad hoc Committee on QEEG" of the American Medical EEG Association – AMEEGA. Clin EEG **25**, 6-22 (1994)

DUMERMUTH, G.: Zur Quantifizierung und Analyse des EEG. Schweiz. Arch. Neurol. Neurochir. Psychiat. **115**, 175 - 192 (1974)

DUTERTRE, F.: Catalogue of the main EEG patterns, 11A-40 - 11A-79. In: Handbook of Electroencephalography and Clinical Neurophysiology, vol. 11 - Clinical EEG, O, Part A. Remond, A. (ed.). Elsevier, Amsterdam 1978

EBERT, D.: Psychopathologie und Verlauf leichter affektiver Psychosen. Fundamenta Psychiatrica **4**, 119-123 (1990)

ECKMANN, J.P. RUELLE, D.: Ergodic theory of chaos and strange attractors. Rev. Mod. Phys. **57**, 617-656 (1985)

EDELMAN, G. M.: The Remembered Present. A Biological Theory of Consciousness. Basic Books, New York, 1989

EEG-OLOFSSON, O.: The development of the electroencephalogram in normal children from the age of 1 through 15 years. Neuropädiatrie **2**, 247-304 and 405-427 (1971)

EDDINGTON, A.: The Philosophy of Natural Sciences Camb. Univ Press Cambridge, 1939

EHLERS,C.L., HAVSTADT, J.W., PRICHARD, D.: Low doses of ethanol reduce evidence for nonlinear structure in brain activity. J. Neurosci. **18**, 7474-7486 (1998)

EIGEN, M, WINKLER-OSWAITITSCH, R.: Das Spiel, Piper München, 1975

EIGEN, M., SCHUSTER, P.: The Hyper Cycle. A Principle of Natural Self Organization Part A Emergence of the Hypercycle. Naturwiss **64**, 541-565 (1977)

ELBERT, T., RAY,W.J., KOWALIK, J. et al.: Chaos and physiology. Physiol. Rev. **74**,1-47 (1994)

D' ELIA, G., PERRIS, C.: Cerebral functional dominance and depression. Acta psychiat. scand. **49**, 191-197 (1973)

ELLINGSON, R. J.: The incidence of EEG abnormality among patients with mental disorders of apparently non-organic origin: a critical review. Am. J. Psychiat. **111**, 263-275 (1954)

ELLIOTT, F. A.: The dyscontrol syndrome. The Practitioner **217**, 51 - 60 (1976)

ELSON, B. D., HAURI, P., CUNIS, D.: Physiological changes in Yoga meditation. Psychophysiology **14**, 52 - 57 (1977)

EMDE, R. N., METCALF, D. R.: EEG signs of toxicity in schizophrenics on phenothiazines. Behav. Neuropsychiatry **1**, 31 - 36 (1969)

ENDO, K.: Experimental study of Mescalin intoxication on relation between clinical picture and EEG in man. Folia psychiat. neurol. jap. **6**, 104-113 (1952)

ENGEL, J., LUDWIG, B.I., FETELL, M.: Prolonged partial complex status epilepticus: EEG and behavioral observations. Neurology **28**, 863 - 869 (1978)

EPSTEIN, A., KING, H. E.: Behavior of epileptic and nonepileptic patients with "temporal spikes". Arch. Neurol. Psychiat. **74**, 488-497 (1955)

EPSTEIN C. ,E. Editorial: Computerized EEG in the courtroom. Neurology **44,** 1566-1569 (1994)

ERESHEFSKY, L., WATANABE, M. D., TRAN-JOHNSON, T. K.: Clozapine: an atypical antipsychotic agent. Clin. Pharmacy **8**, 691 - 707 (1989)

ERKINJUNTTI, T., LARSEN,T., SULKAVA, R. et al.: EEG in the differential diagnosis between Alzheimer's disease and vascular dementia. Acta neurol scand **77**, 36-42 (1988)

ÉTEVENON, P., PIDOUX, B., COTTEREAU, M. J. et al.: Quantiative EEG analysis of high dose haloperidol effects in therapy-resistant schizophrenic patients. Adv. biol. Psychiat. .4, 175-187 (1980). Karger

ÉTEVENON, P., PERON-MAGNAN, P., RIOUX, P. et al.: Schizophrenia assessed by computerized EEG. Adv. biol. Psychiat., **6**, 29-34 (1981). Karger

ETTLIN, T. M., STAEHELIN, B., KISCHKA, U. et al.: Computed tomography, electroencephalography, and clinical features in the differential diagnosis of senile dementia. A prospective clinicopathologic study. Arch. Neurol. **46**, 1217 - 1220 (1989)

EY, H.: Grundlagen einer organo-dynamischen Auffassung der Psychiatrie. Fortschr. Neurol. Psychiat. **20**, 195 - 209 (1952)

EY, H.: Études Psychiatriques, vol.3 (p.693 ff.). Desclee de Brouwer, Paris 1954

EY, H.: Epilepsie. In: Manuel de Psychiatrie. Ey, H., Bernard, P., Brisset, Ch. (eds.). Masson, Paris 1963

FAEHNDRICH, E., GEBHARDT, R., NEUMANN, H.: Zum Problem der Diagnosesicherung des hirnorganischen Psychosyndroms. Arch. Psychiat. Nervenkr. **229**, 239 - 248 (1981)

FAURE, J., DROOGLEEVER-FORTUYN, J., GASTAUT, H. et al.: De la genese et de la signification des rhythmes recueillis a distance dans les cas de tumeurs cerebrales. EEG Clin. Neurophysiol. **3**, 429-434 (1951)

FAZEKAS, J., KLEH, J., WITKIN, L.: Cerebral hemodynamics and metabolism in subjects over 90 years of age. J. Amer. Geriat. Soc. **1**, 836-839 (1953)

FEIGENBERG, I. M.: Comparative electroencephalographic characteristics of various clinical groups of schizophrenic patients. Zh. Nevropatol. Psikhiatr. (russ., franz. Zusammenfassung) **64**, 567 - 574 (1964)

FELL, J. Classification of mental states with nonlinear deterministic and stochastic EEG measures: a combined strategy.Acta Neurobiol Exp **60**, 87-109 (2000)

FILLEY, CH. M., HEATON, R. K., NELSON, L. M. et al.: A comparison of dementia in Alzheimer's disease and multiple sclerosis. Arch. Neurol. **46**, 157-161 (1989)

FINGER, S.. Lesion momentum and behaviour (p. 135-169). In: Finger S (ed) Recovery from Brain Damage: Research and Theory, Plenum New York 1998

FINGER, S. STEIN, D. Brain Damage and Recovery: Research and Clinical Perspectives. Acad Press, Orlando, FL 1982

FINK, M.: EEG and human psychopharmacology. Ann. Rev. Pharmacol. **9**, 241-258 (1969)

FINK, M.: Why quantitative EEG? S. 643-644. In: Quantitative Analysis of the EEG. Matejcek, M., Schenk, K. (Hrsg.). Proc. of the 2nd symposium of the study groups for EEG-methodology. Jongny sur Vevey 1975

FINK, M.: Effects of acute and chronic inhalation of hashish, marijuana, and Delta-9-tetrahydrocannabinol on brain electrical activity in man: evidence for tissue tolerance. Ann. N. Y. Acad. Sci. **282**, 387-398 (1976)

FINK, M., IRWIN, P., WEINFELD, R. E. et al.: Blood levels and electroencephalographic effects of diazepam and bromazepam. Clin. Pharmacol. Ther. **20**, 184-191 (1977)

FINK, M., IRWIN, P, WEINHOLD, P.: EEG profile studies of clozapine in volunteers and psychiatric patients. Pharmakopsychiat. **12**, 184-190 (1979)

FIRNHABER, W., ARDJOMANDI, M. E.: Epileptische Psychosen ohne epileptische Anfälle. Der Nervenarzt **39**, 175-178 (1968)

FISCHGOLD, H., SCHWARTZ, A., DREYFUS-BRISAC, C.: Indicateur de l'etat de presence et traces electroencephalographiques dans le sommeil nembutalique. EEG Clin. Neurophysiol. **11**, 23-33 (1959)

FISH B.J.:Coping with progress: invited comment on topographic EEG mapping. A. J. EEG Technol. **27**, 246-246 (1987)

FISH, B.J.,PEDLEY, T.A. :The risk of quantitative topographic EEG mapping or "Neurometrics" in the diagnosis of psychiatric disorders : the cons.EEG Clin. Neurophysiol. **73**, 5-9 (1989)

FLECK, L.: Entstehung und Entwicklung einer wissenschaftlichen Tatsache Schwabe, Basel, 1935

FLOOD, R. A., SEAGER, C. P.: A retrospective examination of psychiatric case records of patients who subsequently committed suicide. Brit. J. Psychiat. **114**, 443-450 (1968)

FLOR-HENRY, P.: Psychiatric syndromes considered as manifestations of lateralized temporal-limbic dysfunction, S. 22-26. In: Surgical Approaches in Psychiatry. Laitinen, L. V., Livingston, K. E. (Hrsg.). MTP, St. Leonhard's Gate 1973

FLÜGEL, F., BENTE, D.: Das akinetisch-abulische Syndrom und seine Bedeutung für die pharmakologisch psychiatrische Forschung. Dtsch. med. Wschr. **81**, 2071-2074 (1956)

FLÜGEL, F., BENTE, D.: Klinische und electroencephalographische Erfahrungen mit einer neuen und zentral wirksamen anticholinergischen Droge (Bayer WH 4849). Med. exp. **5**, 215-233 (1961)

FODOR, J. A.: The Modularity of Mind - An Essay on Faculty Psychology. MIT Press, Cambridge MA, 1984

von FOERSTER, H.: Sicht und Einsicht. Versuch zu einer operativen Erkenntnistheorie, Vieweg, Braunschweig-Wiesbaden, 1975

FOLSTEIN, M,F., FOLSTEIN, S.E., Mc HUGH, P.R.: 'Mini-Mental State'. A practical method for grading the cognitive state of patients for the clinician. J Psychiat Res **12** 189-198 (1975)

FOSTER, N.L., CHASE,T.N., MANSI, J. et al. : Cortical abnormalities in Alzheimer's disease. Ann. Neurol **16**, 649-654 (1984)

FOLEY, J. M., WATSON, C. W., ADAMS, R. D.: Significance of the electroencephalographic changes in hepatic coma. Trans. Am. Neurol. Assoc. **75**, 161-164 (1950)

FOURNET, A., LANGTERNIER, M.: Constations electroencephalographiques dans 17 cas de Gayet-Wernicke. Rev. Neurol. **94**, 644-645 (1956)

FOX, N.C,,SCAHILL, R.I., CRUM, W.R. et al.: Correlation between rates of brain atrophy and cognitive decline in AD. Neurology **52**,1687-1689 (1999)

FOX, N.C., COUSENS, S., SCAHILL, R., et al.: Using serial registered nuclear magnetic resonance imaging to measure disease progression in Alzheimer's disease: power calculation and estimates of sample size to detect treatment effects. Arch. Neurol. **57** 339-344 (2000)

FOX, N.C., CRUMB,W.R.,SCAHILL, R.I.et al.: Imaging of onset and progression in Alzheimer's disease with voxel-compression mapping of serial magnetic resonance images. Lancet **358** 201-205 (2001)

FOX, N.C., SCHOTT, J.M., SCAHILL, R.I.: Measuring progression in Alzheimer's disease using serial MRI: 4DMRI (p.61-74) In: The Living Brain, Hyman B, Demonet JF, Christen Y(eds.) Springer, Berlin-Heidelberg-New York 2004

FRANZ, A .: Chemie für die Seele. http://zeit.de/2005/41P-Holsboer?page=all

FREAL, J. E., KRAFT, G. H., CORYELL, J. K.: Symptomatic fatigue in multiple sclerosis. Arch. Phys. Med. Rehabil. **65**, 135-138 (1984)

FREEDMAN, D. X.: The search: body, mind, and human purpose. Am. J. Psychiatry **149,** 858-866 (1992)

FREEMAN, W. J.: Mass Action in the Nervous System. Acad. Press, New York - San Francisco - London 1975

FREEMAN, W.J.: Chaos in psychiatry - Editorial. Biol. Psychiat. **31**, 1079-1081 (1992)

FREEMAN, W.J., SKARDA, C.H.: Mind/Brain Science. Neuroscience and philosophy of mind. In: John Searle and His Critics, LePore E, Gulick R (eds.) Cambridge. Blackwell 1991

FREY, T. S., SJÖGREN, H.: The electroencephalogram in elderly persons suffering from neuropsychiatric disorders. Acta psychiat. scand. **34**, 438-450 (1959)

FREYHAN, F. A.: Psychomotilität, extrapyramidale Syndrome und Wirkungsweisen neuroleptischer Therapien. Der Nervenarzt **28,** 504-509 (1957)

FROST, J. D.: Beta rhythms. Amer. J. EEG Technol. **3**, 71-76 (1963)

FUNDERBURK, W. H: Electroencephalographic studies in chronic alcoholism. EEG Clin. Neurophysiol. **1**, 369-370 (1949)

FUNKHOUSER, J. B., NAGLER, B., WALKE, N. D.: The electroencephalogram of chronic alcoholism. Southern Med. J. **46**, 423-428 (1953)

GABRIELLI, W. F., MEDNICK, S. A., VOLAVKA, J. et al.:Electroencephalograms in children of alcoholic fathers. Psychophysiology **19**, 404-407 (1982)

GABUZDA, D. H., LEVY, S. R., CHIAPPA, K. H.: Electroencephalography in AIDS and AIDS-related complex. Clin. EEG **19**, 1 - 16 (1988)

GACHES, J.: Etude statistique sur les traces < alpha largment developpe > en fonction de l'age. Press med. **68**, 1620-1622 (1960)

GALLAIS, P., COLLOMB, H., MILETTO, G. et al.: Confrontations des donnees de l'electroencephalogramme et de l'examen psychologique chez 113 jeunes soldats. EEG Clin. Neurophysiol., pp. 294-303, **Suppl. 6**, 1957

GARBER, H. J., WEILBURG, J. B., DUFFY, F. H., MANSCHRECK, T. C.: Clinical use of topographic brain electrical activity mapping in psychiatry. J. Clin. Psychiatry **50**, 205-211 (1989)

GARMEZY, N. Process and reactive schizophrenia: some conceptions and issues. Schizophrenia Bull. **1**, 30-74 (1970)

GARVEY, M.J., HWANG, S., TEUBNER-RHODES, D. et al.: Dextroamphetamin treatment in mania. J. Clin Psychiat **48**, 412-413 (1987)

GASSER, T., MÖCKS, J., LENARD, H. G. et al.: The EEG of mildly retarded children: developmental classifcatory and topographic aspects. EEG Clin. Neurophysiol. **55**, 131-144 (1983)

GASTAUT, H.: Correlations between the electroencephalographic and the psychometric variables. EEG Clin. Neurophysiol. **12**, 226-227 (1960)

GASTAUT, H., ROGER, J., ROGER, A.: Sur la signification de certaines fugues epileptiques. A propos d'une observation electro-clinique de etat de mal temporal. Rev. neurol. **94**, 298-301 (1956)

GASTAUT, H., DONGIER, M., JEST, C.: Confrontation entre les donnees de l'electroencephalogramme et des examens psychologiques chez 522 sujets repartis en trois groupes differentes, pp.283-293. In: Conditionnement et Reactivite en Electroencephalographie. EEG Clin. Neurophysiol., **Suppl. 6**, 1957

GASTAUT, H., DONGIER, S., DONGIER, M.: Electroencephalography and neuroses: study of 250 cases. EEG Clin. Neurophysiol. **12**, 233 (1960)

GAWIN, F., KLEBER, H.: Abstinence symptomatology and psychiatric diagnosis in cocaine abusers. Arch. Gen. Psychiat. **43**, 107-113 (1986)

GENGERELLI, J. A., PARKER, C. E.: Spectrographic analysis of electroencephalograms under conditions of alertness and relaxation. J. Psychol. **63**, 67-72 (1966)

GIANNITRAPANI, D., KAYTON, L.: Schizophrenia and EEG spectrum analysis. EEG Clin. Neurophysiol. **36**, 377-386 (1974)

GIAQUINTO, S., NOLFE, G.: The EEG in the normal elderly: a contribution to the interpretation of aging and dementia. EEG Clin. Neurophysiol. **63**, 540-546 (1986)

GIBBS, F. A.: Editor's corner: how to read EEG. Clin. EEG **13**, 67 - 70 (1982)

GIBBS, F. A., GIBBS, E. L.: Atlas of Electroencephalography, vol. 1, Methodology and Controls (2nd ed.). Addison-Wesley Publ. Comp., Reading, MA 1950

GIBBS, E. L., RICH, C. L., FOIS, A. et al.: Electroencephalographic study of mentally retarded persons. Amer. J. Ment. Defic. **65**, 236 - 247 (1960)

GIBBS, F. A., GIBBS, E. L.: Atlas of Eectroencephalography, vol.3, Neurological and Psychiatric Disorders. Addison-Wesley Publ. Comp., Reading, MA 1964

GIBBS, F. A., BECKA, D.: Reappraisal of the electroencephalogram in multiple sclerosis. Dis. Nerv. Syst. **29**, 589 - 592 (1968)

GLASER, G. A.: The problem of psychosis in psychomotor temporal lobe epileptics. Epilepsia **5**, 217 - 278 (1964)

GLASER, G. H., NEWMAN, R. J., SCHAFER, R.: Interictal psychosis in psychomotor-temporal lobe epilepsy. In: EEG and Behavior. Glaser, G. H. (eds.). Basic Books, New York & London 1963

GLAZE, D. G.: Drug effects, pp.489-512. In: Current Practice of Clinical Electroencephalography, 2nd ed. Daly, D. D., Pedley, T. A. (eds.). Raven Press, New York 1990

GLATZEL, J.: Die Abschaffung der Psychopathologie im Namen des Empirismus. Der Nervenarzt **61**, 276 - 280 (1990)

GLOOR, P., KALABAY, O., GIRARD, N.: The electroencephalogram in diffuse encephalopathies: electroencephalographic correlates of grey and white matter lesions. Brain **91**, 779-802 (1968)

GLOOR, P.: The EEG and differential diagnosis of epilepsy, pp. 9 – 21; In: Current Concepts in Clinical Neurophysiology. van Duijn, H., Donker D. N., van Huffelen, A. C. (eds.). N. V. Drukkerij Trio, Amsterdam 1977

GLUECK, B., STROBEL, C.: Biofeedback and meditation in the treatment of psychiatric illnesses. Compr. Psychiatry **16**, 303-321 (1975)

GODBOLT, A.K.,CIPOLOTTI, L. WATT, E. et al. The natural history of Alzheimer disease. Arch Neurol **61** 1743-1748 (2004)

GOLDSTEIN, K.: Der Aufbau des Organismus Nijhof, Den Haag, 1934

GOLDSTEIN, K.: The modification of behaviour consequent to cerebral lesions (p 586-610). Psychiat Quart **10**, 586-610 (1936)

GOLDSTEIN, K.: The two ways of adjustment of the organism to cerebral defects.
J Mt Sinai Hosp **9** 4-16 (1942)

GOLDSTEIN, L.: Time domain analysis of the EEG. The integration method, pp. 251 - 270. In: CEAN-Computerized EEG Analysis. Dolce, A., Künkel, H. (eds.). Fischer, Stuttgart 1975

GOLDSTEIN, L.: Is a man, a man, a man? (or: is an EEG, an EEG?). Some remarks on the homogeneity of "normal subjects". Pharmakopsychiatrie **12**, 74-82 (1979)

GOLDSTEIN, L.: Some EEG correlates of behavioral traits and states in humans. Res. Com. Psychol., Psychiat., Behav. **8**, (1983) No. 2

GOLDSTEIN, L., MURPHREE, H., SUGARMAN, A. et al.: Quantitative electroencephalographic analysis of naturally occurrlng (schizophrenic) and drug-induced psychotic states in human males. Clin. Pharmacol. Ther. **4**, 10-21 (1963)

GOLDSTEIN, L., SUGARMAN, A., STOLBERG, H. et al.:
Electro-cerebral activity in schizophrenics and non-psychotic subjects: quantitative EEG amplitude analysis. EEG Clin. Neurophysiol. **19**, 350-361 (1965)

GOLDSTEIN, L., SUGARMAN, A.: EEG correlates of psychopathology, p. 1-19. In: Neurobiological Aspects of Psychopathology. Zubin, J. and Shagass, C. (eds.). Gruner und Stratton, New York 1969

GOMEZ-ISLA, T., HOLISTER, R., WEST, H., et al.: Neuronal loss correlates with but exceeds neurofibrillary tangles in Alzheimer's disease. Ann Neurol **41** 17-24 (1997)

GONCALVES, S.I., de MUNCK J.C., POUWELS, P.J. W. et al.: Correlating the alpha rhythm to BOLD using simultaneous EEG/fMRI: Inter-subject variability. NeuroImage **30**, 203-213 (2006)

GONCHAROVA, I. I., BARLOW, J. S.: Changes in EEG mean frequency and spectral purity during spontaneous alpha blocking. EEG Clin. Neurophysiol. **76**, 197-204 (1990)

GOODIN, D. S., AMINOFF, M. J.: Does the interictal EEG have a role in the diagnosis of epilepsy? Lancet **1**, 837-839 (1984)

GOODWIN, B.: How the Leopard Changed It's Spots. Touchstone, New York, 1994

GOODWIN, F. K., MURPHY, D. L., BRODIE, H. K. et al.: L-dopa catecholamines and behavior: a clinical and biochemical study in depressed patients. Biol. Psychiat. **2**, 341-366 (1970)

GORDON, E. B.: Serial EEG studies in presenile dementia. Br. J. Psychiat. **114**, 779-780 (1968)

GORDON, E. B., SIM, M.: The EEG in the presenile dementia. J. Neurol. Neurosurg. Psychiat. **30**, 285-291 (1967)

GRASSBERGER, P., SCHREIBER, T., SCHAFFRATH, C. et al.: Nonlinear time sequence analysis. Int. J. Bifurcation Chaos. **1**, 521-547 (1991)

GREEN, J., REILLY, A., HAZELWOOD, C.: Observations of the electroencephalogram in seven centenarians. Clin. EEG **17**, 146-151 (1986)

GREENBERG, G.: After the decade of the brain: now what? Review of the New Phrenology: The Limits of Localizing Cognitive Processes in the Brain Behav. Proc. **58** 111-114 (2002)

GREENBLATT, M., HEALY, M. M., JONES, G. A.: Age and electroencephalographic abnormality in neuropsychiatric patients. Am. J. Psychiat. **101**, 82-90 (1944)

GREGORY, R. P., OATES, T., MERRY, R. T. G.: Electroencephalogram epileptiform abnormalities in candidates for aircrew training. EEG Clin. Neurophysiol. **86**, 75-77 (1993)

GREGSON, R.A., BRITTON, A.L., CAMPBELL, E.A. et al.: Comparisons of the nonlinear dynamics of electroencephalograms and various task loading conditions: a preliminary report. Biol Psychol. **31**, 173-191 (1990)

GRIESINGER, W.: Die Pathologie und Therapie der psychischen Krankheiten. Nachdruck der Ausgabe Stuttgart 1867. E. J. Bonset, Amsterdam, 1962

GRÜNEBERG, F., HELMCHEN, H.: Impulsiv-petit mal-status und paranoide Psychose. Der Nervenarzt **40**, 381 - 385 (1969)

GRUHLE, H. W.: Uber den Wahn bei Epilepsie. Z. ges. Neurol. Psychiat. **154**, 395-399 (1936)

GRUNZE, H., GOUZOULIS, E., WALDEN, J. et al.: Clozapin (Leponex) -EEG-Veränderungen und Provokation von Anfällen. EEG-Labor **14**, 167-175 (1992)

GSCHWEND, J., KARBOWSKI, K.: Der Normbereich des Alters-Elektroenzephalogramms. Schweiz. Arch. Neurol. Neurochir. Psychiat. **106**, 269-281 (1970)

GUNN, J.: Affective and suicidal symptoms in epileptic prisoners. Psychol Med. **3**, 108-114 (1973)

HAKEN, H: Synergetik. Springer, Berlin—Heidelberg - New York, 1982

HALL, R. C. W., GARDNER, E. R., STICKNEY, S. K. et al.: Physical illness manifesting as a psychiatric disease, II: analysis of a state hospital inpatient population Arch. Gen. Psychiatry **37**, 989-995 (1980)

HALLER, E., BINDER, R.L.: Clozapine and seizures. Am J. Psychiat. **147**, 1069-1071 (1990)
HARDING, G., JEAVONS, P. M., JENNER, F. A. et al.: The electroencephalogram in three cases of periodic psychosis. EEG Clin. Neurophysiol. **21**, 59 - 66 (1966)

HARRISON, A., NETCHINE, S., ROUZIERES, J.: Étude electroencephalographique de l'enfant d'intelligence superieure. Rev. neurol. **119**, 301-304 (1968)

HARTUNG, M. L., BENTE, D., SCHNEEWIND, K.: Vergleichende Untersuchungen über die Wirkung antidepressiver und neuroleptischer Pharmaka auf die Konzentrationsleistung. Arzneimittelforschg./Drug Res. **14**, 584-587 (1964)

HARVALD, B.: EEG in old age. Acta psychiat. scand. **33**, 193 - 196 (1958)

HASSENSTEIN, B.: Biologische Kybernetik Quelle & Meyer Heidelberg, 1973

HAWKES, C.H., PRESSCOT, R.J.: EEG variation in healthy subjects. EEG Clin. Neurophysiol. **34** 197-199 (1973)

HEAD, H.: The conception of nervous and mental energy - vigilance: a physiological state of the nervous system. Brit. J. Psychol. **14**, 126-147 (1923)

HEBERT, R., LEHMANN, D.: Theta bursts: an EEG pattern in normal subjects practising the transcendental meditation technique. EEG Clin. Neurophysiol. **42**, 397-405 (1977)

HEDENSTRÖM, J. v., SCHORSCH, G.: EEG-Befunde bei epileptischen Dämmer- und Verstimmungszuständen. Arch. Psychiat. ges. Neurol. **199**, 311-329 (1959)

HEGERL, U.,STEIN.,M., MULERT,C. et al. EEG vigilance differences between patients with borderline personality disorders, patients with obsessive-compulsive disorders and healthy controls. **258** 137-143 (2008)

AN DER HEIDEN, U., ROTH, G., SCHWEGLER, H.: Die Organisation der Organismen: Selbstherstellung und Selbsterhaltung. Funkt. Biol. Med. **5**, 330-346 (1985)

HEIMANN, H.: Prüfung psychotroper Substanzen am Menschen. Arzneimittelforsch./Drug Res. **24(9)**, 1341-1346 (1974)

HEIMANN, H.: Changes of psychophysiological reactivity in affective disorders Arch Psychiat Nervenkr **225** 223-231(1978)

HEIMANN, H.: Die Stimme der Psychiatrie im Konzert der medizinischen Fächer. Der Nervenarzt **62**, 391-397 (1991)

HEINEMANN, L. G.: Der mehrtägige Schlafentzug in der experimentellen Psychoseforschung: Psychoathologie und EEG. Arch. Psychiat. Z. ges. Neurol. **208**, 117-197 (1966)

HEINTEL, H.: Die 4/sec. EEG-Grundrhythmusvariante. Z. EEG-EMG **6**, 82-87 (1975)

HEISENBERG, W.: Physik und Philosophie, Hirzel Stuttgart, 1956

HELLER, G. L., KOOl, K. A.: The electroencephalogram in hepatolenticular degeneration (Wilson's disease). EEG Clin. Neurophysiol. **14**, 520 - 526 (1962)

HELMCHEN, H.: Bedingungskonstellationen paranoid-halluzinatorischer Syndrome. Monographien aus dem Gesamtgebiet der Neurologie und Psychiatrie, Heft 122. Springer, Berlin - Heidelberg - New York 1968

HELMCHEN, H.: Zerebrale Bedingungskonstellationen psychopathologischer Syndrome bei Epileptikern, S. 125-148. In: Entwicklungstendenzen biologischer Psychiatrie. Helmchen, H., Hippius, H. (Hrsg.). G.Thieme, Stuttgart 1975

HELMCHEN, H., KÜNKEL, H.: Der Einfluß von EEG-Verlaufsuntersuchungen unter psychiatrischer Pharmakotherapie auf die Prognostik von Psychosen. Arch. Psychiat. Z. Ges. Neurol. **205**, 1-18 (1964)

HELMCHEN, H., KÜNKEL, H.: The EEG in psychiatric pharmacology. EEG Clin. Neurophysiol. **20**, 276 (1966)

HELMCHEN, H., KANOWSKI, S., KÜNKEL, H.: Die Altersabhängigkeit der Lokalisation von EEG-Herden. Arch. Psychiat. Z. Ges. Neurol. **209**, 474-483 (1967)

HELMCHEN, H., HOFFMANN, I., KANOWSKI, S.: Dämmerzustand oder Status fokaler sensorischer Anfälle? Der Nervenarzt **40**, 389-392 (1969)

HELMCHEN, H., KANOWSKI, S.: EEG-Veränderungen unter Lithium-Therapie. Der Nervenarzt **42**, 144-148 (1971)

HERPER, C.G., KRIL, J.J., DALY, J.M.: Brain shrinkage in alcoholics is not caused by changes in hydration. A pathological study. J. Neurol. Neurosurg. Psychiat. **51** (1988) 124-127

HERRINGTON, R. N.: The personality in temporal lobe epilepsy, S. 70-76. In: Current Problems in Neuropsychiatry. Herrington, R. N. (eds.). Headly, Ashford 1969

HERRMANN, W. M.: Development and critical evaluation of an objective procedure for the electroencephalographic classification of psychotropic drugs, pp.249 - 351. In: Herrmann, W. M. (eds.). Electroencephalography in Drug Rescarch. G. Fischer, Stuttgart - New York 1982

HES, J.P.: Manic depressive psychosis. EEG Clin. Neurophysiol. 12, 193-195 (1960) HESS, R.: Das EEG bei endokrinen Stbrungen. In: Endokrinologische Psychiarrie. Bleuler, M. (Hrsg.). Thieme, Stuttgart 1954

HESS, W.R.: Diskussionsbemerkung. Schweiz. Arch. Neurol. Neurochir. Psychiat.76, 342 (1955)

HESS, W. R.: Psychologie in Biologischer Sicht. Thieme, Stuttgart 1962

HESS, R., SCOLLO-LAVIZZARI, G., WYSS, F. E.: Borderline cases of Petit mal Status. Europ. Neurol. 5, 137 - 154 (1971)

HEYCK, H., HESS, R.: Zur Narkolepsiefrage. Klinik und Elektroencephalogramm. Fortschr. Neurol. Psychiat. 22, 531-579 (1954)

HILL, D.: The EEG in episodic and psychopathic behaviour. EEG Clin. Neurophysiol. 4, 419-442 (1952)

HILL, D.: Das Elektroencephalogramm bei Schizophrenie, S. 30 - 47. In: Schizophrenie - Somatische Gesichtspunkte. Richter, D. (Hrsg.). G.Thieme, Stuttgart 1957

HILL, D., WATTERSON, D.: Electroencephalographic studies of psychopathic personalities. J. Neurol. Psychiat. 5, 47-65 (1942)

HILL, D., POND, D. A.: Reflections on 100 capital cases submitted to EEG. J. Ment. Sci. 98, 23-43 (1952)

HIRAI, T.: Electroencephalographic study on the Zen meditation (Zazen) - EEG changes during the concentrated relaxation.Folia psychiat. neurol. jap. 62, 76-105 (1960)

HJORTH, B.: Source derivation simplifies topographic EEG interpretation. Am. J. EEG Technol. 20, 121 - 132 (1990)

HOCHE, A.: Die Bedeutung der Symptomenkomplexe in der Psychiatrie. Z. ges. Neurol. Psychiat. 12, 540-551 (1912)

HOLDER, G. E., JONES, A., HARDING, G. F. A.: A quantitative investigation into the effects of carbamazepine, diazepam and quinalbarbitone on the EEG and visual evoked potential in man. EEG Clin. Neurophysiol. 39, 430 (1975)

HOLLISTER, L. E., OVERALL, J. E., JOHNSON, M. H. et al.: Amitriptyline alone and combined with perphenazine in newly admitted depressed patients. J. nerv. ment. Dis. 142, 460-469 (1966)

HOLLISTER, L. E., OVERALL, J. E., SHELTON, J. et al.: Drug therapy in depression. Amitriptyline, perphenazine and their combination in different syndromes. Arch. gen. Psychiat. 17, 486-493 (1967)

HOLLISTER, L., SHERWOOD, S., CAVASINO, A.: Marijuana and the human electroencephalogram. Pharmacol. Res. Comm. 2, 305 - 308 (1970)

v. HOLST, E., MITTELSTAEDT, H.: Das Reafferenzprinzip. Naturwiss. 20, 464-476 (1950)

HOPKINS, A., SCRAMBLER, G.: How doctors deal with epilepsy. Lancet 1, 183-186 (1977)

HUBBARD, O., SUNDE, D., GOLDENSOHN, E. S.: The EEG in centenerians. EEG Clin. Neurophysiol. **40,** 407-417 (1976)

HUBBARD, B.M., ANDERSSEN, J.M.: A quantitative study of cerebral atrophy in old age and in senile dementia. J Neurol. Sci. **50** 135-145 (1989)

HUBER, G.: Psychiatrie. Schattauer, Stuttgart-New York, 1974
HUBER, H.P.: Single-case analysis. Eur J Beh Anal Modif **2** 1-15 (1977)

HUBER, G., PENIN, H.: Klinisch-elektroenzephalographische Korrelationsuntersuchungen bei Schizophrenen. Fortschr. Neurol. Psychiat. **36**, 641-659 (1968)

HUGHES, J. R.: A statistical analysis on the location of EEG abnormalities. EEG Clin. Neurophysiol. **12**, 905-909 (1960)

HUGHES, J. R.: EEG in uremia. Am. J. EEG Technol. **24**, 1-10 (1984)

HUGHES J.R.: Coping with progress: invited comment on topographic EEG mapping. Am J. EEG Technol. **27**, 239-242 (1987)

HUGHES, J.R.: A review of the usefulness of the standard EEG in psychiatry
Clin. EEG **27** 35-39.(1996)

HUGHES, J. R., SCHREEDER, M. T.: EEG in dialysis encephalopathy. Neurology **30**, 1148-1154 (1980)

HUGHES, J. R., OLSON, S. F.: An investigation of eight different types of temporal lobe discharge. Epilepsia **22**, 421-435 (1981)

HUGHES, J.R., WEINER, R.D., Burchfield, L. et al. Auseinandersetzung mit neuen Entwicklungen- EEG Mapping. EEG-Labor **11**, 56-65 (1989)

HUGHES, J.R., JOHN, E.R.:Conventional and quantitative electroencephalography in psychiatry. J Neuropsychiatry Clin Neurosci **11**, 190-207 (1999)

HURST, L. A., MUNDY-CASTLE, A. C.: The electroencephalogram in manic-depressive psychosis. J. ment. Sci. **100**, 220-240 (1954)

HYMAN, B.T.: The Living Brain and Alzheimer's Disease (p. 25-30) In: The Living Brain and Alzheimer's Disease, Hyman BT, Demonet JF, Christen Y (eds.) Springer- Berlin-Heidelberg-New York, 2004

IGERT, C., LAIRY, G. C.: Interet pronostique de l'EEG au cours de l'evolution des schizophrenes. EEG Clin. Neurophysiol. **14**, 183-190 (1962)

IHL, R., MAURER, K., DIERKS, T. et al.: Effects of pyritinol on the distribution of electrical brain activity. Pharmacopsychiat. **21**, 343-345 (1988a)

IHL, R., DIERKS, T., MAURER, K., FRÖLICH, L.: Lokalisation kognitiver Störungen bei Demenz vom Alzheimer-Typ. Psycho **14**, 381 - 382 (1988b)

INGVAR, D.H., SJOLUND, B., ARDO, A.: Correlation between dominant EEG frequency, cerebral oxygen uptake and blood flow. EEG Clin. Neurophysiol **41**, 405–420 (1976)

ISBELL, H, EISENMAN, H. J., WIKLER, A. et al.: The effect of single doses of 6-dimethylamino-4,4-diphenyl-3-heptanone (amidone, methadon or "10820") on human subjects. J. Pharmacol. exp. Ther. **92**, 83-89 (1948)

ISERMANN, H.: Über die Bedeutung des EEG bei Schizophrenien. Dtsch. med. Wschr. **98**, 1074-1076 (1973)

ISERMANN, H., HAUPT, R.: Auffällige EEG-Veränderungen unter Clozapin-Behandlung bei paranoid-halluzinatorischen Psychosen. Der Nervenarzt **47**, 268 (1976)

ITIL, T. M.: Electroencephalography and pharmacopsychiatry, S. 163 - 194. In: Modern Problems of Pharmacopsychiatry. Freyhan, F. A. et al. (ed.), Vol. 1. Karger, Basel - New York 1968

ITIL, T. M.: Quantitative pharmaco-electroencephalography. Use of computerized cerebral biopotentials in psychotropic drug research, pp. 43-75. In: Psychotropic Drugs and the Human EEG. Itil, T. M. (eds.). Karger, Basel, 1974

ITIL, T. M.: Qualitative and quantitative EEG findings in schizophrenia. Schiz. Bull. **3**, 61-78 (1977)

ITIL, T. M.: The significance of quantitative pharmaco-EEG in the discovery and classification of psychotropic drugs, S.131-157. In: Herrmann, W. M. (ed.). Electroencephalography in Drug Research. G.Fischer, Stuttgart - New York 1982

ITIL, T., KESKINER, A., FINK, M.: Therapeutic studies in "therapy resistant" schizophrenic patients. Compr. Psychiatry **7**, 488-493 (1966)

ITIL, T. M., FINK, M.: EEG and behavioral aspects of the interaction of anticholinergic hallucinogens with centrally active compounds. Progr. Brain Res. **28**, 149 - 168 (1968)

ITIL, T., AKPINAR, S.: Lithium effect on human electroencephalogram. Clin. EEG **2**, 89 - 102 (1971)

ITIL, T. M., ULETT, G., HSU, W. et al.: The effect of smoking withdrawal on quantitatively analyzed EEG. Clin. EEG **2**, 44-51 (1971)

ITIL, T., SALETU, B., DAVIS, S.: EEG findings in chronic schizophrenics basod on digital computer period analysis. and analog power spectra. Biol. Psyciat. **5**, 1-13 (1972)

ITIL,T.M., POVLAN, N. HSU, W.: Clinical and EEG effects of GB-94, a tetracyclic antidepressant. Curr Ther Res **14**, 395-413 (1972b)

ITIL, T., MARASA, J., SALETU, B. et al.: Computerized EEG: predictor of outcome in schizophrenia. J.Nerv. Ment Dis. **160**, 188-203 (1975)

ITIL, T. M., SOLDATOS, C.: Epileptogenic side effects of psychotropic drugs: practical recommendations. J. Am. Med. Ass. **244**, 1460-1463 (1980)

JACK, C.R. Jr. : Validating MRI measures of disease stage and progression in Alzheimer's disease (p. 75-83) In: The Living Brain and Alzheimer's Disease, Hyman BT, Demonet JF, Christen Y (eds.) Springer Berlin-Heidelberg-New York, 2004

JACKEL, R.A., HARNER, R.N.: Computed EEG topography in acute stroke Neurophysiol Clin **19**, 185-197 (1989)

JACKSON, J.H.: On affections of speech from disease of the brain. Brain **12**, 323-356 (1879)

JACKSON, J.H.: Croonian Lectures on the evolution and dissolution of the nervous system. The Lancet, March 29, 1884, übersetzt und eingeleitet von O. Sittig, Karger, Berlin. 1927

JACKSON, J.H.: Remarks on evolution and dissolution on the nervous system. J. ment. sci. **23**, 25-48 (1887)

JACKSON, J.H.: The factors of mental insanity. Med Press and Circ **II**: 615-625, (1894)

JANDL, E.: Die Bibliothek Gedichte, H. Luchterhand , Darmstadt, 1978

JANOWSKY, D., EL-YOUSEF, M., DAVIS, J.M.: Provocation of schizophrenic symptoms by intravenous administration of methylphenidate Arch. Gen. Psychiat. **28** 185-191 (1973)

JACOB, M.D., GLOOR, P., ELWAN, O.H. et al.: Electroencephalographic changes in chronic renal failure. Neurology **15**, 419-429 (1965)

JANATI, A., KIDAWI, S., NOWACK, W. J.: Episodic anterior drowsy theta in adults. Clin. EEG **17**, 135-138 (1986)

JANKE, W., EHRHARDT, K.J., MÜNCH, U.: Behavioral effects of carbamazepin after single and repeated administration in emotionally labile subjects. Neuropsychobiology **10**, 217-227 (1983)

JANZ, D.: Die Epilepsien. G.Thieme, Stuttgart 1969

JANZARIK, W.: Der Wahn schizophrener Prägung in den psychotischen Episoden der Epileptiker und die schizophrene Wahnwahrnehmung. Fortschr. Neurol. Psychiat. **23**, 533-545 (1955)

JANZARIK, W.: Dynamische Grundkonstellationen in endogenen Psychosen. Springer, Berlin -Göttingen- Heidelberg 1959

JANZEN, R., MÜLLER, E.: Über Indikation, Möglichkeiten und Grenzen der hirnelektrischen Untersuchung beim gedeckten Schädel-Hirntrauma. Mschr. Unfallheilk. **58**, 225-228 (1955)

JASPER, H. H., FITZPATRICK, C. A., SOLOMON, P.: Analogies and opposites in schizophrenia and epilepsy. Amer. J. Psychiat. **95**, 835-851 (1939)

JASPER, H. H., VAN BUREN, J.: Interrelationship between cortex and subcortical structures: clinical electroencephalographic studies. EEG clin. Neurophysiol. **suppl. 4**, 168-202 (1953)

JASPERS, K.: Allgemeine Psychopathologie, 4. Aufl. Springer, Berlin-Heidelberg, 1946

JELLES, J., van BIRGELEN, J.H., SLAETS, J.P.J. et al.: Decrease of nonlinear structure in the EEG of Alzheimer's patients, compared to healthy control subjects. Clin. Neurophysiol. **110**, 1159-1167 (1999)

JENNEKENS-SCHINKEL, A., LABOYRIE, P. M., LANSER, J. B. K. et al.: Cognition in patients with multiple sclerosis. J. Neurol. Sci. **99**, 229 - 247 (1990)

JEONG, J.: EEG dynamics in patients with Alzheimer's disease. Clin Neurophysiol. **115**, 1490-1505 (2004)

JEONG, J., CHAE, J.-H., KIM, S. Y. et al.: Non-linear dynamic analysis of the EEG in patients with Alzheimer's disease and vascular dementia. J. Clin. Neurophysiol. 18, 58-67 (2001)

JINDROVA, M., ROTH, B., STEIN, J. et al: Etudes electroencephalographiques des tumeurs suprasellaires comprimant ou infiltrant la region mesodiencephalique, avec consideration speciale des rhythmes de sommeil - tschechisch mit franz. Zus. Csl. Neurol. **23**, 79-89 (1960)

JOHN, E.R.: The role of quantitative EEG topographic mapping or "Neurometrics" in the diagnosis of psychiatric and neurological disorders: the pros. EEG Clin. Neurophysiol. **73** 2-4 (1989)

JOHN, E.R.: Principles of neurometrics. Am. J. EEG Technol. **30**, 251-266 (1990)

JOHN, E.R., PRICHEP, L.S., EASTON, P.: Normative data banks and Neurometrics: basic concepts, methods and results of norm constructions (pp 449-495) In: Remond A (ed). Handbook of EEG and Clinical Neurophysiology, vol III, Amsterdam, Elsevier, 1987

JOHN, E. R., PRITCHEP, L. S., FRIDMAN, J. et al.: Neurometrics: computer-assisted differential diagnosis of brain dysfunctions. Science **239**, 162-169 (1988)

JOHN, E.R., PRICHEP, L.S.: Neurometric studies of aging and cognitive impairment (pp. 545-555). In: Uylings HB et al. (eds) Progr In Brain Res: The Prefrontal Cortex, its Structure, Function and Pathology Elsevier, Amsterdam, 1990

JOHN, E. R., PRITCHEP, L. S., ALMAS, M.: Toward a quantitative electrophysiological classification system for psychiatry, pp.401-406. In: Biological Psychiatry, vol.2, Racagni G. et al. (eds.). Elsevier Science Publ. 1991

JOHN, E.R., PRICHEP,L.S., ALMAS, M.: Subtyping of psychiatric patients by cluster analysis of QEEG Brain Topogr. **4** 321-326 (1992)

JOHNSON, G. M., MACCARIO, M., GERSHON, S. et al.: The effects of lithium on electroencephalogram, behavior and serum electrolytes. J. Nerv. and Ment. Dis. **151**, 273-289 (1970)

JONAS, H.: The Phenomenon of Life: Towards a Philosophical Biology Univ of Chicago Press, Chicago, 1980

JONES, R., STONE, G.: Psychological studies of marijuana and alcohol in man. Psychopharmacologia (Berlin) **18**,108-117 (1970)

JONES, F. W., HOLMES, D. S.: Alcoholism, alpha production and biofeedback. J. consult. clin. Psychol. **44,** 224-228 (1976)

JORDAN, S.E., NOWACKI, R., NUWER,.R.: Computerized electroencephalography in the evaluation of early dementia Brain Topogr 1 (1989) 271-282

JUDD, L.L., HUBBARD, D.S., JANOWSKY, L.Y. et al.: The effect of lithium carbonate on the cognitive function of normal subjects. Arch. Gen. Psychiat. **34**, 355-357 (1977)

JUNG, R.: Die praktische Anwendung des Elektroencephalogramms in Neurologie und Psychiatrie. Med. Klin. **45**, 257-266 u. 289 - 295 (1950)

JUNG, R.: Neurophysiologische Untersuchungsmethoden, S.1206-1420. In: Handbuch der inneren Medizin, Bd. V/1, Bergmann, G. v., Frey, W., Schwiegk, H. (Hrsg.). Springer, Berlin-Göttingen-Heidelberg, 1953

JUNG, R.: Neurophysiologie und Psychiatrie, S.325 - 928. In: Psychiatrie der Gegenwart, Bd. IA. Gruhle, H. W., Jung, R., Mayer-Gross, W. (Hrsg.). Springer, Berlin-Heidelberg—New York 1967

JURKO, M.F., COLLE, G.M.: An EEG-psychological study of a family. Clin. EEG **13**, 108-115 (1982)

JUSTISS, W. A.: The electroencephalogram of the frontal lobes and abstract behavior in old age, pp.566-574. In: Medical and Clinical Aspects of Aging. Blumenthal, H.T. (ed.). Columbia Univ. Press, New York-London, 1969

KAISER, D.A.: QEEG: state of the art, or state of confusion. J. Neurotherapie **4**, 57-75 (2001)

KANT, I.: Kritik der Urteilskraft. Werksausgabe, Vol. 10, Suhrkamp, Frankfurt a.M. !977 (reprint)

KANOWSKI, S.: Klinische und electroencephalographische Untersuchungen zur basalen Dysrhythmie. Inaug.-Diss., Freie Univ. Berlin, 1966

KAPLAN, A., ROESCHKE, J. DARKHOVSKY, B. et al.: Macrosteructural EEG characterization based on nonparametric change point segmentation: application to sleep analysis. J. Neurosci. Meth. **106**, 81-90 (2001)

KARBOWSKI, K.: Sixty years of clinical electroencephalography. Eur. Neurol. **30**, 170 -175 (1990)

KARNAZE, D. S., BICKFORD, R. G.: Triphasic waves: a reassessment of their significance. EEG Clin. Neurophysiol. **57**, 193-198 (1984)

KASAMATSU, A., OKUMA, T., TAKENAKA, S. et al: The EEG of „Zen" and „Yoga" practitioners. EEG Clin. Neurophysiol., **Suppl. 9**, 51 - 52 (1957)

KASAMATSU, A., HIRAI, T. : An electroencephalographic study on the Zen meditation (Zazen). Folia Psychiat. Neurol. Jap. **20**, 315-336 (1966)

KASPER, S., KICK, H.: Occipital betonte Asymmetrie im EEG schizophrener Patienten. Der Nervenarzt **58**, 369-373 (1987)

KATZ, R.I., HOROWITZ, G. R.: Electroencephalogram in the septuagenerian: studies in a normal geriatric population. J Amer. Geriat. Soc. **30**, 273-275 (1982)

KELLAWAY, P.: Diskussionsbemerkung. EEG Clin. Neurophysiol. **10**, 767 (1958)

KELLAWAY, P.: An orderly approach to visual analysis: parameters of the normal EEG in adults and children, pp.69-147. In: Current Practice of Clinical Electroencephalography.

KELLAWAY, P., FOX, B. J.: Electroencephalographic diagnosis of cerebral pathology in infants during sleep. J.Pediatr. **41**, 262-287 (1952)

KEMALI, D., VACCA, L., MARCIANO, F. et al.:CEEG findings in schizophrenics, depressives, obsessives, heroin addicts and normals.. Adv. Biol. Psychiatr. **6**, 17-28 (1981)

KENNARD, M.: Diskussionsbemerkung, (S.440). In Hill, D.: EEG in episodic psychotic and psychopathic behaviour. EEG clin. Neurophysiol. **4,** 419-442 (1952)

KETZ, E.: Wirkung von Antikonvulsiva und psychotropen Drogen auf das EEG. Z. EEG-EMG **5**, 99-106 (1974)

KIEFER, M., EYMANN, R., STEUDEL, W.I.: LOVA-Hydrozephalus. Eine neue Entität des chronischen Hydrozephalus Nervenarzt **73** 972-981 (2002)

KLIESER, E.: Psychopharmakologische Differentialtherapie endogener Psychosen Thieme, Stuttgart-New York, 1990

KNAPP, M.J., KNOPMAN, D.S., SOLOMON, P.R. et al.: A 30-week randomized controlled trial of high-dose tacrine in patients with Alzheimer's disease. J. Am. Med. Assoc. **271,** 985-991 (1994)

KLASS, D., W., DALY, D.D.: (eds.) Klinische Elektroenzephalographie, G. Fischer Suttgart-New York, 1984

KNOPMAN, D.S.: The initial recognition and diagnosis of dementia. Am. J. Med. **104**, 2S-12 (1998)

KNORRING, L.von, PERRIS, C., GOLDSTEIN, L. et al.: Intercorrelation between different computer-based measures of the EEG alpha amplitude and its variability over time and their validity in differentiating healthy volunteers from depressed patients. Adv. Biol. Psychiat. **13**, 172-181 (1983)

KNOTT, V., BAKISH, D., LUSK, S. et al. Quantitative EEG correlates of panic disorder. Psychiat. Res. **68**,310-339 (1996)

KOEHLER, G. K.: Epileptische Psychosen. Fortschr. Neurol. Psychiat, **43**, 99-153 (1975)

KOEHLER, G. K., PETZOLD, J.: Klinisch-elektroenzephalographische Verlaufsuntersuchung einer Psychose nach Jauchgrubengasvergiftung. Nervenarzt **11**, 607-612 (1974)

KOEHLER, K., SASS, H.: Deutsche Bearbeitung und Einführung in das Diagnostic and Statistical Manual of Mental Disorders (DSM III), 3. Aufl. Beltz, Weinheim 1984

KOOI, K. A., GÜVENER, A. M., TUPPER, C. J. et a.: Electroencephalographic patterns of the temporal region in normal adults. Neurology **14**,1029-1035 (1964)

KOLARIK, J., SEVCIK, M., DUBANSKY, B. et al.: Comparison of EEG desynchronisation and the optical hallucinogenic effect after psilocybin in organic brain lesions. Activ. Nerv. Suppl. (Prag) **8**, 350 (1966)

KOREIN, J., MUSACCHIO, J. M.: LSD and focal cerebral lesions. Neurology **18**, 147 - 152 (1968)

KOSHINO, Y., MURATA, I., MURATA,T. et al.: Frontal intermittent delta activity in schizophrenic patients receiving antipsychotic drugs. Clin. EEG **24**,13-18 (1993)

KOUFEN, H., BECKER, W.: Klinische und EEG-Untersuchungen zum Problem der sogenannten Alkoholepilepsie. Der Nervenarzt **51**,100 -105 (1980)

KOUFEN, H., GAST, C.: Zur Frage der Alters- und Diagnoseabhängigkeit der Links-Lateralisation und Lokalisation von EEG-Herden. Arch. Psychiat. Nervenkr. **229**, 227-237 (1981)

KOUKKOU-LEHMANN, M.: Hirnmechanismen normalen und schizophrenen Denkens. Springer, Berlin etc. 1987

KOUKKOU, M., ANGST, J., ZIMMER, D.: Paroxysmal EEG activity and psychopathology during the treatment with clozapine. Pharmakopsychiat. **12**, 173-183 (1979)

KOUKKOU, M., LEHMANN, D., WACKERMANN, J. et al.: Dimensional complexity of EEG brain mechanism in untreated schizophrenia. Biol. Psychiat. **33**, 397-407 (1993)

KOYAMA, K., HIRASAWA,H., OKUBO,Y. et al.: Quantitative EEG correlates of normal aging in the elderly. Clin EEG **28**,160-165 (1997)

KRAEPELIN, E.: Lehrbuch der Psychiatrie, 5. Aufl. Barth, Leipzig, 1896

KRAEPELIN, E.: Zur Epilepsiefrage. Z. Neurol. **52**, 107 - 116 (1919)

KRAEPELIN, E. Die Erscheinungsformen des Irreseins. Z. ges. Neurol. Psychiat. **62** *1-29 (1920)*

KRANKENHAGEN, B., PENIN, H., ZEH, W.: Prä- und postoperative EEG-Untersuchungen bei Patienten mit Cushing-Syndrom. EEG-EMG **1**, 14-19 (1970)

KRANKENHAGEN, B., KÖHLER, G.-K.: Die Alzheimersche Erkrankung. Fortschr. Neurol. Psychiat. **41**, 141-165 (1973)

KRETSCHMER, E.: Über psychogene Wahnbildung bei traumatischer Hirnschwäche. Z. ges. Neurol. Psychiat. **45**, 272-300 (1919)

KRAUSS, G. L., FISHER, R S.: Alcohol and the EEG. Am. J. EEG Technol. **32**, 118-126 (1992)

KUBICKI, S., HÖLLER, L., PASTELAK-PRICE, C.: Subvigil beta activity: a study of fast EEG patterns in drowsiness. Am. J. EEG Technol. **27**, 15-31 (1987)

KÜNKEL, H.: Quantitative EEG-Analyse und schizophrene Psychosen, p.41-50. In: Entwicklungstendenzen der Biologischen Psychiatrie. HELMCHEN, H. & HIPPIUS, H. (Hrsg.). G.Thieme, Stuttgart, 1975

KüNKEL, H.: Historical review of principal methods, p.9-25. In: EEG Informatics: A Didactic Review of Methods and Applications of EEG Data Processing. Rémond, A. (ed.). Elsevier/North-Holland Biomedical Press, 1977

KÜNKEL, H.: Elektroenzephalographie und Psychiatrie, S. 115-196.
In: Psychiatrie der Gegenwart, Bd. 1. Kisker, K. P., Meyer, J. E., Müller, C., Strömgren, E. (Hrsg.). Springer, Berlin-Heidelberg-New York, 1980

KUGLER, J., LORENZONI, E., SPATZ, R. et al.: Drug-induced paroxysmal EEG activities. Pharmacopsychiat. **12**, 165 - 172 (1979)

KUGLER, J.: Elektroenzephalographie in Klinik und Praxis. Thieme, Stuttgart-New York, 1981

KUHLO, W.: The beta rhythm, 6A-29 - 6A-45. In: Handbook of Electroencephalography and Clinical. Neurophysiology, vol.6. The Normal EEG Throughout Life, Part. A. Rémond, A. (ed.). Elsevier, Amsterdam, 1976

KUHLO, W., LEHMANN, D.: Das Einschlaferlebnis und seine neurophysiologischen Korrelate. Arch. Psychiat. Nervenkr. **205**, 687-716 (1964)

KUHLO, W., HEINTEL, H., VOGEL, F.: The 4-5 c/sec rhythm. EEG. Clin. Neurophysiol. **26**, 613-618 (1969)

KUHN, T. S.: The Structure of Scientific Revolution. Univ. of Chicago Press, Chicago, (1962)

KUROIWA, Y., CELESIA, G. G.: Clinical significance of periodic EEG patterns. Arch. Neurol. **37**, 15-19 (1980)

KURZWEIL, R.: Homo Sapiens – Leben im 21. Jahrhundert; Kiepenheuer &Witsch, 1999

KURZWEIL, R.: The singularity is near: When humans transcend biology; Penguin, 2009

Kurtzke JF: Rating neurologic impairment in multiple sclerosis. Neurology 33 1444-1452 (1983)

LADER, M.: The Psychophysiology of Mental Illness. Routlege & Kegan Paul, London-Boston, 1975

LAIRY, G. C.: .The Normal EEG Throughout Life (p 543 cf), Vol 6. In: Handbook of Electroencephalography and Clinical Neurophysiology, Elsevier, Amsterdam, 1976

LAIRY, G.C.: The EEG of the waking adult (preface) 6A-3 – 6-A5. In: Handbook of Electroencephalography and Clinical. Neurophysiology, vol.6. The Normal EEG Throughout Life, Part A. Remond, A. (ed.). Elsevier, Amsterdam, 1978

LAIRY, G.C., FISCHGOLD, H.: Reactions electroencephalographiques diffuses aux stimulations psychosensorielles interet clinique. EEG Clin. Neurophysiol. **5**, 343-362 (1953)

LAIRY, G.C., BENBANASTE, J.V.: Some EEG aspects of subjective posttraumatic syndromes. EEG Clin. Neurophysiol. **6**, 162 (1954)

LAIRY, G.C., DELL, P.: La regulation de l'activite corticale: aspects psychophysiologiques et psychopathologiques, pp. 341-390. EEG Clin. Neurophysiol., **Suppl. 6**, 1957

LAIRY, G.C., NETCHINE, S.: Signification psychologique et clinique de l'organisation spatiale de l'EEG chez l'enfant. Rev. neurol. **102**, 380-388 (1960)

LANDOLT, H.: Über Verstimmungen, Dämmerzustände und schizophrene Zustandsbilder bei Epilepsie. Schweiz. Arch. Neurol. Neurochir. Psychiat. **76**, 313 - 321 (1955)

LANDOLT, H.: Elektroenzephalographische Untersuchungen bei nicht katatonen Schizophrenien. Schweiz. Z. f. Psychol. **16**, 26-30 (1957)

LANDOLT, H.: Die Temporallappenepilepsie und ihre Psychopathologie. Karger, Basel, 1960

LANDOLT, H.: Psychische Störungen bei Epilepsie. Klinische und elektroenzephalographische Untersuchungen. Dtsch. med. Wschr. **87**, 446-452 (1961)

LANDOLT, H.: Die Dämmer- und Verstimmungszustände bei Epilepsie und ihre Elektroencephalographie. Dtsch. Z. Nervenheilk. **185**, 411-430 (1963)

LA VECK, G. D., DE LA CRUZ, F.: Electroencephalographic and etiologic findings in mental retardation. Pediatrics **31**, 478-485 (1963)

LAZARUS, L.W., NEWTON, N., COHLER, B. et al.: Frequency and presentation of depressive syndromes in patients with primary degenerative dementia. Am. J. Psychiat. **144**, 41-45 (1987)

LAZLO, E.: Introduction to Systems Philosophy. Gordon & Breach, New York-London-Paris, 1972

LECHNER, H.: Zur Objektivierbarkeit der Commotio cerebri. Wiener klin. Wschr. **38/39**, 749-755 (1957)

LEHMANN, E.I., HOPES, H.: Effects of imipramine and lofepramine on EEG and their dependence on relative alpha-intensity. Pharmakopsychiatrie **11**, 128-135 (1978)

LEHRER, P.M., SCHOICKET, S., CARRINGTON, P. et al.: Psychophysiological and cognitive responses to stressful stimuli in subjects practicing progressive relaxation and clinically standardized meditation. Beh. Res. Ther. **18**, 293-303 (1980)

LENNOX, W. G., GIBBS, E. L., GIBBS, F. A.: Inheritance of cerebral dysrhythmia and epilepsy. Arch. Neurol. Psychiat. (Chic.) **44**, 1155-1183 (1940)

LETEMENDIA, F., PAMPIGLIONE, G.: Clinical and EEG observations in Alzheimer's disease. J. Neurol. Neurosurg. Psychiat. **21**,167-172 (1958)

LEUCHTER, A.F., SPAR, J.E., WALTER, D.O. et al.: Electroencephalographic spectra and coherence in the diagnosis of Alzheimer's type and multiinfarct dementia. A pilot study. Arch.Gen.Psychiatry **44**, 993-998 (1987)

LEIBNIZ, G.W. F.: (1714) Monadologie, Reclam Stuttgart, 1998

LEWIN, R.: Is your brain really necessary? Science **210**, 1332-1334 (1980)

LIBERSON, W.T.: Functional electroencephalography in mental disorders. Dis. Nerv. Syst. **5**, 357-364 (1944)

LIBERSON, W.T.: Problems of sleep and mental disease. Digest of Neurol. Psychiat. **13**, 93-108 (1945)

LIBERSON, W. T.: Electroencephalographie differentielle: principes, methodes, perspectives. Biotypologie **17**, 1-17 (1956)

LIBERSON, W. T.: Diskussionsbemerkung. Am. J. Psychiat. **115**, 54 (1958)

LIBERSON, W.T., LIBERSON, C.W.: EEG records, reaction times, eye movements, respiration and mental content during drowsiness, pp. 295-302. In: Recent Advances in Biological Psychiatry, vol. Vlll. Wortis, J. (ed.). Plenum Press, New York, 1965

LIENERT, G.A.: Verteilungsfreie Methoden in der Biostatistik. Bd. I (S.538 ff.) Hain, Meisenheim, 1973

LINN, R.T., WOLF,. P. A., BACHMANN, D.L. et al.: The „preclinical phase" of probable Alzheimer's disease: a 18 years prospective study of the Framington cohort. Arch. Neurol. **52**, 485-490 F(1995)

LIFSHITZ, K., GRADIJAN, J.: Relationship between measures of the coefficient of variation of the mean absolute EEG voltage and spectral intensities in schizophrenic and control subjects. Biol. Psychiat. **5**, 149-163 (1972)

LINDSLEY, D.B.: Psychological phenomena and the electroencephalogram. EEG Clin. Neurophysiol. **4**, 443-456 (1952)

LINDSLEY, D.B.: Attention, consciousness, sleep and wakefulness, pp.1553-1593. In: Handbook of Physiology - Neurophysiology. American Physiological Soc., Washington D.C., 1960

LINDSLEY, D.B., HENRY, C.E.: The effect of drugs on behavior and the electroencephalograms of children with behavior disorders. Psychosom. Med. **4**, 140 - 149 (1942)

LIPMAN, J.J., HUGHES, J.R.: Rhythmic mid-temporal discharges. An electro-clinical study. EEG Clin. Neurophysiol. **27,** 43 - 47 (1969)

LISHMAN, W.A., RON, M., ACKER, W.: Computed tomography of the brain and psychometric assessment of alcoholic patients – a British study. Psychopharmacol. Alcohol 23 33-41 (1980)

LITTLE, S. C., Mc AVOY, M.: Electroencephalographic studies in alcoholism. Quart. J. Stud. Alcohol. **13**, 9-15 (1952)

LIUKKONEN, J., KOPONEN, H.J., NOUSIAINEN, U.: Clinical picture and long-term course of epileptic seizures that occur during clozapine treatment. Psychiatry Res. **44**, 107–112 (1992)

LIVANOV, M.N.: Spatial Organization of Cerebral Processes Wiley, New York, 1977

LOEW, R. Philosophie des Lebendigen. Der Begriff des Organischen bei Kant, sein Grund und seine Aktualität. Suhrkamp, Frankfurt/M, 1980

LLOPIS, B.: Das allen Psychosen gemeinsame Axialsyndrom. Fortschr. Neurol. Psychiat. **28**, 106-129 (1960)

LOGSDAIL, S. ., TOONE, B.K.: Post-ictal psychoses. A clinical and phenomenological description. Brit. J. Psychiatry **152**, 246 - 252 (1988)

LONG, M. T., JOHNSON, L. C.: Fourteen-and six-per-second positive spikes in a nonclinical male population. Neurology (Minneap.) **18**, 714-716 (1968)

LOOMIS, A.L., HARVEY, E.N., HOBART, G.A.: Cerebral states during sleep as studied by human brain potentials. J. exp. Psychol. **21**, 127-144 (1937)

LOOMIS, A. L., HARVEY, E. N., HOBART, G. A.: Distribution of disturbance patterns in the human EEG with special reference to sleep. J. Neurophysiol. **1**, 413 - 430 (1938)

LOPES DA SILVA, F. H.: Neural mechanisms underlying brain waves: from neural membranes to networks. EEG Clin. Neurophysiol. **79**, 81 - 93 (1991)

LOPES DA SILVA, F. H., LIERTOP, T. H. M. T., van SCHRIJER, C. F.: Organization of the thalamic and cortical alpha rhythms: spectra and coherences. EEG Clin. Neurophysiol. **35**, 627 - 639 (1973)

LOPES DA SILVA, F. H., VAN ROTTERDAM, A., BARTS, P. et al.: Models of neuronal populations: the basic mechanisms of rhythmicity, pp.281 -308. In: Perspectives of Brain Research. Corner M. A., Swaab D. F. (eds.) series: Progress in Brain Research, 1976

LORBER, J.: Is your brain really necessary? Nursing Mirror **152** (1981) 29-30

LORENTZ DE HAAS, A. M., MAGNUS, O.: Clinical and electroencephalographic fndings in epileptic patients with episodic mental disorders, pp.134-167. In: Lectures in Epilepsy. Lorentz de Haas, A. M. (ed.). Elsevier, Amsterdam, 1958

LORENZ, K.: Gestaltwahrnehmung als Quelle wissenschaftlicher Erkenntnis. Z. exp. angew. Psychol. **6**, 118 (1959)

LORENZONI, E.: Das EEG im posttraumatischen Koma. Fortschr. Neurol. Psychiat. **43**, 155-191 (1975)

LOW, M. D.: Psychology, psychophysiology, and the EEG, pp.541-548. In: Electroencephalography. Niedermeyer, E., Lopes da Silva, F. (eds.). Urban und Schwarzenberg, Baltimore-Munich ,1987

LU, S.T., KAJOLA M., JOUTSINIEMI, S. L.: Generator sites of spontaneous MEG activity during sleep. EEG Clin. Neurophysiol. **82,** 182-196 (1992)

LUGARESI, E., PAZZAGLIA, P., TASSINARI, C.A.: Differentiation of absence status and temporal lobe status. Epilepsia **12**, 77-87 (1971)

LUTZENBERGER, W., ELBERT,T., BIRBAUMER, N. et al.: The scalp distribution of the fractal dimension of the EEG and ist variation with mental tasks. Brain Topogr. **5**, 27-34 (1992 a)

LUTZENBERGER, W., BIRBAUMER, N., FLOR, H. et al.: Dimensional analysis of the human EEG and intelligence. Neurosci. Lett. **143**, 10-14 (1992 b)

MAAS, J.W., KATZ, M.M.: Neurobiology and psychopathological states: are we looking in the right place? Biol. Psychiatry **31**, 757-758 (1992)

MACKWORTH, N.H.: The breakdown of vigilance during prolonged visual search. Quart. J exp Psycho **1**, 6-21(1948)

MAKEIG, S., INLOW, M.: Lapses in alertness; coherence of fluctuations in performance and EEG spectrum. EEG Clin, Neurophysiol, **86** (1993) 23-35

MANN, K., SCHROTH, G., STETTER, F. et al.: Thiamine deficiency and brain atrophy in alcoholic patients. Der Nervenarzt **62**, 177-181 (1991)

MANN, K, BARTELS, M.: What are the psychiatrists' expectations for nuclear magnetic resonance tomography and spectroscopy ? Fortschr. Neurol. Psychiat. **60**, 308-314 (1992).

MARCIANI, M.G., STEFANI, F., STEFANI, N. et al.: Effect of carbamazepine treatment on EEG changes induced by different cortical activation patterns in newly referrend epileptic patients. Neuropsychobiology **25**, 221-226 (1992)

MARJERRISON, G., KRAUSE, A., KEOGH, R.: Variability of the EEG in schizophrenia: quantitative analysis with a modulus voltage integrator. EEG. Clin. Neurophysiol. **24**, 35-41 (1967)

MARJERRISON, G., JAMES, J., REICHERT, H.: EEG findings in a comparative study of unilateral and bilateral ECT. Paper presented at the Canadian Psychiatric Association's Meeting, Ottawa, 1974

MATEJCEK, M.: Cortical correlates of vigilance regulation and their use in evaluating the effects of treatment, pp.339-348. In: Ergot compounds and Brain Function: Neuroendocrine and neuropsychiatric aspects. Goldstein, M. et al. (eds.). Raven Press, New York, 1980

MATEJCEK, M., POKORNY, R., FERBER, G. et al: The effect of morphine on the EEG and on other physiological and behavioural parameters. Vortrag beim Symposium der International Pharmaco-EEG Group (IPEG) in Santa Margeritha Ligure, 1986

MATOUSEK, M., PETERSEN, I.: Frequency analysis of the EEG in normal children (1-15 years) and in normal adolescents (16-21 years) pp.75-102. In: Automation of Clinical Electroencephalography. Kellaway, P., Petersen, I. (eds.). Raven Press, New York, 1973

MATOUSEK, M., PETERSEN, I.: Automatic measurement of the vigilance level and its possible application in pharmacology. Pharmakopsychiat. **12**, 148-154 (1979)

MATOUSEK, M., ARVIDSON, A., FRIBERG, S.: Serial quantitative electroencephalography. EEG Clin. Neurophysiol. **47** 614-622 (1979)

MATOUSEK, M., PETERSEN, I.: A method for assessing alertness-fluctuations from EEG spectra. EEG Clin. Neurophysiol. **55**, 108-113 (1983)

MATOUSEK, M., HJALMARSON, A., KOCH, J. et al.: The use of the EEG for assessment of vigilance changes. Neuropsychobiol. **12**, 55-59 (1984)

MATTHEWS, W.B.: The clinical value of routine electroencephalography. J.Coll. Physicians Lond. **7**, 207-212 (1973)

MATURANA, H. R.: Erkennen: Die Organisation und Verkörperung von Wirklichkeit. Vieweg, Braunschweig-Wiesbaden, 1982

MAULSBY, R. L.: An illustration of emotionally evoked theta rhythm in infancy: hedonic hypersynchrony. EEG Clin. Neurophysiol. **31**, 157-165 (1971)

MAULSBY, R.L., KELLAWAY, P., GRAHAM, M. et al: The normative electroencephalographic data reference library. Final Report Contract NAS 9 - 1200, National Aeronautics and Space Administration, Washington D.C. 1968

MAYER-KRESS, A. (ed.) Dimensions and Entropies in Chaotic Systems. Vol **32**, Springer, Berlin, 1986

MAYEUX, R, (editorial) : Finding the beginning or predicting the future. Arch Neurol **67** 783-784 (2000)

McLEAN, D.R., KLASS, D.W., WAKIM, K.G.: Factors responsible for EEG alterations in dogs undergoing hemodialysis. EEG Clin. Neurophysiol. **31**, 298 Abstr. (1971)

MEDALIA, A., MERRIAM, A., BARNETT, J. et al.: Neuropsychological sequelae of partial complex status epilepticus. Arch. clin. Neuropsychol. **3**, 303-311 (1988)

MEEHL, P. E.: Schizotaxia, schizotypy, schizophrenia. Am. Psychol., **17**, 827-838 (1962)

MENDELSON, J. H.: Marijuana, S. 1565-1571. In: Psychopharmacology: The Third Generation of Progress. Meltzer H.Y. (ed.). Raven Press, New York 1987

MENGOLI, G.: L'ettroencefalogramma nei vecci. Riv. Neurol. **22**, 166-193 (1952)

MERRIN, E. L., MEEK, P., FLOYD, T. C. et al.: Topographic segmentation of waking EEG in medicationfree schizophrenic patients. Int. J. Psychophysiol. **9**, 231-236 (1990)

MEYER-MICKELEIT, R. W.: Das Elektroencephalogramm nach gedeckten Kopfverletzungen. Dtsch. med. Wschr. **78**, 480-484 (1953).

MILLER, H., BLUME, W.T.: Primary generalized seizure disorder: correlation of epileptiform discharges with seizure frequency. Epilepsia **34**, 128-132 (1993)

MILSTETN, V., SMALL, J. G.: Psychological correlates of 14 and 6 positive spikes, 6/sec spike wave, and small sharp spike transients. Clin. EEG **2**, 206-212 (1971)

MIRAS, C. J.:Experience with chronic hashish smokers, pp.191-198. In: Drugs and Youth. Wittenborn, R. et al. (Hrsg.). C.C.Thomas, Springfleld ILL. 1969

MOELLER, A.A., SIMON, O., JAEGER, H.: EEG-Ableitung bei HIV Enzephalopathie. Dtsch. Med. Wsch. **111**, 1090-1091 (1986)

v. MONAKOW, C.: Die Lokalisation im Grosshirn und der Abbau der Funktion durch kortikale Herde. Bergmann, Wiesbaden, 1914

MONOD, N., THARP, B.: Activite electro-encephalographique normale du nouveau - ne et du premature au cours des etats de veille et de sommeil. Rev. EEG Neurophysiol. **7**, 302-312 (1977)

MORIHISIA, J, M., DUFFY, F. H., WYATT, R. J.: Brain electrical activity mapping (BEAM) in schizophrenic patients. Arch. Gen. Psychiatry **40**, 719-728 (1983)

MORRISON, J.H., HOFF, P.R.: Life and death of neurons in the aging brain. Science **278**, 412-419 (1997)

MORSTYN, R., DUFFY, F.H., McCARLEY, R.W.: Altered topography of EEG spectral content in schizophrenia. EEG Clin. Neurophysiol. **56**, 263-271 (1983)

MÜLLER, D. , KOCH, R. D. , v. SPECHT, H. et al.: Neurophysiologische Befunde beim chronischen Alkoholmissbrauch. Psychiat. , Neurol. med. Psychol., **37**, 129-132 (1985)

MÜLLER-KÜPPERS, M., VOGEL, F.: Über die Erblichkeitsstruktur von Trägern einer seltenen erblichen EEG-Variante. Jahrbuch f. Psychologie **12**. 75-101 (1965)

MÜLLER-OERLINGHAUSEN, B., BAUER, H., GIRKE, W. et al.: Impairment of vigilance and performance under lithium-treatment. Pharmakopsychiat. **10**, 67-78 (1977)

MÜLLER-OERLINGHAUSEN, B., HAMANN, S., HERRMANN, W.M. et al.: Effects of lithium on vigilance, performance, memory, and mood. Pharmakopsychiat. **12**, 388-396 (1979)

MUNDY-CASTLE, A.C.: Theta and beta rhytm in the electroencephalograms of normal adults. EEG Clin. Neurophysiol. **3**, 477-486 (1951)

MUNDY-CASTLE, A.C.: Central excitability in the aged, pp.575-595. In: Medical and Clinical Aspects of Aging. Blumenthal, H. T. (ed.). Columbia Univ. Press, New York 1962

MUNDY-CASTLE, A.C., HURST, L.A., BEERSTECHER, D.M. et al.: The EEG in the senile Psychoses. EEG Clin. Neurophysiol. **6**, 245-252 (1954)

MURPHREE, H., JENNEY, E., PFEIFFER, C.: Quantitative electroencephalographic analysis of the effects of Iysergic and diethylamide (LSD-25) and d-amphetamine in man. Fed. Proc. 21 337 (1962)

NAGATA, K.: Topographic EEG in brain ischemia with blood flow and metabolism. Brain Topogr **1**, 97-106 (1988)

NAGAKUBO, S., KUMAGAI, N., KAMEYAMA, T. et al.: Diagnostic reliability and significance of irregular beta patterns. Jpn. J. Psychiatr. Neurol. **45**, 631 -640 (1991)

NAITOH, P.: The value of electroencephalography in alcoholism. Ann. New York Aacd. Sci. **215**, 303 -320 (1973)

NEIL, J. F., MERIKANGAS, J. R., DAVIES, R. K. et al.: Validity and clinical utility of neuroleptic-facilitated electroencephalography in psychotic patients. Clin. EEG **9**, 38-48 (1978)

NELSON, J. C., CHARNEY, D. S.: The symptoms of major depressive illness. Amer. J. Psychlat. **138**, 1-13 (1981)

NESTOR, P.J. SCHELTENS, P., HODGES, .J.R.: Advances in the early detection of Alzheimer's disease. Nature Rev Neurosci **5**, S34-S41 (2004)

NEUNDÖRFER, B.: Uber die 4 - 5/sec-EEG-Grundrhythmus-Variante. Der Nervenarzt **41**, 321-326 (1970)

NEWMANN, S. E.: The EEG manifestations of chronic ethanol abuse: relation to cerebral cortical atrophy. Ann. Neurol. **3**, 299 - 304 (1978)

NIEDERMEYER, E.: Electroencephalographic studies on the anticonvulsive action of intravenous diazepam. Eur. Neurol. **3**, 88-96 (1970)

NIEDERMEYER, E. : Engpässe und Ausblicke in der klinischen Elektroenzephalographie. Der Nervenarzt **57**, 555 - 557 (1986)

NIEDERMEYER, E., FREUND, G., KRUMHOLZ, A.: Subacute encephalopathy with seizures in in alcoholics: a clinicial electroencephalographic study. Clin. EEG **12**, 113 - 129 (1981)

NOEL, M. G.: L'EEG dans l'arteriosclerose cerebrale. Rev. neurol. **87**, 198-199 (1952)

NUNEZ, P.L. (ed.) : Neocortical Dynamics and Human EEG Rhythms. Oxford Univ. Press, New York, 1995

NUWER, M.R.: Assessment of digital EEG, quantitative EEG and EEG brain mapping Neurology **49,** 277-292 (1997)

NUWER, M.R., SHELDON, E., JORDAN, E. et al.: Evaluation of stroke using EEG frequency analysis and topographic mapping Neurology **37**, 1153-1159 (1987)

NYSTRÖM, C., MATOUSEK, M., HÄLLSTRÖM, T.: Relationships between EEG and clinical characteristics in major depressive disorder. Acta psychiat. scand. **73**, 390-394 (1986)

OBRIST, W.D.: The electroencephalogram of normal aged adults. EEG Clin. Neurophysiol. **6**, 235-244 (1954)

OBRIST, W.D.: Cerebral physiology of the aged: relation to the psychological function, pp. 421-430. In: Behavior and Brain Electrical Activity. Burch, N. and Altshuler, H. l. (eds.).Plenum Press, New York-London, 1975

OBRIST, W. D.: Problems of aging, pp.275-295. In: Handbook of Electroencephalography and Clinical. Neurophysiology, vol.6, The EEG of the Waking Adult, Part A. Remond, A. (ed.). Elsevier, Amsterdam 1976

OBRIST, W.D., HENRY,C.E.: Electroencephalographic frequency analysis of aged psychiatric patients. EEG Clin. Neurophysiol. **10**, 621-632 (1958)

OBRIST, W. D., BUSSE, E.W., HENRY, C. E.: Relation of electroencephalogram to blood pressure in elderly persons. Neurology **11**, 151-158 (1961)

OBRIST, W. D., BUSSE, E. W.: The electroencephalogram in old age, pp. 185-205. In: Applications of Electroencephalography in Psychiatry. Wilson, W. P. (ed.). Duke Univ. Press, Durham, N.C. 1965

OHM, T.G., MUELLER, H., BRAAK, H. et al.: Close-meshed prevalence rates of different stages of a tool to uncover the Alzheimer's disease related neurofibrillary changes. Neurosci. **64**, 209-212 (1995)

OI, S., SHIMODA, M., SHIBATA, M. et al.: Pathophysiology of long- standing overt ventriculomegaly in adults. J. Neurosurg. **92**, 933-940 (2000)

OKADA, S., INOUE, R.: Frontal spindle activity that appears in conjunction with nontraumatic diffuse encephalopathy. Clin. EEG **23**, 196-202 (1992)

OKEN, B,S., CHIAPPA, K.H.: Short-term variability in EEG frequency analysis EEG Clin Neurophysiol **69,** 191-198 (1988)

OKEN, B. S., CHIAPPA, K. H., SALINSKY, M.: Computerized EEG frequency analysis: sensitivity and specifity in patients with focal lesions. Neurology **39**, 1281-1287 (1989)

OKEN, B.S., KAYE, J.A.: Electrophysiologic function in the healthy, extremely old. Neurology **42,** 519-526 (1992)

OKEN, B.S., SALINSKY, M.C., ELSAS, R.D. et al.: Vigilance, alertness, or sustained attention: physiological basis and measurement Clin. Neurophysiol. **117**, 1885-1909 (2006)

OLBRICH, S., MULERT, C. KARCH, S. et al.: EEG-vigilance and BOLD effect during simultaneous EEG/fMRI measurement. NeuroImage **45**) 319-332 (2009)

OSTOW, M.: Psychic functions and the electroencephalogram. Arch. Neurol. Psychiat. (Chic.) **65**, 385-400 (1950)

PAKKENBERG, B., PELVING, D., MAMER, L. et al.: Aging and the human cortex.
Exp. Geronto **38**, 95-99 (2003)

PALEM, R.M., FORCE, L., ESVAN, J.: Hallucinations critiques epileptiques et délire. Ann. med.-psychol. **128**, 161-190 (1970)

PAMPIGLIONE, G.: EEG studies after cardiac arrest. Proc. Roy. Soc. Med. **55**, 653-657 (1962)

PARISI, A., STROSSELLI, M., DI PERRI, G. et al.: Electroencephalography in the early diagnosis of HlV-related subacute encephalitis: analysis of 185 patients. Clin. EEG **20**, 1-5 (1989)

PASCUAL-MARQUI, R.D.: Standardized low resolution brain electromagnetic tomography. Methods, Find., Exp., Clin.,Pharmacol. **24 D**, 5-12 (2002).

PASCUAL- MARQUI, R.D., MICHEL, C.M., LEHMANN, D.: Low resolution electromagnetic tomography: a new method for localizing electric activity in the brain. Int. J. Psychophysiol. **18**, 49-65 (1994).

PASSOUANT, P., DUC, N., MAUREL, H.: L'electroencephalographie au cours du traitment par le carbonate de lithium. Montpellier Med. **A96**, 38 (1953)

PENIN, H.: Das EEG der symptomatischen Psychosen. Der Nervenarzt **42,** 242-252 (1971)

PENIN, H.:Psychische Störungen bei Epilepsie. Vortrag bei der 14.Jahrestagung der Deutschen Sektion der Int. Liga gegen Epilepsie. Schattauer, Stuttgart-New York, 1973

PERRIS, C.: Central measures of depression, pp.183-223. In: Handbook of Biological Psychiatry, part II van Praag, H. M., Lader, M. H., Rafaelsen, O. J., Sachar, E. J. (eds.). M. Dekker, New York – Basel, 1980

PETERS, U. H.: Bewußtseinstrübung - Vigilität-Vigilanz. Der Nervenarzt **47**, 173-175 (1976)

PETERSEN, I., SÖRBYE, R.: Slow posterior rhythm in adults. EEG Clin. Neurophysiol. **14**, 161-170 (1962)

PIAGET, J.: Weisheit und Illusionen der Philosophie (S. 86); Suhrkamp, Frankfurt a.M. 1974

PIAGET, J.: Biologie und Erkenntnis. Über die Beziehungen zwischen organischen Regulationen und kognitiven Prozessen. Fischer, Frankfurt a. M. 1983

PICARD, P., NAVARRANNE, P., LABOUREUR, G. et. al.: Confrontations des donnees de l'electroencephalogramme et de l'examen psychologique chez 309 candidats pilots a l'aeronautique. EEG Clin. Neurophysiol., Suppl. **6**, 304-314 (1957)

PIJN, J.P., van WERVEN, H., NOEST, A. et al.: Chaos or noise in EEG signals: dependence on state and brain site. EEG Clin. Neurophysiol. **79**, 371-382 (1991)

PILLAY, S.S., STOLL, A.L., WEISS, M.K. et al.: EEG abnormalities before clozapine therapy predict a good clinical response to clozapine. Ann. Clin. Psychiat. **8,**
1-5 (1996)

PILLMAN, F., SCHLOTE, K. BROICH, K. et al. Electroencephalogram alterations during treatment with olanzapine. Psychopharmacology 150, 216-219 (2000)

PINE, I., PINE, H. M.: Clinical analysis of patients with low voltage EEG. EEG clin. Neurophysiol. **3**, 104 (1951)

PLOTKTN, W. B., COHEN, R.: Occipital alpha and the attributes of the "alpha experience". Psychophysiology **13**, 16-21 (1976)

POLLOCK, V. E., SCHNEIDER, L. S.: Topographic electroencephalographic alpha in recovered depressed elderly. J. abnorm. Psychol. **98**, 268-273 (1989)

POST, R. M., GERNER, R. H., CARMAN, J. S. et al.: Effects of a dopamine agonist piribedil in depressed patients. Arch. Gen. Psychiat. **35**, 609-615 (1978)

POVLSEN, U. J., NORING, U., FOG, R. et al.: Tolerability and therapeutic effect of clozapine. Acta psychiat. scand. **71**, 176-185 (1985)

van PRAAG, H. M.: A critical investigation of the importance of monamine oxidase inhibition as a therapeutic principle in the treatment of depression. Thesis, Utrecht 1962

van PRAAG, H.M.: Biological Psychiatry audited (Editorial). J.Nerv.Ment. Dis. **176** 195-199 (1988)

van PRAAG, H.M.: Moving ahead yet falling behind. Neuropsychobiol. **22** 181-193 (1989)

van PRAAG, H.: Editorial: The DSM-IV (Depression) Classifcation: to be or not to be? J. Nerv. Ment. Dis. **178**, 147-149 (1990)

van PRAAG, H.M.: "Make-Believes" in psychiatry or the perils of progress. Brunner/Mazel Publ. New York, 1993

van PRAAG, H. M., KORF, J., LAKKE, J. P. et al.: Dopamin metabolism in depressions, psychoses and Parkinson's disease: the problem of the specifity of biological variables in behavior disorders. Psychol. Med. **5**, 138-146 (1975)

van PRAAG, H. M., KAHN, R. S., ASNIS, G. M. et al.: Denosologization of biological psychiatry or the specifity of 5-HT disturbances in psychiatric disorders. J.Aff. Dis. **13**, 1 - 8 (1987)

PRAETORIUS, H.M., BODENSTEIN, G., CREUTZFELDT, D.O.: Adaptive segmentation of EEG records; a new approach to automatic EEG analysis. EEG clin. Neurophysiol. **42**, 84-94 (1977)

PRICE, R. W., NAVIA, B. A., CHO, E.-S.: AIDS encephalopathy. Neurol. Clin. **4**, 404 - 418 (1986)

PRICHEP, L.: Neurometric quantitative EEG features of depressive disorders, pp.55-69. In: Cerebral Dynamics, Laterality and Psychopathology. Takahashi, R., Flor-Henry, P., Gruzelier, J., Niwa, S. (eds.). Elsevier, Amsterdam-New York-Oxford 1987

PRICHEP, L., GOMEZ-MONT, F., JOHN, E. R. et al.: Neurometric electroencephalographic characteristics of dementia, pp. 252-257, In: Alzheimer's Disease, Reisberg, B. (ed.). The Free Press, New York 1983

PRICHEP, L.S., JOHN, E.R, FERRIS, S.H. et al. Quantitative EEG correlates of cognitive deterioration in the elderly. Neurobiol Aging **15** (1994) 85-90

PRIGOGINE, I.: Structure, dissipation and life. Vortrag bei der "First International Conference on Theoretical Physics and Biology (p. 23-52) in Versailles, North Holland Publ Comp, Amsterdam, 1969

PRIGOGINE, I.: Vom Sein zum Werden Piper, München, 1985

PRINZ, P.N., PESKIND, E.R., VITALIARIO, P.P. et al.: Changes in the sleep and waking EEGs of nondemented and demented elderly subjects. J. Amer. Geriat. Soc. **30**, 86-92 (1982)

PRITCHARD, W. S., DUKE, D. W.: Dimensional analysis of no-task human EEG using the Grassberger-Procaccia method. Psychophysiology **29**, 182-192 (1992)

PRITCHARD, W.S., DUKE, D.W., COBURN K.L. et al.: EEG-based neural-net predictive classification of Alzheimer's disease versus control subjects is augmented by non-linear EEG measures. EEG Clin. Neurophysiol. **91**, 118-130 (1994)

PROPPING, P.:Genetic control of ethanol action on the central nervous system: an EEG study in twins. Human Genetics 35, 309-334 (1977)

PRÜLL, G.: Formen des Petit mal Status. Vortr. bei den 8.Treysaer Fortbildungstagen, Mai 1976

RAO, S.M.: Neuropsychology of multiple sclerosis: a critical review. J.Clin. Exp. Neurophysiol. **8**, 503-542 (1986)

RAO, S. M., LEO, G. J., BERNARDIN, L. et al.: Cognitive dysfunction in multiple sclerosis. Neurology **41**, 685 - 691 (1991)

REIHER, J., KLASS, D. W.: Two common EEG patterns of doubtful clinical significance. Med. Clin. North Am. **52**, 933-940 (1968)

REILLY, E., HALMI, K. A., NOYES, R.: Electroencephalographic responses to lithium. Int. Pharmacopsychiat. **8**, 208-213 (1973)

RÉMOND, A., LESEVRE, N.: Remarques sur l'activite cerebrale des sujets normeaux. EEG Clin. Neurophysiol., Suppl. **6**, 235-255 (1957)

RENSING, L.: Biologische Regulation. G. Fischer, Stuttgart, 1973

RICE, D.M., BUCHSBAUM, M.S., STARR, L. et al.: Abnormal EEG slow activity in left temporal areas in senile dementia of the Alzheimer type. J.Gerontol. **45**, M 145 - M 151 (1990)

RIEDEL, R. R., HELMSTAEDTER, C., BÜLAU, P. et al.: Early signs of cognitive deficits among human immunodeficiency virus-positive hemophiliacs. Acta psychiatr. scand. **85**, 321-326 (1992)

RIEGER, H., KUGLER, J., ANGSTWURM, H.: Abnorme EEG-Befunde bei Multipler Sklerose. Z. EEG-EMG **1**, 141 - 149 (1970)

RIEHL, J.-L., MC INTYRE, H. B.: A quantitative study of the acute effects of diphenylhydantoin on the electroencephalogram of epileptic patients. Neurology **18**, 1107 - 1112 (1968)

RITACCIO, A. L., MARCH, G.: The signifcance of PLEDs in complex partial status epilepticus. Am. J. Technol. **33**, 27-34 (1993)

RODIN, E. A.: Uber die Aussagekraft des EEG in Bezug auf die Prognose der Epilepsie. EEG-EMG **1**, 65-68 (1970)

RODIN, E.A., LUBY, E.D., GOTTLIEB, J.S.: The electroencephalogram during prolonged experimental sleep deprivation. EEG Clin. Neurophysiol. **14**, 544-551 (1962)

RODIN, E.A., DOMINO, E.F., PORZAK, J.P.: The marihuana-induced "social high". JAMA **213**, 1300 -1302 (1970)

ROESCHKE, J., BASAR, E.: The EEG is not a simple noise: strange attractors in intracranial structures, pp.203-216.In: Dynamics of Sensory and Cognitive Processing by the Brain, Vol. l. Basar, E. (ed.). Springer, Berlin, 1988

ROESCHKE, J., BASAR, E.: Correlation dimensions in various parts of cat and human brain in different states, pp.132-148.In: Dynamics of Sensory and Cognitive Processing by the Brain, Vol.2. Basar, E., Bullock, T. H. (eds.) Springer, Berlin 1989

ROESCHKE, J., ALDENHOFF, J.: The dimensionality of human's electroencephalogram during sleep. Biol. Cybern. **64**, 307-313 (1991)
ROESCHKE, J., ALDENHOFF, J. B.: Estimation of the dimensionality of sleep-EEG data in schizophrenics. Eur. Arch. Psychiatry Clin. Neurosci. **242**, 191-196 (1993)

ROGER, J., SOULAYROL, R. A propos des accidents neurologiques du traitement de l'epilepsie par les hydantoines. Rev. neurol. **100**, 783-785 (1959)

ROGERS, S.L., FARLOW, M.R., DOODY, R.S. et al.: A 24-week, double-blind, placebo-controlled trial of donepzil in patients with Alzheimer's disease Neurology **50** 136-145 (1998)

ROGERS, S.L., FRIEDHOFF, L.T.: Long term efficacy and safety of donepzil in the treatment of Alzheimer's disease: an interim analysis of the results of a US multicentre open extension study. Eur. Neuropsychopharmacol **8** 67-75 (1998)

RON, M. A., ACKER, W. SHAW, G. K. et al.: Computerized tomography of the brain in chronic alcoholism : a survey and follow-up study. Brain, **105**, 497-514 (1982)

ROSEMAN, E.: Dilantin toxicity. A clinical and electroencephalographic study. Neurology **11**, 912-921 (1961)

ROSENBERG, G.A., APPENZELLER, O.: Amantadine, fatigue and multiple sclerosis. Arch. Neurol. **45**, 1104-1106 (1988)

ROTH, B.: Beitrag zum Studium der Narkolepsie. Analyse eines persönlichen Beobachtungsgutes von 155 Kranken. Schweiz. Arch. Neurol. Psychiat. **84**, 181-210 (1959)

ROTH, B.: The clinical and theoretical importance of EEG rhythms corresponding to states of lowered vigilance. EEG Clin. Neurophysiol. **13**, 395-399 (1961)

ROTH, G.: Biological systems theory and the problem of reductionism, pp. 106-120. In: Self-organizing Systems. Roth, G., Schwegler, H. (eds.). Campus, Frankfurt-New York, 1981

ROWNTREE, D.W., KAY, W.W.: Clinical, biochemical and physiological studies in cases of recurrent schizophrenia. J. ment. Sci. **98**, 100-121 (1952)

RUBIN, E.H., STORANDT, M., MILLER, . et al.: A prospective study of cognitive function and onset of dementia in cognitive healthy elders Arch. Neurol. **55**, 395-401 (1998)

SACHDEO, R., CHOKROVERTY, S.: Increasing epileptiform activities in the EEG in the presence of decreasing clinical seizures after carbamazepine. Epilepsia **26**, 522 (1985)

SACHDEV, P.S., SNITH J.S., ANGUS-LEPAN H. et al.: Pseudodementia twelve years on. J. Neurol. Neurosurg. Psychiat. **53**, (254-259 (1990)

SACKS, B., FENWICK, P. B. C., MARKS, I.: An investigation of the phenomenon of autocontrol of the alpha rhythm and possible associated feeling states using visual feedback. EEG clin. Neurophysiol. **32**, 461 (1972)

SAINO, K., STENBERG,D., KESKIMÄKI, A. et al.: Visual and spectral EEG analysis in the evaluation of the outcome in patients with ischemic brain infarction. EEG Clin. Neurophysiol. **56**, 117-124 (1983)

SALETU, B.: Pharmaco-EEG profiles of typical and atypical antidepressants. Adv. Biochem. Psychopharmacol. **32**, 257-268 (1982)

SALETU, B., GRÜNBERGER J., RAJINA, P.: Pharmaco-EEG profiles of antidepressants. Pharmacodynamic studies with Fluvoxamine. Br. J. clin. Pharmac. **15** 369S-384S (1983)

SALETU, B., ANDERER, P., PAULUS, E. et al.: EEG brain mapping in SDAT and MIT patients before and during placebo and xantinolnicotinate therapy: reference considerations, pp.251-275. In: Statistics and Topography in Quantitative EEG. Samson-Dollfus, D. (eds.). Elsevier, Paris 1988

SALETU B., ANDERER P., SALETU-ZYHLARZ G.M.: EEG topography and tomography (LORETA) in the classification of psychotropic drugs. J. Clin. EEG Neurosci. **37** 66-81 (2006)

SALINSKY, M.C., OKEN, B.S., MOREHEAD, L.: Test-retest reliability in EEG frequency analysis. EEG Clin. Neurophysiol. **79**, 382 - 392 (1991).

SANNITA, W. G., RAPPALINO, M. V., RODRIGUEZ, G. et al.: EEG effects and plasma concentrations of phenobarbital in volunteers. Neuropharmacology **19**, 927-930 (1980)

SANTAMARIA, J., CHIAPPA, K. H.: The EEG of Drowsiness. Demos, New York, 1987

SAUL, L.J., DAVIS, H., DAVIS, P.A.: Psychological correlations with the electroencephalogram. EEG Clin. Neurophysiol. **1,** 515 (1949)

SAUNDERS, M.G.: EEG changes in metabolic disorders. Am. J. EEG Technol. **8**, 41-57 (1968)

SAUNDERS, M.G., WESTMORELAND, B.F.: Das EEG bei diffusen Funktionsstörungen des Gehirns, S.311 -344. In: Klinische Elektroenzephalographie. Klass, D. W., Daly, D. D. (Hrsg.). G. Fischer, Stuttgart-New York, 1984

SAUNDERS, J., WHITMAN, R., SCHAUMANN, B.: Sleep disturbance, fatigue, and depression in multiple sclerosis. Neurology **41**, (Suppl. 1) 728 (1991)

SCAHILL, R.L., FROST, C.,JENKINS, R. et al.: A longitudinal study of brain volume changes in normal aging serial registered magnetic resonance imaging. Arch. Neurol. **60,** 989-994 (2003)

SCHAFFER, C., DAVIDSON, R.J., SARON, C.: Frontal and parietal EEG asymmetries in depressed and non-depressed subjects. Biol. Psychiatry **18**, 753-762 (1983)

SCHAUL, N., GLOOR, P., GOTMAN, J.: The EEG in deep midline lesions. Neurology **31**, 157-167 (1981a)

SCHAUL, N., LUEDERS, H., SACHDEV, K.: Generalized, bilaterally synchronous bursts of slow waves in the EEG. Arch. Neurol. **38**, 690-692 (1981b)

SCHEAR, H. E.: The EEG pattern in delirium tremens. Clin. EEG **16**, 30-32 (1985)

SCHELLING, F.W.J. : Einleitung zu dem Entwurf eines Systems der Naturphilosophie oder über den Begriff der speculativen Physik und die innere Organisation eines Systems dieser Wissenschaft (1799) In KFA Schelling (Hrsg.) Friedrich Wilhelm Joseph von Schellings sämtliche Werke, Bd.III Stuttgart, 1856-1861

SCHENK, G. K.: A geometric model for the analysis of antagonistic activation and deactivation in electroencephalograms, pp.337-356. In: Quantitative Analysis of the EEG. Matejcek, M., Schenk, G. K. (eds.). Proceedings of the 2nd Symposium of the Study Group for EEG-Methodology, Jongny sur Vevey 1975. AEG-Telefunken, Konstanz, 1975

SCHEULER, W., KUBICKI, S., PASTELAK-PRICE, C.: Steile Wellen und Spitzen in der Okzipitalregion bei Gesunden und Patienten ohne Epilepsie. EEG-Labor **10**, 61-105 (1988)

SCHLENSKA, G. K., WALTER, G. F.: Temporal evolution of electroencephalographic abnormalities in Creutzfeld-Jakob-disease. J.Neurol. **236**, 456- 60 (1989)

SCHMICKLAY, R., NICKEL, B., JÄRISCH, M. et al.: Elektrolytstörungen, EEG-Veränderungen und epileptische Anfälle beim Alkoholentzugsdelir. Psychiat. Neurol. med. Psychol. **41**, 722-729 (1989)

SCHMIDT, S., GREIL, W.: Carbamazepin in der Behandlung psychiatrischer Erkrankungen. Der Nervenarzt **58**, 719-736 (1987)

SCHMITT, F.A., DAVIS, D.G., WEKSTEIN, D.R.: "Preclinical" AD revisted. Neurology **55**, 370-376 (2000)

SCHNEIDER, C.: Über Geistesstörungen bei perniciöser Anämie, Der Nervenarzt **2**, 286-293 (1929)

SCHNEIDER, C.: Die Schizophrenen Symptomverbände. Springer, Berlin, 1939

SCHNEIDER, K.: Klinische Psychopathologie. Thieme, Stuttgart, 1959

SCHNEIDER, J., RÉMOND, A.: Notes preliminaires concernant l'action de la morphine a doses variables sur le trace EEG. EEG Clin. Neurophysiol. **1**, 372 (1949)

SCHORSCH, G., HEDENSTRÖM, J. v.: Die Schwankungsbreite hirnelektrischer Erregbarkeit in ihrer Beziehung zu epileptischen Anfällen und Verstimmungszuständen. Arch. Psychiat. ges. Neurol. **195**, 393-407 (1957)

SCHOTT, J., SIMON, J.E., WHITWELL, J.L. et al.: Global brain atrophy as a surrogate marker of progress in Alzheimer's disease: a one year, prospective, longitudinal MRI study using the brain boundary shift integral. Neurology **60**, Suppl 1:A 16, (2003)

SCHROTH, G., NAEGELE, T., Klose, U.: Reversible brain shrinkage in abstinent alcoholics, measured by MRI. Neurology, **30**, 383-390 (1988)

SCHULD A., KUHN M., HAACK M. et al.: A comparison of the effects of clozapine and olanzapine on the EEG in patients with schizophrenia. Pharmacopsychiatry **33**, 109-111 (2000)

SCHULZ, H., MÜLLER, J., ROTH, B. et al.: Die bioelektrisch kontrollierte Krampfbehandlung der endogenen Psychosen in Narkose und Relaxation. Arch. Psychiat. Nervenkr. **211**, 414-432 (1968)

SCHUPP, H.T., LUTZENBERGER, W., BIRBAUMER, N. et al.: Neurophysiological differences between perception and imagery. Cogn. Brain Res. **2**, 77-86 (1999)

SCHUSTER, H. G.: Deterministic Chaos. An Introduction. Physik Verlag, Weinheim, 1984

SCOTT, D.F., HEATHFIELD, K.W.G., TOONE, B. et al.: The EEG in Huntington's chorea: a clinical and neuropathological study. J. Neurol. Neurosurg. Psychiat. **35**, 97-102 (1972)

SEARLE, J.R.: Geist: eine Einführung Suhrkamp, Frankfurt a. M. 2006

SELBACH, H.: Das Kippschwingungsprinzip, S.300-332. In: Klinische Pathologie des vegetativen Nervensystems. Sturm, A. und Birkmayer, W. (Hrsg.). G. Fischer, Stuttgart, 1976

SELYE, H.: The General Adaptation Syndrome J. clin. endocrine. **14**, 117-123 (1946)
SELYE, H.: The Story of the Adaptation Syndrome. Acta Inc. Med. Publ., Montreal, 1952

SHAGASS, C.: An electrophysiological view of schizophrenia. Biol. Psychiat. **11**, 3-30 (1976)

SHAGASS, C., ROEMER, R. A., STRAUMANIS, J. J.: Relationship between psychiatric diagnosis and some quantitative EEG variables. Arch. Gen. Psychiat. **39**, 1433-1435 (1982)

SHAGASS, C., ROEMER, R.A., STRAUMANIS, J. et al.: Psychiatric diagnostic discriminations with combinations of quantitative EEG variables. Brit. J. Psychiat. **144**, 581-592 (1984)

SHANNON, C.E., WEAVER, W.: The Mathematical Theory of Communication. Univ, Ill Press, Urbana, 1949

SHAW, J. C.: The ubiquitous alpha rhythm - a selective review. J. Electrophysiol. Technol. **18**, 5-27 (1992)

SHERRIDAN, P.H:, SATOS, S, FOSTER, N. et al.: Relation of EEG alpha background to parietal lobe function in Alzheimer's disease as measured by positron emission tomography and psychometry Neurology **38** 747-750 (1988)

SHERRINGTON, C.S.: The Integrative Action of the Nervous System. Yale Univ. Press, New Haven Connecticut, 1906

SIFFERMANN, A., SPIELMANN, J. P., PERRIN, J.: Contribution a l'etude electroencephalographique des aures neuroleptiques phenothiazinique. Med. exp. (Basel) **5**, 391-395 (1961)

SILBERMAN, E. K., REUS, V., JIMERSON, D. C. et al.: Heterogeneity of amphetamine response in depressed patients. Amer. J. Psychiat. **138,** 1302-1307 (1981)

SILBERMAN, E. K., WEINGARTEN, H., POST, R. M.: Thinking disorder in depression. Arch. Gen. Psychiat. **40**, 775-780 (1983)

SILVERMAN, D.: Diskussionsbemerkung. EEG Clin. Neurophysiol. **10**, 767 (1958)

SILVERMAN, D.: Retrospective study of EEG in coma. EEG clin. Neurophysiol. **15**, 486-505 (1963)

SILVERMAN, A.J., BUSSE, E.W., BARNES, R.H.: Studies in the processes of aging: electroencephalographic findings in 400 elderly subjects. EEG Clin. Neurophysiol. **7**, 67-74 (1955)

SIMON, C. W., EMMONS, W. H.: EEG - consciousness and sleep. Science **124**, 1066-1069 (1956)

SINGER, W.: Coherence as an organizing principle of cortical function. Int. Rev. Neurobiol. **37**, 153-183 (1997)

SINGER, W.: Consciousness and neuronal synchronization (pp. 43-52) In S. Laureys, G. Tononi (eds.) The Neurology of Consciousness, Elsevier, Amsterdam, 2002

SITTIG, O: Hughlings Jacksons Hirnpathologie. Nervenarzt **4**, 473-482 (1931)

SLATER, E., BEARD, A. W., GLITHERO, E.: The schizophrenia-like psychoses of epilepsy. Brit. J. Psychiatry **95**, 109-150 (1963)

SMALL, J. G.: Photoconvulsive and photomyoclonic responses in psychiatric patients. Clin. EEG **2**, 78-88 (1971)

SMALL, J. G.: EEG and lithium CNS toxicity. Am. J. EEG Technol. **26**, 225-239 (1986)

SMALL, J. G.: Psychiatric disorders and EEG, pp.523-539. In: Electroencephalography: Niedermeyer, E., Lopes da Silva, F. (eds.). Urban and Schwarzenberg, Baltimore-Munich, 1987

SMALL, J.G., STERN, J A.: EEG indicators of prognosis in acute schizophrenia. EEG Clin. Neurophysiol. **18**, 526 (1965)

SMALL, J. G., SHARPLEY, P., SMALL, I. F.: Positive spikes, spike wave phantoms, and psychomotor variants. Arch. Gen. Psychiatry **18**, 232-238 (1968)

SMALL, J.G., MILSTEIN, V., SHARPLEY P.H. et al.: Electroencephalographic findings in relation to diagnostic constructs in psychiatry. Biol. Psychiatry **19** (1984) 2294-2306

SMALL, J.G., MILSTEIN, V., MEDLOCK, C.E.: Clinical EEG findings in mania. Clin EEG 28 (1997) 229-235

SMITH, J. R.: The electroencephalogram during normal infancy and childhood. J. genet. Psychol. **53**, 431-482 (1938)

SMITH, C.D., CHEBROLU, H., WEKSTEIN, D.R.: Brain structural alterations before mild cognitive impairment. Neurology **68** 1268-1278 (2007)

SMITH, J. B., WESTMORELAND, B. F., REAGAN, T. J. et al.: A distincive clinical EEG profile in herpes simplex encephalitis. Mayo Clin. Proc. **50**, 469-474 (1975)

SMITH, S.J.M., KOCEN, R.S.: A Creutzfeldt-Jakob-like syndrome due to lithium toxicity. J. Neurosurg. Psychiatry **51**, 120-123 (1988)

SO, N. K., ANDERMANN, F., OLIVER, A. et al.: Acute postictal psychosis: a stereo EEG study. Epilepsia **31**, 188-193 (1990)

SOININEN, H., PARTANEN, J., LAULUMAA, V.: et al. Longitudinal EEG spectral analysis in early stage of Alzheimer's disease. EEG Clin. Neurophysiol. **72**, 290-297 (1989)

SOKOLOFF, L.: Cerebral circulatory and metabolic changes associated with aging. Res. Publ. Assoc. Nerv. Ment. Dis. **41**, 237-254 (1966)

SOONG, A., STUART, C.: Evidence of chaotic dynamics underlying the human alpha-rhythm electroccephalogram. Biol. Cybern. **62**, 55-62 (1989)

SOUCACHET, P.: Étude EEG de l'endormissement spontane et des reactions d'eveil. Leur interet dans certains pathologiques domaines. Theses, Paris 1952

SPATZ, R., LORENZONI, E., KUGLER, J. et al.: Häufigkeit und Form von EEG-Anomalien bei Clozapintherapie. Arzneimittelforsch./Drug Res. **28**, 1449 - 1450 (1978)

SPITZER, R.L., ENDICOTT, J., ROBINS, E.: Forschungs-Diagnose-Kriterien (RDC). Beltz, Weinheim, 1982

SPITZER, R. L., WILLIAMS, J. B. W., FIRST, M. B. et al.: A proposal for DSM-IV: solving the "organic/nonorganic problem" (editorial). J. Neuropsychiatry Clin. Neurosciences **1**, 126-127 (1989)

SPITZER, R.L., FIRST, M., TUCKER, G.: Organic mental disorders and DSM-IV. Am. J. Psychiatry **148,** 396 (1991)

STAM, C.J., PIJN, J.P.M., SUFFCZYNSKI, P.: Dynamics of the human alpha rhythm: evidence for non-linearity? Clin. Neurophysiol. **110**, 1801-1813 (1999)

STAM, C.J., JELLES, B., ACHTEREEKTE, H.A.M, et al.: Investigations of the EEG nonlinearity in dementia and Parkinson's disease. EEG Clin. Neurophysiol. **95**, 309-317 (1998)

STAM, C.J., van der MADE, Y., PIJNENBERG, Y.H.L.: EEG synchronization in mild cognitive impairment and Alzheimer's disease. Acta neurol. Scand. **108**, 90-96 (2003)

STASSEN, H.H.: Computerized recognition of persons by EEG spectral pattern. EEG clin. Neurophysiol. **49**, 190-194 (1980)

STEINERT, T. BAIER H., FRÖSCHER W. et al. Epileptische Anfälle unter der Behandlung mit Antidepressiva und Neuroleptika. Fortschr. Neurol. Psychiat. **79**, 138-143 (2011)

STERIADE, M., GLOOR, P., LLINAS, R.R. et al.: Basic mechanisms of cerebral rhythmic activities. EEG Clin. Neurophysiol. **76**, 481-508 (1990)

STIGSBY, B., JJOHANNESON, G., INGVAR, D.H.: Regional EEG analysis and regional cerebral flow in Alzheimer's and Pick's disease. EEG Clin. Neurophysiol. **51**, 537-547 (1981)

STOLLER, A.: Slowing of the alpha rhythms of the electroencephalogram and its association with mental deterioration and epilepsy. J. ment. Sci. **95**, 972-984 (1949)

STORM van LEEUWEN, W.: The Alpha Rhyhthm, Suppl. No.34. In: Contemporary Clinical Neurophysiology. Cobb, W. A., van Duijn, H. (eds.). Elsevier, Amsterdam, 1978

STRAUSS, H.: Clinical and electroencephalographic studies: the electroencephalogram in psychoneurotics. J.Nerv. Ment. Dis. **101**, 19-27 (1945)

STROBOS, R. J., KARALLINIS, G. P.: Changes in repeat electroencephalograms in epileptics. Neurology (Minneap.) **18**, 622 - 633 (1968)

STRÖMGREN, E.: The concept of schizophrenia: the conflict between nosological and symtomatological aspects. J. Psychiat. Res. **26**, 237 - 246 (1992)

STRÖMGREN, L.S., JUUL-JENSEN, P.: EEG in unilateral and bilateral electroconvulsive therapy. Acta psychiat. scand. **51**, 340-360 (1975)

STRUVE, F.A.: The necessity and value of screening routine EEG in psychiatric patients: a preliminary report on the issues of referrals. Clin. EEG **7**, 115-130 (1976)

STRUVE, F. A.: Electroencephalographic relationship to suicidal behavior: qualitative considerations and a report on a series of completed suicides. Clin. EEG **14**, 20-26 (1983)

STRUVE, F. A.: Selective referral versus routine screening of clinical EEG assessment of psychiatric inpatients. Psychiatr. Med. **1**, 317-343 (1984)

STRUVE, F. A., KLEIN, D. F., SARAF, K. R.: Electroencephalographic correlates of suicide ideation and attempts. Arch. Gen. Psychiat. **27**, 363 - 365 (1972)

STRUVE, F. A., SARAF, K. R., ARKO, R. S. et al.: Relationship between paroxysmal electroencephalographic dysrhythmia and suicide ideation and attempts in psychiatric patients, pp. 199-221. In: Psychopathology and Brain Dysfunction. Shagass, C., Gershon, S., Friedhoff, A.J. (eds.). Raven Press, New York, 1977

STRUVE, F. A., STRAUMANIS, J. J., PATRICK, G. et al.: Topographic mapping of quantitative EEG variables in chronic heavy marihuana users: empirical fTndings with psychiatric patients. Clin. EEG **20**, 6-23 (1989)

SUGARMAN, A., GOLDSTEIN, L., MURPHY, C. et al.: EEG and behavioral changes in schizophrenia. Arch.gen.Psychiat. **10**, 340-344 (1964)

SUGARMAN, A., GOLDSTEIN, L., MARJERRISON, G. et al.: Recent research in EEG amplitude analysis. Dis. nerv. syst. **34**, 162-166 (1973)

SWARTZBURG, M., CHOWDREY, S.: On the informational value of quantitated interhemispheric EEG data for the appraisal of the mental status of patients. 6. World Congress of Psychiatry, Honolulu. Abstr. No.205, 1977

van SWEDEN, B.: The EEG in hypnosedative drug withdrawal and dependence. Eur. Arch. Psychiat. Neurol. Sci. **234**, 268-274 (1984)

van SWEDEN, B.: Disturbed vigilance in mania. Biol. Psychiat. **21**, 311-313 (1986)

TAKAHASHI, T., NIEDERMEYER, E., KNOTT, J.: EEGs in younger and older adult groups with convolsive disorder. EEG Clin. Neurophysiol. **15**, 724 (1963)

TAKENS, F.: Detecting strange attractors in turbulence (pp. 366-381). Lecture Notes in Mathematics **898**, Springer, Berlin, 1981

TARTER, R. E., ALTERMAN, A.U. , EDWARDS, K.L.: Alcoholic denial : a biopsychological interpretation. J. of Studies on Alcohol, **45**, 214-220 (1984)

TAYLOR, J.: Selected Wrltings of John Hughlings Jackson. Vol. 1: On Epilepsy and Epileptiform Convulsions. Vol.2: Evolution and Dissolution of the Nervous System, Taylor, J. (ed.). Basic Books, New York, 1958

TAYLOR, M.A., SIERLES, F., ABRAMS, R.: The neuropsychiatric evaluation, pp.109-141. In: Psychiatry Update: The American Psychiatric. Association Annual Review, vol.4. APA, Washington DC, 1985

TELLENBACH, H.: Epilepsie als Anfallsleiden und als Psychose. Uber alternative Psychosen paranoider Prägung bei „forcierter Normalisierung" (Landolt) des Elektroenzephalogramms Epileptischer. Der Nervenarzt **36**, 190-202 (1965)

TELLENBACH, H.: Zur Psychopathologie und Klinik der Psychosen bei forcierter Normalisierung des Elektroenzephalogramms Epileptischer. Z. Neurol. **3**, 185 (1966)

TERRY, R.D., De THERESA, R., HANSEN, L. A.: Neocortical cell counts in normal human adult aging. Ann Neurol **21** 530-539 (1987)

THATCHER. R.W.: Neuropsychiatry and quantitative electroencephalography (qEEG) in the 21st century. Neuropsychiatry **33** 722-758 (2011)

THATCHER, R.W., WALKER, R.A., GERSON, I. et al. EEG discriminant analyses of mild head trauma. EEG Clin. Neurophysiol **73** 93-106 (1989)

THATCHER, R.W., MOORE, J.,JOHN, E.R. et al.: QEEG and traumatic brain injury: rebuttal of the American Academy of Neurology (Report of 1997 by the EEG and Clinical Neuroscience Society) Clin. EEG **30** (1999) 94-98

THATCHER, R.W., NORTH, D., CURTIN, R. et al. An EEG severity index of traumatic brain injury . J. Neurophysiol. Clin. Neurosci. **13** 77-87 (2001)

THOMPSON, L. W., WILSON, S.: Electrocortical reactivity and learning in the elderly. J. Gerontol. **21**, 45-51 (1966)

THOMPSON, P.M.,HAYSHI, K.M., de ZUBICARAY, G. et al.: Dynamic mapping of Alzheimer's disease (p. 87-112) In: The Living Brain and Alzheimer's Disease. Hyman BT. Demonet JF, Christen Y (eds.) Springer Berlin-Heidelberg-New York. 2004

TIIHONEN, J., HARI, R., KAJOLA, M. et al.: Magnetencephalographic 10-Hz rhythm from the human auditory cortex. Neurosci. Lett. **129**, 303-305 (1991)

TINUPER, P., DE CAROLIS, P., GALEOTTI, M. et al.: Electroencephalogram and HIV infection: a prospective study in 100 patients. Clin. EEG **21**, 145-150 (1990)

TOLONEN, U., SULG, I.A.: Comparison of quantitative EEG parameters from four different analysis techniques in evaluation of relationship between EEG and rCBF in brain infarction. EEG Clin. Neurophysiol. **51** 177–185 (1981)

TOLONEN, U., AHONEN, A., SULG, I.A. et al.: Serial measurement of quantitative EEG and cerebral blood flow and circulation time after brain infarction. Acta neurol. scand. **63** (1983) 145-155

TOONE, B.: Psychoses of epilepsy, pp.113 - 137. In: Epilepsy and Psychiatry. Reynolds E. H., Trimble, M. R. (eds.) Churchill Livingstone, London, 1981

TORRES, F., FAORO, A., LOEWENSON, R. et al.: The electroencephalogram of elderly subjects revisted. EEG Clin. Neurophysiol. **56**, 391-389 (1983)

TOWNSEND, R.E., JOHNSON, L.C.: Relation of frequency-analyzed EEG to monitoring behavior EEG Clin. Neurophysiol. **47,** 272-279 (1979)

TRABERT, W., BETZ, T., NIEWALD, M. et al.: Significant reversibility of alcoholic brain shrinkage within 3 weeks of abstinence. Acta Psychiat. scand. **92** 87-90 (1995)

TRAVIS, T., KONDO, C. Y., KNOTT, J. R.: Alpha enhancement research: a review. Biol. Psychiat. **10,** 69-89 (1975)

TREFFERT, D. A.: The psychiatric patient with an EEG temporal lobe focus. Am. J. Psychiat. **120**, 765-771 (1964)

TUCKER, G.J., DETRE, T., HARROW, W. et al.: Behavior and symptoms of psychiatric patients and the electroencephalogram. Arch. Gen. Psychiat. **12**, 278-286 (1965)

v. UEXKÜLL, J. Theoretische Biologie, Paetel, Leipzig, 1920

UEXKÜLL, Th. v., WESIACK, W.: Theorie der Humanmedizin. Grundlagen ärztlichen Denkens und Handelns. Urban & Schwarzenberg, München, 1988

ULETT, J. A, ITIL, T. M.: Quantitative electroencephalogram in smoking and smoking deprivation. Science **164**, 969-970 (1969)

ULRICH, G.: Zur Wirkung von Nimodipin auf die topische Verteilung der absoluten Alpha-Leistung im EEG sowie die aktuelle Befindlichkeit gesunder Probanden. Arzneimittelforsch./Drug Res. **37**, 541-545 (1987)

ULRICH, G.: The importance of the concept of vigilance for psychophysiological research. Medical Hypotheses **27**, 227-229 (1988)

ULRICH, G.: Ist global gleich multifokal? Das Ganze und seine Teile in Psychiatrie und Neurologie. Der Nervenarzt **63**, 14- 20 (1992)

ULRICH, G.: Psychiatrische Elektroenzephalographie. G. Fischer, Jena, 1994

ULRICH, G.: QUEIDA – Quantitative Electroencephalographic Ipsative Difference Assessment. Books on Demand, Hamburg, 2001

ULRICH, G.: ITA – ein verhaltensphysiologisches Verfahren zur Messung von Änderungen des unspezifischen Anteils von Krankheiten. WischSoft, 1. Aufl. Heidenrod, 2003

ULRICH, G.: Vigilance regulation in psychiatric patients; A summing up of the controversial discussion of EEG-*vigilance* at the Symposium "Vigilance regulation in Psychiatric Patients," Leipzig, 3./4. April 2008

ULRICH, G.: Das Spontane Ruhe-EEG: Die Physiologische Basis der Psychiatrie – Vergangenheit, Gegenwart und Zukunftsperspektiven. Königshausen & Neumann, Würzburg, 2012

ULRICH, G., SCHEULER, W., MÜLLER-OERLINGHAUSEN, B.: Zur visuell-morphologischen Analyse des hirnelektrischen Verhaltens bei Patienten mit manisch-depressiven und schizoaffektiven Psychosen unter Lithiumprophylaxe. Fortschr. Neurol. Psychiat. **51**, 24-36 (1983)

ULRICH, G., OTTO, W.: Zur Bedeutung intermittierender rechts-posterior betonter langsamer Wellen im EEG psychiatrischer Patienten. Fortschr. Neurol. Psychiat. **52**, 48-61 (1984a)

ULRICH, G., OTTO, W.: Intermittierend rechts-posterior betonte langsame Wellen (IRP) im EEG psychiatrischer Patienten und das theoretische Konstrukt des Maturationsdefizits. Der Nervenarzt **55**, 179-187 (1984b)

ULRICH, G., FRICK, K.: A new quantitative approach to the assessment of stages of vigilance as defined by spatiotemporal EEG-patterns. Percept. Mot. Skills **62** 567-576 (1986)

ULRICH, G., BECKER, E., ZELLER, G. et al.: The lateralization of occipital alpha-power under resting conditions in the EEG of healthy volunteers. Pharmacopsychiat. **18**, 246-251 (1985)

ULRICH, G., GAEBEL, W.: Zur Psychophysiologie schizophrener Aufmerksamkeitsstörung - Konzepte, Befunde und Arbeitshypothesen. Fortschr. Neurol. Psychiat. **55**, 273-278 (1987)
ULRICH, G., KRIEBITZSCH, R. Ein rechnergestütztes visuomotorisches Tracking-Verfahren zur trennscharfen Objektivierung zentralnervöser Pharmakoneffekte. Arzneimittelforsch. Drug Res. **37**, 472 - 475 (1987)

ULRICH, G., FRICK, K., STIEGLITZ, R.-D.: Interindividual variability of lithium-induced EEG changes in healthy volunteers. Psychiatry Res. **20**, 117-127 (1987)

ULRICH, G., SUCHY, I.: Zur Wirkung von Tergurid auf Vigilanzdynamik und mittleres Vigilanzniveau - eine kontrollierte elektroenzephalographische Studie an Altersprobanden. Arzneimittelforsch./Drug Res. **37**, 472-475 (1987)

ULRICH, G., BOHN, D.: Intermittently occurring right-posterior slow waves (IRP) in psychiatric patients. Eur. Arch. Psychiat. Neurol. Sci. **237**, 258-263 (1988)

ULRICH, G., STIEGLITZ, R D.: Effect of nimodipine upon electroencephalographic vigilance in elderly persons with minor impairment of brain functions. Arzneimittelforsch./Drug Res. **38**, 392 - 396 (1988)

ULRICH, G., GAEBEL, W., PIETZCKER, A. et al: Prediction of neuroleptic on-drug respanse in schizophrenic in-patients by EEG. Eur. Arch. Psychiatr. Neurol. Sci. **237**, 144 - 155 (1988)

ULRICH, G., GSCHWILM, R.: Vigilanz - Ordnungszustand oder ordnende Kraft? Fortschr. Neurol. Psychiat. **56**, 398-402 (1988)

ULRICH, G., FÜRSTENBERG, U.: Quantitative assessment of dynamic electroencephalogram (EEG) organization as a tool for subtyping depressive syndromes Eur Psychiat **14** 217-229 (1999)

ULRICH, G., HEGERL, U.: The observing subject and psychophysiological research: an epistemological discourse. Theoretical Medicine **10**, 59-65 (1989)

ULRICH, G., KRIEBITZSCH, R.: Visuomotor tracking performance and task-induced modulation of Alpha activity. Int. J. Psychophysiol. **10** 199-202 (1990)

ULRICH, G., HERRMANN, W. M., HEGERL, U.: Effect of lithium on the dynamics of electroencephalographic vigilance in healthy subjects. J. Aff. Dis. **20**, 19-25 (1990)

ULRICH, G., FRICK, K., LEWINSKY, M.: Lithium and the theoretical concept of "dynamic restriction": a comparison of the effects on different levels of quantitative EEG analysis. Lithium **3**, 33-44 (1993)

ULRICH, G., HAUG, H-J., FÄHNDRICH, E.: Acute vs. chronic effects in maprotiline and in clomipramine treated depressive inpatients and the prediction of therapeutic outcome. J. Aff. Dis. **32**, 213-217 (1994)

ULRICH, G., BRAND, K.: Dynamically rigid EEG and subtyping of depressive syndromes. Eur. Psychiatry, **8**, 25-34 (1993)

UPTON, A., GUMPERT, J.: Electroencephalography in diagnosis of herpes simplex encephalitis. Lancet **1**, 650-652 (1970)
USUI, M., SHIGETA, M., JELIC, V. et al.: Shift of EEG model source location in Alzheimer's disease and mild cognitive impairment Neuropsychobiol **35** 17(1997)

UTTAL, W.R.: The New Phrenology. The Limits of Localizing Cognitive Processes in the Brain. Bradford MIT Cambridge, MA ,2001

VACCA, L., KEMALI, D., MARCIANO, F. et al.: Quantitative EEG analysis in schizophrenia and depressed patients. Adv. Biol. Psychiat. **4**, 111-118 (1980)

VAN DIS, H., CORNER, M., DAPPER, R. et al.: Individual differences in the human electroencephalogram during quiet wakefulness. EEG Clin. Neurophysiol. **47**, 87-94 (1979)

VALSINER, J.: The individual subject and scientific psychology J. Valsiner (ed) Plenum Press New York-Oxford, 1979

VENABLES, P.H: Mechanisms, instrumentation, recording techniques, and quantification of responses. In: Prokasy W.F. Raskin D.C. (eds) New York Acad. Press, 1975

VIRCHOW, R.: Über das Bedürfnis und die Richtigkeit einer Medizin vom mechanischen Standpunkt. Arch. Path. Anat. **188**, 7 (1907)

VARGA, B., NAGY, T.: Analysis of alpha-rhythm in the EEG of alcoholics (abst.). EEG Clin. Neurophysiol. **12**, 933 (1960)

VISSER, S.L.: EEG and senescence; structural and behavioral correlates, pp.403-407, In: The London Symposia (EEG Suppl. 39). Ellingson, R.J., Murray, N. M. F., Halliday, A. M. (Hrsg,), Elsevier. 1987

VISSER, S. L., VAN DER HORST, L., HERNGREEN, H.: Clinical observations and pathophysiological aspects concerning the organic origin of the paradoxical reaction to neuroleptics. Neuropsychopharmacol. **4**, 463-467 (1964)

VISSER, S.L., HOOIGER, C., JONKER, C. et al.: Anterior temporal focal abnormalities in EEG in normal aged subjects: correlations with psychopathological and CT brain scan findings. EEG Clin. Neurophysiol. **66**, 1-7 (1987)

VOGEL, F.: Ergänzende Untersuchungen zur Genetik des menschlichen Niederspannungs-EEG. Dtsch. Z. Nervenheilk. **184**, 105-111 (1962)

VOGEL, F.: The genetic basis of the normal human electroencephalogram (EEG). Humangenetik **10**, 91-114 (1970)

VOGEL, F., GÖTZE, W.: Statistische Betrachtungen über die beta-Wellen im EEG des Menschen. Dtsch Z. Nervenheilk. **184**, 112-136 (1962)

VOGEL, F., FUJIYA, Y.: The incidence of some inherited EEG-Variants in normal Japanese and German males, Humangenetik **7**, 38-42 (1969)

VOLAVKA, J., ZAKS, A., ROUBICEK, J. et al.: Electroencephalographic effects of diacetylmorphine (heroin) and naloxon in man. Neuropharmacology **9**, 587-593 (1970)

VOLAVKA, J. S., FELDSTEIN, S., ABRAMS, R.: EEG and clinical change after bilateral and unilateral electroconvulsive therapy. EEG Clin. Neurophysiol. **32**, 631 - 639 (1972)

VOLAVKA, J., CROWN, P., DORNBUSH, R. et al.: EEG, heart rate and mood change ("high") after Cannabis. Psychopharmacologia (Berlin) **32**, 11-25 (1973a)

VOLAVKA, J., MATOUSEK, M., FELDSTEIN, S. et al.: The reliability of EEG assessment. EEG-EMG **4**, 123 - 130 (1973b)

VOLAVKA, J., MATOUSEK, M., ROUBICEK, J. et al.: The reliability of visual EEG assessment. EEG Clin. Neurophysiol. **31**, 294 (1975)

VOLKOW, N. D., HITZEMANN. R., WANG, G.-J. et al.: Decreased brain metabolism in neurologically intact healthy alcoholics. Am. J. Psychiatry, **149**, 1016-1022 (1992)

VOLOW, M. R., ZUNG, W. W. K., GREEN, R. L.: Electroencephalographic abnormalities in suicidal patients. J. Clin. Psychiat. **40**, 213-216 (1979)

WADDINGTON, C. H.: Die Biologischen Grundlagen des Lebens. Vieweg & Sohn, Braunschweig – Wiesbaden,1966

WAEHRENS, J., GERLACH, J.: Bromocriptine and imipramine in endogenous depressions: a double-blind controlled trial in outpatients. J.Affect. Dis. **3**, 193-202 (1981)

WAGNER, R.: Probleme und Beispiele biologischer Regelung. G.Thieme, Stuttgart, 1954

WAGNER, D.: Elektroenzephalographisch gekennzeichnete Psychosen. Schweiz. Arch. Neurol., Neurochir. Psychiat. **103**, 377-397 (1969)

WALLACE, R. K.: Physiological effects of transcendental meditation. Science **167**, 1751-1754 (1970)

WALLACE, R. K., BENSON, H., WILSON, A. F.: A wakeful hypometabolic physiologic state. Am. J. Physiol. **221**, 795-799 (1971)

WALLACE, R. K., BENSON, H.: The physiology of meditation. Scientific American **226**, 85 - 90 (1972)

WALSH, J. K., SMITSON, S. A., KRAMER, M.: Sleep-onset REM sleep: comparison of narcoleptic and obstructive sleep apnoe patients. Clin. EEG **13**, 57-60 (1982)

WALTER, W. G.: Electroencephalography in cases of mental disorder. J. ment. Sci. **88**, 110-121 (1942).

WANG, H. S., OBRIST, W. D., BUSSE, E. W.: Neurophysiological correlates of the intellectual function of elderly persons living in the community. Am. J. Psychiat. **126,** 1205-1212 (1970)

WARNER, M.D., BOUTROS, N.N., PEABODY, C.A.: Usefulness of screening EEGs in a psychiatric inpatient population. J. Clin. Psychiatry **51**, 363-364 (1990)

WEINER, R.D.: Coping with progress; invited comment on topographic EEG mapping Am. J. EEG Technol. **27** (1987) 242-244

WEINSHENKER, B.G., PENMAN, M., BASS, B. et al.: A double-blind, randomized, crossover trial of pemoline in fatigue associated with multiple sclerosis. Neurology **42**, 1468-1471 (1992)

WEISS, P.: Das lebende System: ein Beispiel für den Schichtendeterminismus, S.13-59. In: Das Neue Menschenbild. Koestler, A., Smythies, J. R. (Eds.). Molden, Wien-München-Zürich, 1969

WEISS, P.A.: Empirische Grundlagen des Systemdenkens. F. Molden, Nova Acta Leopoldina **47**, 325-334 (1978)

v. WEIZSÄCKER, V.: Der Gestaltkreis, 4. Aufl. , Thieme, Heidelberg, 1948

WENDLAND, K.-L., FENZEL, G.: Erhebungen bei Patienten mit einer Theta-Grundrhythmusvariante des EEG. Psychiat. Prax. **19**, 164-170 (1992)

WERNER, G.: The many faces of neuroreductionism, pp.241-257. In: Dynamics of Sensory and Cognitive Processing by the Brain. Basar, E. (ed.). Springer, Berlin-Heidelberg, 1988

WERNER, S. S., STOCKARD, J. E., BICKFORD, R. G.: Atlas of Neonatal Electroencephalography. Raven Press, New York, 1977

WEST, M.J., COLEMAN, P.D., FLOOD, D.G. et al.: Differences in the pattern of hippocampal loss in normal aging and Alzheimer's disease. Lancet **344** 769-772 (1994)

WESTCOTT, M.: Hemispheric asymmetry of the EEG during altered states of consciousness. B.A. Dissertation, Durham Univ., Durham 1974

WESTMORELAND, B. F.: The EEG in cerebral Infection, pp.221-231. In: Electroencephalography: Basic Principles, Clinical Applications and Related Fields, Niedermeyer E., Da Silva, F. L. (eds.), Vol.15,Urban & Schwarzenberg, Baltimore, 1982

WESTMORELAND, B. F., KLASS, D.W., SHARBROUGH, F.W. et al.: "Alpha coma": EEG, clinical, pathologic, and etiologic correlations. Arch. Neurol. **32**, 713-718 (1975)

WEXLER, B. E.: Beyond the Kraepelinean dichotomy (editorial). Biol. Psychiatry **31**, 539-541 (1992)

WICHNIACK, A., SZAFRANSKI, T. WIERZBICKI, A. et al.: Electroencephalographic slowing, sleepiness and treatment response in patients with schizophrenia during olanzapine treatment. Psychopharmacology **20**, 80-85 (2006)

WIENER, N. Cynernetics, Cambridge MA. 1948

WIKLER, A.: Clinical and electroencephalographic studies on the effects of mescaline, N-allylnormophine and morphine in man. J. nerv. ment. Dis. **120**, 157-175 (1954)

WIKLER, A., LLOYD, B. J.: Effect of smoking marihuana cigarettes on cortical electrical activity. Fed. Proc. **4**, 141-142 (1945)

WIKLER, A., ALTSCHUL, S.: Effects of methadone and morphine on the electroencephalogram of the dog. J. pharmac. exp. Ther. **98**, 437-446 (1950)

WIKLER, A., FRASER, H., ISBELL, H. et al.: Electroencephalograms during cycles of addiction barbiturates in man. EEG Clin. Neurophysiol. **7**, 1-13 (1955)

WIKLER, A., PESCOR, F. T., FRASER, H. F. et al.: Electroencephalographic changes associated with chronic alcoholic intoxication and the alcohol abstinence syndrome. Am. J. Psychiat. **113**, 106-114 (1956)

WIKLER, A., ESSIG, C. F.: Withdrawal seizures following chronic intoxication with barbiturates and other sedative drugs, pp. 170 - 184. In: Modern Problems of Pharmacopsychiatry, vol.4: Epilepsy. Niedermeyer, E. (ed.). KARGER, Basel 1970

WIKSWO, J.P., GEVINS, A., WILLIAMSON, S.J.: The future of the EEG and MEG; EEG Clin Neurophysiol **87** (1993) 1-9

WILDER, J.: The law of initial value in neurology and psychiatry. J. Nerv. Ment. Dis. **125**, 73-86 (1956)

WILDER-SMITH, E., KARBOWSKI, K.: Zur Signifikanz einer „intermittierenden EEG-Stille". EEG-Labor **14**, 162 - 166 (1992)

WILKUS, R., DODRILL, C., TROUPIN, A.: Carbamazepine and the electroencephalogram of epileptics: a double blind study in comparison to phenytoin. Epilepsia **19**, 283-291 (1978)

WILLIAMS, D.: Neural factors related to habitual aggression. Brain, **92**, 503-520 (1969)

WILLIAMS, E.G., HIMMELSBACH, C.K., WIKLER, A. et al.: Studies on marijuana and pyrahexyl compound. Publ. Hlth. Rpts. **61**, 1059-1083 (1946)

WILLIAMS, G.W., LÜDERS, H.O., BRICKNER, A. et al.: Interobserver variability in EEG interpretation. Neurology **35**, 1714 - 1719 (1985)

WILLIAMSON, P. C., MERSKEY, H., MORRISON, S. et al.: Quantitative electroencephalographic correlates of cognitive decline in normal elderly subjects. Arch. Neurol. **47**, 1185- 1188 (1990)

WILLNER, P.: Dopamin and depression: a review of recent evidence. Brain Res. Rev. **6**, 211-246 (1983)

WILSON, W.H. Do anticonvulsants hinder clozapine treatment ? Biol. Psychiatry **37** 425-426 (1995)

WINTERER, G., SCHMIDT, L. G., FRICK, K. , ULRICH, G.: "Neuroadaptation" bei langjährigem Cannabiskonsum. Der Nervenarzt **65**, 635-637 (1994)

WINTERER, G., HERRMANN, W.M.: Über das Elektroenzephalogramm in der Psychiatrie: eine kritische Bewertung Z EEG-EMG **26** 19-37 (1995)

WISSFELD, E., KAINDL, E.: Über die Deutung und den Wert abnormer EEG-Befunde bei psychopathischen Persönlichkeiten. Der Nervenarzt **32**, 57-66 (1961)

WOLF, P.: Zur Pathophysiologie epileptischer Psychosen, pp..51-65. In: Psychische Störungen bei Epilepsien. Psychosen, Verastimmungen, Persönlichkeitsveränderungen. Penin, H. (Ed.) Schattauer, Stuttgart, 1973

WOLF, P.: Psychosen bei Epilepsie, Ihre Bedingungen und Wechselbeziehungen zu Anfällen.Habil.-Schrift, FU Berlin 1976

WOLF, P.: Systematik von Status kleiner Anfälle in psychopathologischer Hinsicht, S.32-52. In: Psychopathologische und pathogenetische Probleme psychotischer Syndrome bei Epilepsie. Wolf, P., Köhler, G.-K. (Hrsg.), Huber, Bern-Stuttgart-Wien 1980

WOLPERT, E., NEUNDÖRFER, B., KÖMPF, D. et al.: Untersuchungen zur Psychopathologie bei Merkmalsträgern der 4-5/s-EEG Grundrhythmusvariante. Arch. Psychiat. Nervenkr. **226**, 269-282 (1979)

YAGU, T., WACKERMAN, J., SHIGETA, M. et al.: Global dimensional complexity of multichannel EEG in mild Alzheimer's disease and age-matched control subjects. Dementia **8**, 343-347 (1997)

YAKOVLEV, P.I., LECOURS, A.R.: The myelogenetic cycles of regional maturation of the brain (pp. 3-70) In: A. Minkowski (ed.): Regional Development of the Brain in Early Life. Blackwell, Oxford (1967)

YAMADA, K, ISOTANI, T. IRISAWA, S. et al.: EEG global field power spectrum changes after a single dose of atypical antipsychotics in healthy volunteers. Brain Topography **16**. 281-285 (2004)

YORK, G.K., STEINBERG, D.A.: The philosophy of Hughlings Jackson. J. R. Soc. Med. **95**, 314-318 (2002)

YOSHIMURA, M. KOENIG,T. IRISAWA, S. et al.: A pharmaco-EEG study on antipsychotic drugs in healthy volunteers. Psychopharmacology **192**, 995-1004 (2006)

ZANGEMEISTER, W. H., BUSHART, W.: Statistische und Verlaufs-Untersuchungen zur 4/s Variante der EEG-Grundaktivität. Arch. Psychiat. Nervenkr. **224**, 273-280 (1977)

ZAKS, A., BRUNER, A., FINK, M. et al.: Intravenous diacetylmorphine (heroin) in studies of opiate dependence. Dis.nerv.Syst. **30**, 89 - 92 (1969)

ZEH, W.: Symptomwandel oder Verlaufsgestalt, erläutert am Beispiel der progressiven Paralyse. Fortschr. Neurol. Psychiat. **30**, 113-135 (1962)

ZIMKINA, A. M., ASAFOV, B. D., KISELEVA, A. M. et al.: Pecularities of the electroencephalogram in elderly and aged persons. EEG Clin. Neurophysiol. **18**, 107 (1965)

ZIMMERMAN, M., BLACK, D. W., CORYELL, W.: Diagnostic criteria for melancholia. Arch. Gen. Psychiatry **46**, 361-368 (1989)

ZIPURSKI, R.B., LIM, K.O., PFEFFERBAUM, A.: MRI study of brain changes with short-term abstinence from alcohol. Alcohol. Clin. Exp. Res., **13**, 664-666 (1989)

ZUBIN.J. Symposion on statistics for the clinician. J. clin. Psychol **6**,1-6 (1950)

ZUBIN, J., SPRING, B.: Vulnerability. A new view of schizophrenia. J. Abnorm. Psychiat. **86** 103-125 (1977)

ZUREK, R., SCHIEMANN-DELGADO, J., FROESCHER, W. et al.: Frontal intermittent rhythmical delta activity and anterior bradyrhythmia. Clin. EEG **16**, 1-10 (1985)

Index

A

AAD-event (Abrupt Amplitude Decrease) 342
Abnormalities
  non-specific 17
Absence
  time-accelerated psychosis 220
Abulic-akinetic syndrome 249
Activation
  brain electrical 6
acute brain trauma 173
ADHD
  EEG dynamics 224
  maladaptive control of vigilance dynamics 302
adult minimal brain damage syndrome 92
adversive seizures 220
AIDS-related symptom complex 172
Alcohol 261
  neuroadaptivity 264
Alcoholism 320
  metalcoholic encephalopathies 125
Allgemeinveränderung (JUNG) 18, 19, 21, 23, 148, 166, 259
allopoietic 31
Alpha activity 180
alpha-anteriorization 41
alpha background activity 97
Alpha-blocking 36
Alpha-coma 148
Alpha continuity 308
alternative psychoses 214, 215
Alzheimer's disease 318, 335
  Ipsative Trend Assessment 185
  slowly progressive pathology 178
amisulprid 244
amitriptyline 245
amplitudes 290
anteriorization
  degree of 306
anticholinergic effect 249
anticonvulsants
  prophylaxis after brain lesions 22
apallic syndrome 148
arousal reaction 28
Arterial Pulse Impedance Artifact (APIA) 288
artifact editing
  visual 301
asthenic personality 88
Attention Deficit Hyperactivity Disorder (ADHD) 330
attractor
  convergence of trajectories 335
autochthonous twilight states 213
automatic actions 213

B

Barbituate Addicts
  Withdrawal 263
barbiturates 260
Barycentric Frequency (BF) 305
benzodiazepine addicts 156, 261, 263
  withdrawal 263
biorhythms 292
biperspectivism 338
body-mind problem 100
BOLD (Blood Oxygenation Level Dependent) 284
Borderline Personality Disorder (BPD) 333
Borrelia encephalitis 169
brain electrical patterns 102
"Brain Language" (Laszlo) 181
Brain Physics 300
Burn-out Syndrome 339
burst suppression activity 159

C

cannabis 267
  withdrawl 267
Carbamazepin (CBZ) 325
categorical fallacy 6
c-EEG 266
centenarians 160
Central Limit Theorem 287
central nervous system 228
cerebral compression 176
cerebral electrometry (FINK) 226
Cerebral Global Function 292
Chaotic determination 32
chloroform 260
choppy activity 327
chronospectrograms 34

clomethiazol 229
clozapine 240, 243
cocaine 267
cognitive load 335
coherence 73
compensation capacities 168
complex-partial seizures 213
connectivity 68
correlation dimension D2 221

D

data driven research 178
deflection 34
dehydrobenzperidol 262
Dementia of Alzheimer Type 312
"Denosologization" (VAN PRAAG) 386
depressive syndrome 163
Deterministic chaos (SCHUSTER) 336
detoxification period 29
diazepam 78
diffuse dysrhythmia (DD) 69, 74, 75, 127, 164, 166, 189, 244, 256, 263, 267, 119, 310
disequilibrium state 34
dissociative vigilance shift 245
dissolution 246, 250
  via Stage A 272
  via Stage B 264
"Doctrine of Concomitance" (JACKSON) 293
"Double-sided accounting" (JANZARIK) 214
drowsiness 293, 324
dynamic attractors 68
dynamic equilibrium 35
Dynamic Lability (DL) 63, 96, 97, 99, 119, 120, 123, 162, 164, 167, 169, 175, 197, 199, 209, 210, 222, 250, 251, 303, 323, 331
Dynamic Rigidity (DR) 65, 69, 96, 97, 99, 119, 122, 132, 164, 169, 181, 209, 251, 254, 322, 327, 331
dynamics of transition between patterns 37
dynamic studies 183
dyscontrol syndrome 93

E

Eddington's Parable vi, 277
EEG
  dynamic information 226
  immaturity indicators 70
  mapping 5
  maturation phases 71
  psychophysiological 103
  spontaneous resting 1
  time function 33
  time resolution 297
  vigilance stages 65
  visual pattern recognition 295
electrodes 42, 127
eliminative reductionism 102
embedding dimensions d 336
empirism 33, 102
encephalopathies 125, 176
endocrinous psychosyndromes 174
epilepsy 210, 214
epileptic equivalents 210, 220
Epileptic Psychoses 210
epileptic seizure 210
epistemological fallacy 32
equilibrium state
  stable 34
états subvigile 63
explanatory principle 293

F

fentanyl 263
First Order Cybernetics 31
fluvoxamin 250
f-MRI 297
forced normalization 215
formative tendencies 33, 230
frequency range 121
frontalization 41
functional compensation 168
Functional Electroencephalography (LIBERSON) 300
Funktionskreis 30
Funktionswandel 37

G

Gaches' triad 162
General Adaptation syndrome 302
General Cerebral Function 330
General Systems Theory 30
Global Function 33
graphoelement 22, 342
GRASSBERGER-PROCACCIA algorithm 32

H

Healthy Aging 159
heroine 267

higher structural characteristics 342
homeostasis 30
HPA-Axis 302
hydrocarbons 260
hypersynchronic potentials 20
hyperthyreosis 174
hyperventilation effect 28
hyponoic-hypobulic syndrome 249

I

IBA - Intermittent Bilateral Anterior 27, 124, 125, 255
IBP - Intermittent bilateral posterior 78, 90
ideal smooth control 303
idle state 34
imipramin 188, 245
impulse control impairment 93
Individualized Medicine 333
indivisible organismic unity 338
infantile drowsiness patterns 27
integrated wholeness 67
interhemispheral coordination 73
interictal psychoses 214
intermediary stages 111
intermittent left anterior (ILA) 27, 125, 126, 161, 255
intermittent left posterior (ILP) 90
Ipsative Trend Assessment (ITA) 185, 304, 310, 339

K

K-complex 59
ketamine 262
Krampfbereitschaft 20

L

Law of Initial Value 311
linearity 334, 336
lithium 99
Lithium 336
living systems 102
Logical Positivism 294
Low resolution electromagnetic tomography 385
low voltage EEG 176

M

manic syndrome 200
Manic Syndrome 196
maprotiline 245

mass activity 33
Maturation 69
maturation deficit 73
Medication
 anticonvulsive 156
Meditation 221
melancholia 254
meprobamat 260
mescaline 274
metascience 31
methadon 267
microprecise causality 30
mind language 102
momentum 177
morphine 267
morphodynamics 270
Multiple Sclerosis 222

N

narcolepsy 174
Neophrenology 297
Neuroadaptation 318
neuro-integrative defect 92
neuroleptics 94
neurometrics 106
Neuronal
 rarefication 162
Neuroplasticity 178
neuropsychiatry 278
neurotic decompensation 93
nicotine 268
nimodipine 275
nitrous oxyde 260
nomifensine 245
noninteger correlation dimension 336
nonlinear complexity analysis 336
nonrandomness 287
non-reactive coma 148
Nootropics 275
normal distribution 286
Normative Data Base 313

O

Obsessive Compulsive Disorder 333
olanzapine 244
ontogenetic maturation level 69
Opioids 267

Ordering term 293
overshooting control 301

P

paradoxical alpha-activation 28
paraldehyde 262
paroxysmal activity 22
paroxysmal potentials 20, 21, 22, 23, 24, 159, 215, 220, 263
patent protection 343
pathological dissolution 112
Pathological Dissolution v, 117
pathological functional change 117
pathomorphic organization 118
Patterns
   spatio-temporal 180
Periodic Lateralized Epileptiform Discharges 159
Persistent Vegetative State 339
petit mal status 211
Pharmaco-EEG 5
phase randomization 334
phase space 335
phenomena 337
phrenology 3
Physiomorphic dynamics 120
polyrhythmic frequency dissolution 124
postconcussional syndrome 173
posteriorization 41
postictal psychosis 212
postparoxysmal after-discharge 212
postparoxysmal twilight state 212
predilection types 34
preictal flattening 216
preparoxysmal states 216
Proneness to Epileptic Seizures 20
protrusions of the skull 3
pseudoneurasthenic syndrome 173
psychiatric classification 17
psychiatric diagnoses 105
psychiatric EEG 115
psychiatric syndromes 185
psychiatrie organo-dynamic 110
Psychoanaleptics 267
psychopathology 326
psycho-physic interaction 293
psychophysiology 6
Psychosomatic Disorder 339
Psychotomimetics 274
psychotropic drugs 19

Q

q-EEG 279
qualitative information 36
quantitative evaluation 287
quasi-periodicity 34
quetiapine 244

R

readaptation process 267
Reizgebundenheit 332
repetitive sharp waves 146
Resting Dynamics Assessment 342
rigidly encapsulated moduls 297
risperidone 244
Root-Mean-Squared 342

S

schizophrenia 9
schizophrenic psychoses 91, 98, 106, 202
seizure 212
self-organizing process 3, 292
sensorial reactivity 147
smooth adaptive control 301
somnolence 63
source derivation 163
Spontaneous Resting EEG 32, 33
   dynamics 301
   non-linearity 296
   non-stationarity 305
   process 34
   quantitative reconstruction of the time course 304
   resting conditions 1
   stationarity assumption 287, 296
   systemic motion 36
SR-EEG (Spontaneous Resting EEG) 1, 3
state-dependent 19, 74
states of order 35
status psychomotoricus 213
suicidal acts 94
surrogate method 334
sustained attention 64
synchronization 71
systemic thinking 30
Systems Philosophy 31
systems theory 33

T

tacit assumption 295
target symptoms 232
temporalization 41
temporal lobe epilepsy 217
temporal lobe mythology 217
tergurid 275
terminology 15
test-retest-reliability 311
theoretical construct 340
third dissolution path 124
Thymoleptics vi, 244
thyreotoxic psychosis 174
topographical differentiation 296
tracé alternant 159
trajectories 335
transitional stages 63
Traumatic brain injuries 339
tri-phasic waves 156
trivialization 32

U

Umstellerschwerung 332

V

Verlaufsgestalt 33
vigilance 2, 35, 63, 65, 66, 70, 92, 100, 118, 124,
    168, 174, 200, 245, 251, 264, 266, 286, 292,
    302, 303, 342
visualization techniques 3
vulnerability 19

W

wake-sleep cycle 2
wisdom of age 336
withdrawal phase 20
within-subject measurements of change 299
within-subject stability 41

Z

z-transformation 296

www.ingramcontent.com/pod-product-compliance
Ingram Content Group UK Ltd.
Pitfield, Milton Keynes, MK11 3LW, UK
UKHW050412240426
12048UKWH00020B/1470